Genetic Management of Animals

Genetic Management of Animals

Edited by Dominic Fasso

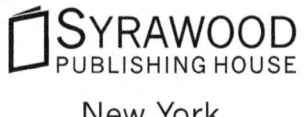
SYRAWOOD
PUBLISHING HOUSE

New York

Published by Syrawood Publishing House,
750 Third Avenue, 9th Floor,
New York, NY 10017, USA
www.syrawoodpublishinghouse.com

Genetic Management of Animals
Edited by Dominic Fasso

International Standard Book Number: 978-1-68286-656-6 (Hardback)

Cataloging-in-Publication Data

Genetic management of animals / edited by Dominic Fasso.
    p. cm.
Includes bibliographical references and index.
ISBN 978-1-68286-656-6
1. Animal genetics. 2. Genetics. I. Fasso, Dominic.
QH432 .G46 2019
591.35--dc23

TABLE OF CONTENTS

PREFACE

Animal genetics is the study of the genes and heredity traits amongst animals. It involves the breeding and genetic manipulation of superior quality animals primarily to achieve disease resistance. It is primarily applied to the areas of animal husbandry and livestock management. Animal genes are also studied to understand the evolution, growth and anatomy of animals. This book is a valuable compilation of topics, ranging from the basic to the most complex advancements in this field. Different approaches, evaluations and methodologies in the area of animal genetics have been included herein. It includes contributions of experts and scientists, which will provide innovative insights into this discipline.

This book unites the global concepts and researches in an organized manner for a comprehensive understanding of the subject. It is a ripe text for all researchers, students, scientists or anyone else who is interested in acquiring a better knowledge of this dynamic field.

I extend my sincere thanks to the contributors for such eloquent research chapters. Finally, I thank my family for being a source of support and help.

Editor

Semi-supervised learning for genomic prediction of novel traits with small reference populations: an application to residual feed intake in dairy cattle

Chen Yao[1*], Xiaojin Zhu[2] and Kent A. Weigel[1]

Abstract

Background: Genomic prediction for novel traits, which can be costly and labor-intensive to measure, is often hampered by low accuracy due to the limited size of the reference population. As an option to improve prediction accuracy, we introduced a semi-supervised learning strategy known as the self-training model, and applied this method to genomic prediction of residual feed intake (RFI) in dairy cattle.

Methods: We describe a self-training model that is wrapped around a support vector machine (SVM) algorithm, which enables it to use data from animals with and without measured phenotypes. Initially, a SVM model was trained using data from 792 animals with measured RFI phenotypes. Then, the resulting SVM was used to generate self-trained phenotypes for 3000 animals for which RFI measurements were not available. Finally, the SVM model was re-trained using data from up to 3792 animals, including those with measured and self-trained RFI phenotypes.

Results: Incorporation of additional animals with self-trained phenotypes enhanced the accuracy of genomic predictions compared to that of predictions that were derived from the subset of animals with measured phenotypes. The optimal ratio of animals with self-trained phenotypes to animals with measured phenotypes (2.5, 2.0, and 1.8) and the maximum increase achieved in prediction accuracy measured as the correlation between predicted and actual RFI phenotypes (5.9, 4.1, and 2.4%) decreased as the size of the initial training set (300, 400, and 500 animals with measured phenotypes) increased. The optimal number of animals with self-trained phenotypes may be smaller when prediction accuracy is measured as the mean squared error rather than the correlation between predicted and actual RFI phenotypes.

Conclusions: Our results demonstrate that semi-supervised learning models that incorporate self-trained phenotypes can achieve genomic prediction accuracies that are comparable to those obtained with models using larger training sets that include only animals with measured phenotypes. Semi-supervised learning can be helpful for genomic prediction of novel traits, such as RFI, for which the size of reference population is limited, in particular, when the animals to be predicted and the animals in the reference population originate from the same herd-environment.

Background

When using whole-genome markers to predict breeding values or future phenotypes, a main challenge is the construction of an effective reference population that includes genotyped and phenotyped individuals for training the prediction model. Both size of the reference population and genetic distance between the reference population and the current pool of selection candidates are critical factors [1, 2]. Given a sufficient number of individuals in the reference population or training set, there are several highly effective "supervised learning" techniques for training prediction models, such as

_____
*Correspondence: cyao5@wisc.edu; chen.yao225@gmail.com
[1] Department of Dairy Science, University of Wisconsin, Madison, Madison, WI, USA
Full list of author information is available at the end of the article

Bayesian regression models, genomic best linear unbiased prediction (BLUP), kernel-based methods, and machine-learning algorithms (e.g., [3–6]). Very large reference populations are available for some traits and species, such as for milk yield in Holstein dairy cattle, but for other traits such as feed efficiency, the size of the reference population is often limited by the exorbitant cost or intensive labor requirements associated with measuring individual phenotypes. For dry matter intake (DMI) in dairy cattle, researchers have collated data from multiple countries to estimate genetic parameters and perform genomic prediction [7, 8]. Alternatively, after several years of genomic selection on traits such as milk yield, hundreds of thousands of dairy cows and bulls have been genotyped, and useful information that can enhance the accuracy of genomic prediction for feed efficiency could be extracted from the available genomic data of animals that have not been measured for the phenotype of interest.

A powerful tool from the machine-learning community has potential for addressing this challenge, i.e. a technique known as semi-supervised learning. As its name suggests, semi-supervised learning refers to models that combine attributes of supervised and unsupervised learning [9]. Most genomic prediction models that are currently popular, such as genomic BLUP and Bayesian regression, rely on supervised model training. In supervised models, a measured phenotype is provided as the desired "label" for an animal, and this phenotype supervises the process of model training to predict future phenotypes from the corresponding genotypes. In contrast, for unsupervised learning no measured phenotype is available to supervise the labeling of an animal's genotype. An example of unsupervised learning is the use of principal component analysis to cluster animals into groups based on the similarity of their genotypes.

In this study, and in the context of genomic selection for enhanced feed efficiency in dairy cattle, we applied a simple but widely used semi-supervised learning algorithm known as the "self-training" model [9]. During the learning process, this model uses its own predictions that are derived from the subset of "labeled" individuals with measured phenotypes, to teach itself on the relationships between genotypes and phenotypes of "unlabeled" individuals with missing phenotypes. The self-training model that can be wrapped around a wide variety of genomic prediction methods. In this study, we extended a typical machine-learning genomic selection model, namely the support vector machine (SVM) [10, 11], which provided higher prediction accuracies of residual feed intake (RFI) using whole-genome molecular markers than the random forests model [12]. In this approach, the training data

consist of a combination of individuals with measured phenotypes and model-derived "self-trained" phenotypes, and both sources of data are used for subsequent prediction of genomic breeding values for RFI. Knowledge about the genomic relationships within the population of animals without phenotypes can contribute to the accuracy of selection, and if this is successful, the resulting prediction accuracy will exceed that of a supervised learner trained with only the animals that have measured phenotypes. The underlying assumptions are that the measurement of additional phenotypes for the novel trait is difficult or expensive, and that additional genotypes of animals without novel trait phenotypes are available at little or no cost.

Although, until now, self-training has not been introduced in an animal breeding context, it has been used for a variety of promising applications in the broader subject area of artificial intelligence. For example, Rosenberg et al. [13] implemented a semi-supervised learning approach as a wrapper around an existing object detector and achieved results that were comparable to a model trained with a much larger set of fully labeled data. McClosky et al. [14] self-trained an effective two-phase parser-re-ranker system using unlabeled data, and the semi-supervised model achieved a 12% reduction in error compared to the best previous result for parsing. Tang et al. [15] proposed the semi-supervised transductive regression forest for real-time articulated hand pose estimation and showed that accuracies could be improved by considering unlabeled data. In genetics, this method has been used to increase the accuracy of gene start prediction, by combining models of protein-coding and non-coding regions and models of regulatory sites near the gene start [16]. In the area of gene identification, a self-training model was used to find genes in eukaryotic genomes in parallel with statistical model estimates that were taken directly from anonymous genomic DNA [17].

In this work, we present the first application of a self-training algorithm in the context of genomic selection of livestock, using RFI as the phenotype of choice for measuring feed efficiency in dairy cattle. A comprehensive evaluation of the model training process was undertaken in order to facilitate effective application of semi-supervised learning techniques to predict a complex trait such as RFI using whole-genome molecular markers. This study focused on determining how performance of the predictor is affected by the number of "labeled" individuals with measured phenotypes and "unlabeled" individuals with self-trained phenotypes. It also aimed at providing new insights in genomic selection by enhancing prediction accuracy through the inclusion of animals without measured phenotypes via semi-supervised learning methods.

Methods

Description of the semi-supervised self-training algorithm

One particular semi-supervised learning strategy, i.e. the self-training model, was used in this study. Animals with measured phenotypes were separated into training and testing sets. The training and testing sets included animals with genotypes, G_1 and G_T, and measured phenotypes, P_1 and P_T. Animals without measured phenotypes only contributed genotypes, denoted as G_2. During self-training, an initial model was trained using the training set of G_1 and P_1 to formulate the base predictor (f). This predictor was then used to predict the self-trained phenotypes, $\hat{P}_2$, for the individuals that lacked measured phenotypes. Next, the individuals comprising G_2 and $\hat{P}_2$ were added to the training set in order to train a new predictor (f^*). In the testing phase, accuracies of f and f^* within the testing set (denoted as R_{SL} and R_{SSL}) were compared. First, phenotypes $\hat{P}_T$ and $\hat{P}_T^*$ were predicted from G_T using f and f^*, respectively. Second, R_{SL} (R_{SSL}) was computed as the correlation between $\hat{P}_T$ ($\hat{P}_T^*$) and P_T. The self-training algorithm is summarized below and illustrated in Fig. 1.

Step 1: Train a base predictor, f, using genotypes G_1 and phenotypes P_1 from animals with measured phenotypes.

Step 2: Predict the self-trained phenotypes ($\hat{P}_2$) from the genotypes G_2 for animals without measured phenotypes.

Step 3: Combine genotypes G_1 and G_2 with phenotypes P_1 and $\hat{P}_2$, in order to train a new predictor, f^*, which is used to compute the final genomic predictions.

An SVM algorithm was used as the genomic prediction model and implemented using the "svm" function of the "e1071" package Version 1.6-1 in R [18] with radial basis kernel and default parameters tuned within the training set.

Definition of the RFI phenotypes

The data consisted of 792 lactating Holstein dairy cows from the Allenstein Dairy Herd at the University of Wisconsin–Madison. Phenotypes used in this study were a subset of the data analyzed by Tempelman et al. [19], in which a detailed description of the data is provided. All animals with measured phenotypes were recorded for daily DMI, daily milk yield, weekly milk composition (fat %, protein %, and lactose %), and weekly body weight (BW) during the period from 50 to 200 days postpartum. Quality control and editing were similar to Yao et al. [12]. Only one lactation record per animal was used.

Residual feed intake was defined as the deviation of an animal's feed intake from the average intake of its cohort, after adjusting for milk production and composition, maintenance of body weight, and known environmental differences. Fixed environmental effects included year-season of calving (YSC) with 19 levels (year: 2007–2013; season: January–March, April–June, July–September, or October–December) and parity-by-age at calving (ParAge) with 20 levels (1st parity: ≤ 23, 24, 25, 26, or ≥ 27 months; 2nd parity: ≤ 35, 36, ..., 40, or ≥ 41 months; 3rd parity or later: ≤ 48, 49, 50, 51, 52–56, 57–61, 62–69, or ≥ 70 months), while medium days in milk for the week (dim) was included as a covariate. A total of 81 rations used in specific nutrition experiments were modeled as random cohort effects. Weekly mean RFI phenotypes were the residuals from this model, calculated as:

$$\mathbf{y} = \mu + \mathbf{YSC} + \mathbf{ParAge} + \beta_1 \mathbf{dim} + \beta_2 \mathbf{MilkE} + \beta_3 \mathbf{MBW} + \mathbf{ration} + \mathbf{RFI},$$

where $\mathbf{y}$ is a vector of DMI phenotypes, μ is the population mean, $\mathbf{YSC}$ is a vector of the fixed effects of year-season of calving, $\mathbf{ParAge}$ is a vector of fixed effects of parity-by-age at calving interaction, $\mathbf{dim}$ is a vector of the fixed covariate of the medium days in milk during the week with regression coefficient β_1, $\mathbf{MilkE}$ is a vector of the fixed covariate of energy expressed in milk (defined in [12]) with regression coefficient β_2, $\mathbf{MBW}$ is a vector of the fixed covariate of the metabolic BW (i.e., $BW^{0.75}$) with regression coefficient β_3, $\mathbf{ration} \sim N(0, \mathbf{I}\sigma_r^2)$ is a vector of the random cohort effects, and $\mathbf{RFI} \sim N(0, \mathbf{I}\sigma_e^2)$ is a vector of random residuals. The mixed model equations were solved with the restricted maximum likelihood (REML) method using the R-package "lme4", Version 0.999999-0 [14]. Then, for each animal, the RFI phenotype was set to the mean of weekly RFI estimates available for that animal.

Genetic marker data

Single nucleotide polymorphism (SNP) genotypes were available for the 792 cows with measured RFI phenotypes and for 3000 cows without measured RFI phenotypes; these 3000 cows included 1127 Holstein cows from four other university research herds (University of Florida, Iowa State University, Michigan State University, and Virginia Tech University) and 1813 Holstein cows born in 2009 and selected randomly from the Council on Dairy Cattle Breeding (CDCB; Bowie, MD) Holstein genotype database. Raw genotypes represented various low-density and medium-density arrays, and missing genotypes were imputed to higher density using genotype information from bulls and cows in the CDCB database [20, 21]. Any remaining missing genotypes (about 2%) were imputed by using rounded allele frequencies from the current US Holstein population. SNPs with minor allele frequencies lower than 5% were removed. A total of 57,491 SNPs per individual were available for the genomic prediction analysis. The SNP genotype at each locus was coded as 0, 1, or 2, counting the number of copies of the minor allele.

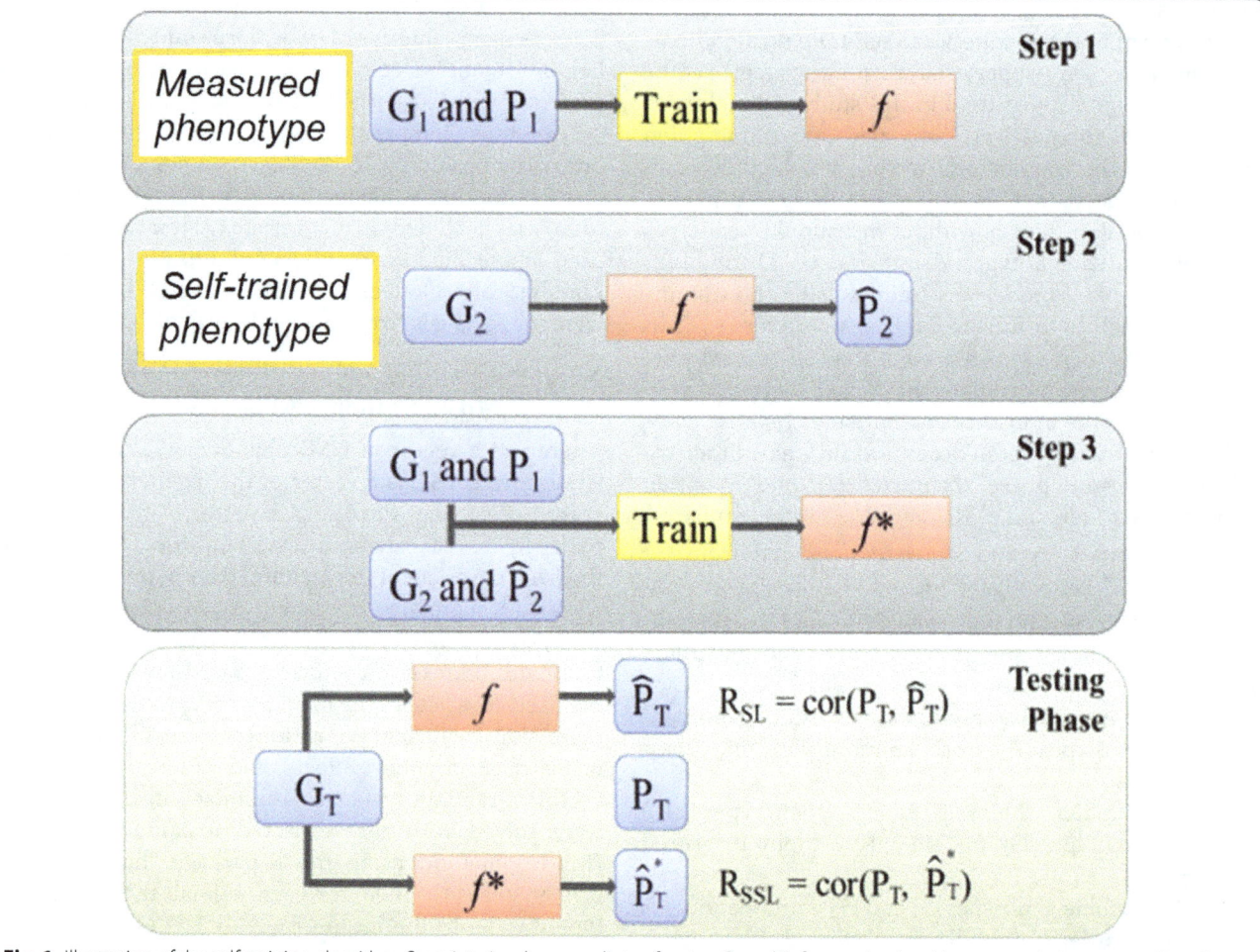

Fig. 1 Illustration of the self-training algorithm. Step 1: train a base predictor, f, using G_1 and P_1 from animals with measured phenotypes. Step 2: predict self-trained phenotypes, $\hat{P}_2$, based on G_2 for animals without measured phenotypes. Step 3: combine G_1, G_2, P_1, and $\hat{P}_2$ to train a new predictor, f^*. In the testing phase, compare accuracies of f and f^* on the testing set (R_{SL} and R_{SSL}). First, predict phenotypes $\hat{P}_T$ and $\hat{P}_T^*$ based on G_T using f and f^*, respectively and second, calculate R_{SL} (R_{SSL}) as the correlation between $\hat{P}_T$ ($\hat{P}_T^*$) and P_T

Design of the validation study

In practical applications of genomic selection in dairy cattle, training is typically carried out using historical animals, and the target population of selection candidates for genomic prediction includes, but is not limited to, offspring and descendants of animals in the training set [22]. In this study, genomic prediction models were trained using 540 animals born before January 1, 2010 and validation of the prediction accuracies was carried out using 252 animals born after January 1, 2010. In order to assess the impact of size of the reference population on the accuracy of genomic prediction with supervised learning, size of the training set was varied from 20 to 540 in increments of 20 (i.e., $n = 20, 40, 60, ..., 540$), and prediction accuracy for a given n was averaged over 100 random samples from the training set. To assess the impact of the relative numbers of animals with measured phenotypes versus self-trained phenotypes in the

training set, the number of animals with measured phenotypes was set to 300, 400, or 500, whereas the number of animals with self-trained phenotypes was set to 200, 400, 600, or 800. Again, the accuracy of genomic prediction was evaluated by averaging over 100 replicates of each scenario, for which reference animals with and without measured RFI phenotypes were sampled from the respective pools of available animals.

Results and discussion
Prediction accuracy of supervised learning

The goal of semi-supervised learning in the context of genomic prediction for novel traits is to train a learner using genotyped animals that may or may not have a measured phenotype for the trait of interest. First, we characterized the sensitivity of the prediction model for supervised learning to the size of the training set, in order to assess the possible gains in prediction accuracy that could be achieved by adding unlabeled animals without measured phenotypes. If performance of the model is already at its maximum, given a training set with measured phenotypes of a specific size, then gains by including additional animals without measured phenotypes are unlikely. Accuracies of prediction for supervised learning with training sets that range in size from 20 to 540 animals are in Fig. 2, where each point represents the correlation (Fig. 2a) and mean squared error (MSE) (Fig. 2b) between genomic predictions and actual RFI phenotypes for cows in the testing set, averaged over 100 replicates. As shown in Fig. 2, accuracy measured as the correlation increased and MSE decreased rapidly until the training set reached about 200 animals, and accuracy changed more slowly thereafter, while 95% of the confidence intervals decreased steadily as the size of the training set increased. Clearly a reference population with less than 200 individuals with measured phenotypes was not sufficient to train the prediction model. The reduction in standard error of the predictive accuracy may be attributed to a greater likelihood that the same individuals would be repeated among different replicates as size of the training set increased. Overall, Fig. 2 shows that the accuracy of genomic prediction increased throughout the range of training sets considered, and therefore opportunities for improvement exist by including animals with self-trained phenotypes. Based on these results, we set the size of the training set with measured phenotypes to 300, 400, and 500 for the subsequent semi-supervised learning analyses.

Prediction accuracy of semi-supervised learning

Second, we assessed how the number and proportion of animals with self-trained phenotypes changed the accuracy of genomic predictions for animals in the testing set. This change was calculated by subtracting the accuracy of the initial supervised learning model from the final accuracy of the corresponding semi-supervised learning model, i.e. $R_{SL} - R_{SSL}$. The average baseline accuracies, measured as the correlation (as the MSE) between predicted and measured RFI phenotypes for supervised SVM models trained with 300, 400, and 500 animals with measured phenotypes were equal to 22.9 (1.41), 27.0 (1.39), and 28.7% (1.37), respectively. The results in Fig. 3a suggest that including animals with self-trained phenotypes can improve prediction accuracy and the degree of improvement tended to increase as the number of additional animals with self-trained phenotypes increased. In addition, a 0% change was not included in any of the 95% confidence intervals in the graph, which suggests that results from semi-supervised and supervised learning models were significantly different. The MSE in Fig. 3b improved when adding 200 animals with self-trained phenotypes and started to decrease at 400 animals with self-trained phenotypes. Although the increases in Fig. 3a were only up to 1.7%, these increases are valuable for traits with an estimated heritability of 0.15 [19]. As shown by Pryce et al. [23], the accuracy (correlation) of genomic prediction of RFI only increased by 2% (from 11 to 13%) when adding 939 heifers from New Zealand to the reference population of 843 Australian

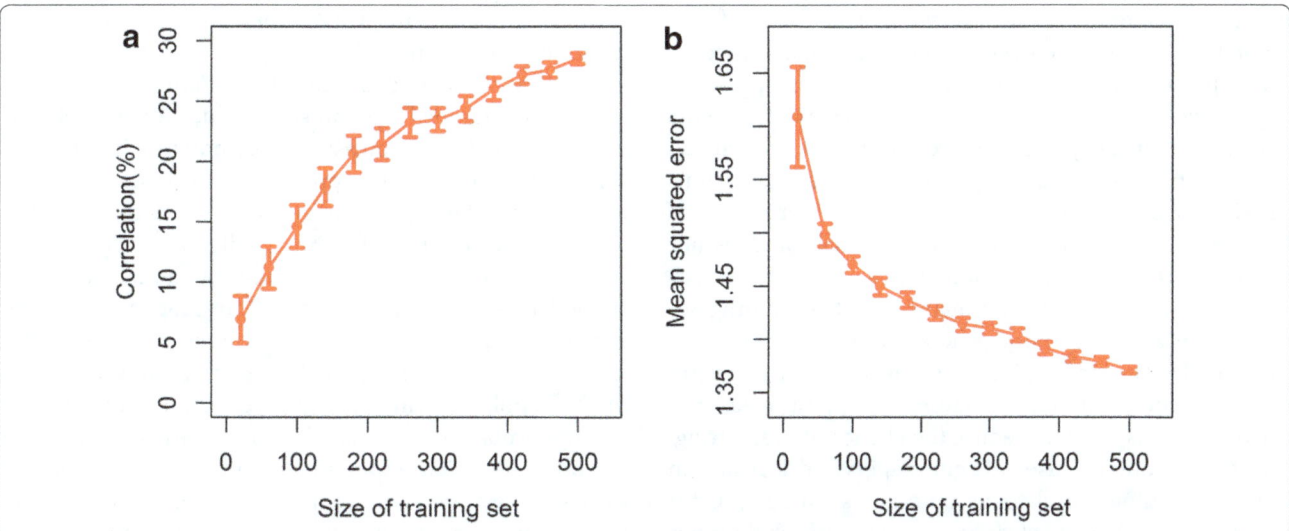

Fig. 2 Average accuracy of genomic prediction for 252 animals in the testing set. Accuracy of genomic prediction was measured as the **a** correlation or **b** mean squared error between predicted and measured residual feed intake phenotypes, plotted against the size of the training set of animals with measured phenotypes. The results for each training set size were based on 100 replicates using $n = 20, 60, \ldots, 500$ random samples from the full training set of 540 individuals with measured phenotypes. *Error bars* indicate the 95% confidence interval for each mean

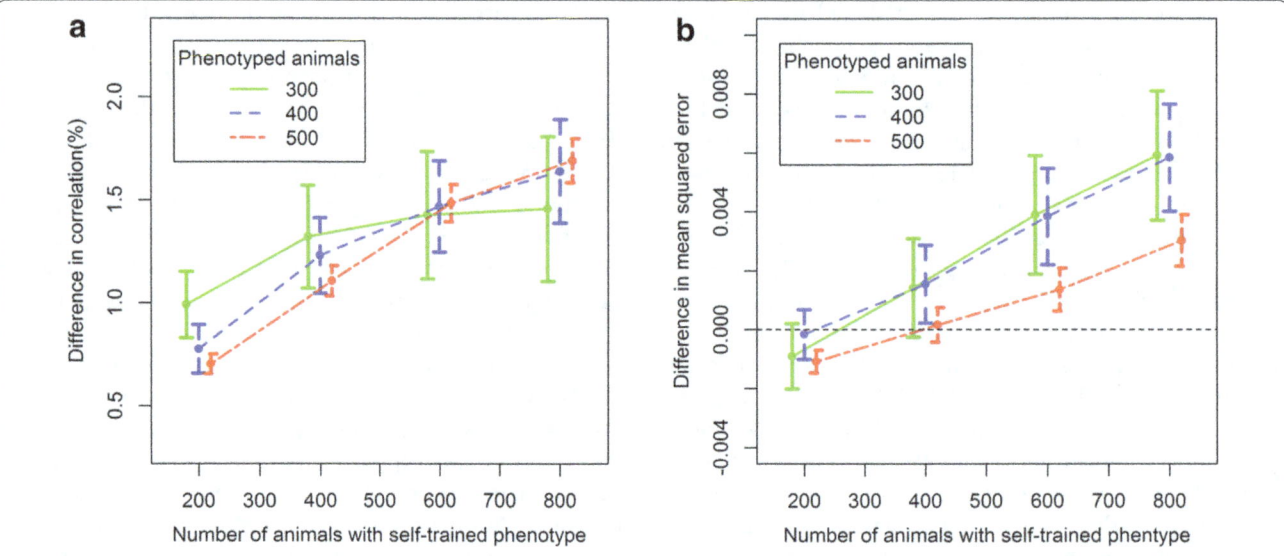

Fig. 3 Difference in accuracies of genomic predictions between the supervised and self-training algorithms. Accuracy of genomic prediction was tested for 252 animals in the testing set, and measured as the **a** correlation or **b** mean squared error between predicted and measured residual feed intake phenotypes. The number of initial reference animals with measured phenotypes was 300, 400, or 500, and a total of 200, 400, 600, and 800 animals with self-trained phenotypes were added to the training set using the self-training algorithm. *Error bars* indicate the 95% confidence intervals for each mean of 100 replicates

heifers. However, the cost to measure the individual feed intake of these 939 extra heifers was not negligible.

Figure 3a also indicates that, for a given number of animals with self-trained phenotypes, the improvement in accuracy measured as the correlation due to semi-supervised learning depends on the number of animals with measured phenotypes. The benefit of adding a given number of animals with self-trained phenotypes was greater for models that included fewer animals with measured phenotypes. A similar outcome was reported by Filipovych et al. [24] when using semi-supervised learning to classify brain images of patients with uncertain diagnoses. The reason is that, in general, semi-supervised learning is used to address situations in which labeled data are scarce [9]. In other words, if the sample of training animals is too small or does not completely represent the genomes of animals in the testing set, over-fitting specific nuances of the training set animals may lead to poor generalization to future testing populations. In semi-supervised learning, the extra genomic information from animals without measured phenotypes may help to reduce the chance of over-fitting. Therefore, potential uses of semi-supervised learning in animal breeding could focus on traits such as RFI, for which the number of reference animals with phenotypes is small. When the number of animals with measured phenotypes is sufficient, the potential gains by adding information from animals with self-trained phenotypes is limited. However, this trend was not clear for the MSE

shown in Fig. 3b. Figure 3a also shows that the slopes of all three curves decreased as the number of animals with self-trained phenotypes increased. In other words, the gain in prediction accuracy (correlation) associated with an increase from 200 to 400 animals with self-trained phenotypes was greater than the gain in accuracy associated with an increase from 400 to 600, and so on. Therefore, we may approach a plateau beyond which inclusion of more animals with self-trained phenotypes provides no additional benefit.

Third, we evaluated the number of animals with self-trained phenotypes that must be added to the training set of animals with measured phenotypes in order to achieve the maximum improvement in prediction accuracy measured using as the correlation. For this purpose, we fixed the number of animals with measured phenotypes, and we increased the number of animals with self-trained phenotypes by 200, until we reached the point at which additional improvements in accuracy were less than 0.01% for a given replicate. Figure 4a shows the ratio of the number of animals with self-trained phenotypes to the number of animals with measured phenotypes at the point at which improvements in accuracy measured as the correlation became negligible, for a given size of the initial training set. These results indicate that the optimal ratio of animals with self-trained to animals with measured phenotypes decreases as the size of the initial labeled training set increases and thus, that more animals with self-trained phenotypes are needed to compensate

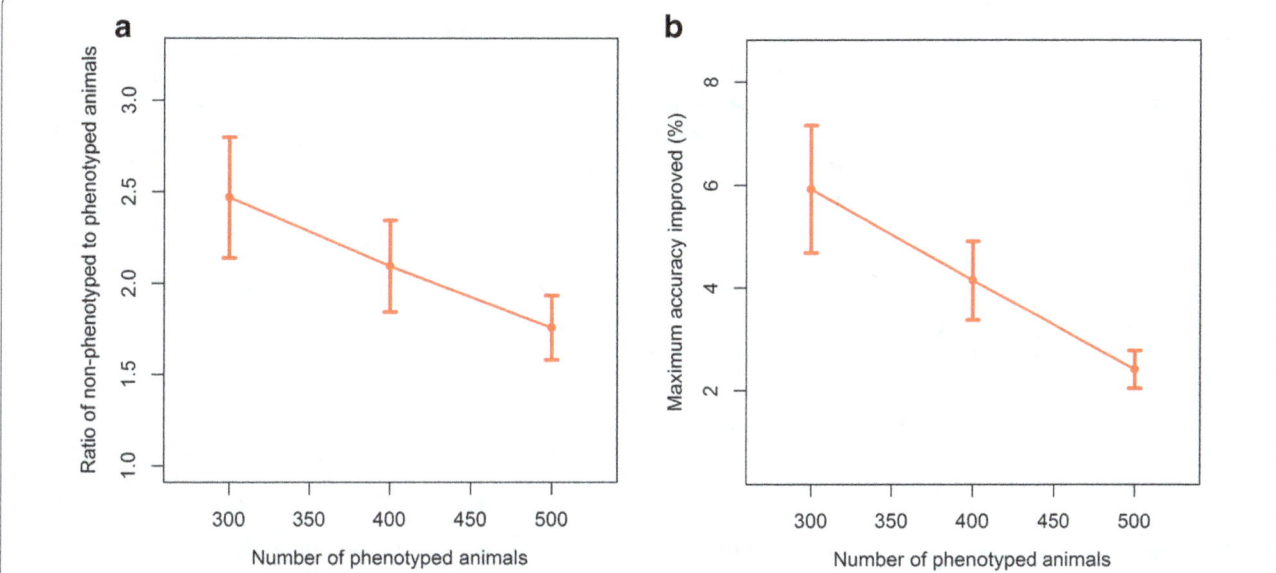

Fig. 4 **a** Ratio of the number of animals with self-trained phenotypes to that with measured phenotypes and **b** maximum improvement of the correlation (%). Incremental improvement in accuracy of prediction measured as the correlation between predicted and actual residual feed intake phenotypes within a replicate due to additional animals with self-trained phenotypes was smaller than 0.01%. The numbers of animals with measured phenotypes were 300, 400, and 500, whereas the numbers of animals with self-trained phenotypes started with 200 and increased in increments of 200 additional animals. *Error bars* indicate the 95% confidence intervals for means of 100 replicates

for the smaller labeled training sets. The highest average accuracies (correlations) achieved by semi-supervised learning were equal to 30.9, 31.4, and 30.9% for initial training sets of 300, 400, and 500 animals with measured phenotypes, respectively. Figure 4b shows that the maximum improvement achieved in prediction accuracy measured as the correlation was equal to 5.9, 4.1, and 2.4% by including animals with self-trained phenotypes in relation to the size of the initial labeled training set. Results show that maximum gains in prediction accuracy decreased as the size of the initial training set increased. In each case, these exceeded the correlation of 29.2% that was achieved using supervised learning with the full training set of 540 animals with measured phenotypes. Thus, in this study, self-training models achieved prediction accuracies measured as correlations that were comparable to those obtained from fully supervised models that were trained using larger reference populations with measured phenotypes.

Prediction accuracy measured as the correlation is an estimator of the linear relationship between predictions and responses and does not address the bias of predictions, in contrast to the MSE, as noted by González-Recio et al. [5]. The optimal number of animals with self-trained phenotypes based on minimizing MSE, was less than 400, as shown in Fig. 3b. This optimal number was smaller than when it was estimated by using the correlation based on minimizing the correlation. Thus,

depending on the purpose and criterion used for the accuracy of the prediction, the optimal number of animals with self-trained phenotypes may differ. If only the linear relationship is important, it is likely that a larger number of animals with self-trained phenotypes could be used compared with a situation where the bias of the predictions is critical.

Advantages and limitations of self-training models

The major advantages of self-training models for semi-supervised learning are threefold. First, implementation of the algorithm is simple. Second, self-training can be wrapped around any prediction model, such as SVM, genomic BLUP, or Bayesian regression. Third, if additional genotypes of animals without phenotypes are readily available (which is almost always the case), the additional costs are negligible. However, a potential disadvantage is that a self-training model is allowed to learn from its own predictions. Thus, a mistake that is made early in the learning process may reinforce itself in the self-trained phenotypes, and this could lead to poorer predictions from the final genomic prediction model. Such mistakes can occur, for example, if assumptions in the prediction model are inappropriate for a given dataset, or if the number of animals with measured phenotypes in the first step is inadequate to construct a useful predictor. As an example, we explored the use of a random forests model with a set-up that is similar to that in

Yao et al. [12] instead of using SVM in the self-training model, and found no improvement from using self-training model. As shown in [12], SVM resulted in substantially better prediction accuracy (correlation) than that obtained with the random forests model when predicting RFI (20.5 vs. 8.876%). Therefore, choosing an appropriate prediction model for the self-training method is essential. Various heuristics have been introduced to address this problem [9], and, in practice, many researchers have noted that semi-supervised learning does not always improve the accuracy of prediction or classification [25, 26]. Therefore, additional studies in animal breeding or livestock production beyond this initial application to genomic prediction of RFI in Holstein dairy cattle are needed.

Conclusions

We introduced a self-training model, chosen from the class of semi-supervised learning strategies, as a novel method to achieve potential improvements in the accuracy of genomic prediction, with a specific application to RFI in dairy cattle. Our results suggest that a self-training algorithm wrapped around a SVM prediction model may increase the accuracy of genomic prediction by collecting additional genomic information about the population from animals without measured phenotypes. For a given training set of animals with measured phenotypes, improvements in prediction accuracy measured as the correlation associated with semi-supervised learning increased as the number of additional animals with self-trained phenotypes increased, and eventually reached a plateau. In addition, improvements in accuracy measured as the correlation between predicted and measured RFI phenotypes from adding animals with self-trained phenotypes to the reference population were smaller when more animals with measured phenotypes were available in the initial testing set. The optimal number of animals with self-trained phenotypes can be smaller when predictions are evaluated based on MSE, rather than based on a correlation. Semi-supervised learning may be helpful to enhance the accuracy of genomic prediction for novel traits that are difficult or expensive to measure, and hence for small reference populations, but potential gains for other traits beyond RFI in dairy cattle should be studied.

Authors' contributions
CY designed the study, performed the data analyses and drafted the manuscript; XZ helped design the experiment; KW contributed to the data analysis and helped draft the manuscript. All authors read and approved the final manuscript.

Author details
[1] Department of Dairy Science, University of Wisconsin, Madison, Madison, WI, USA. [2] Department of Computer Science, University of Wisconsin, Madison, Madison, WI, USA.

Acknowledgements
This project was supported by Agriculture and Food Research Initiative Competitive Grant Nos. 2008-35205-18711 and 2011-68004-30340 from the USDA National Institute of Food and Agriculture (Washington, DC). Support from Hatch Grant No. MSN139239 from the Wisconsin Agricultural Experiment Station (Madison, WI) is acknowledged, and K. A. Weigel acknowledges partial financial support from the National Association of Animal Breeders (Columbia, MO).

Competing interests
The authors declare that they have no competing interests.

References
1. Clark SA, Hickey JM, Daetwyler HD, van der Werf JH. The importance of information on relatives for the prediction of genomic breeding values and the implications for the makeup of reference data sets in livestock breeding schemes. Genet Sel Evol. 2012;44:4.
2. Habier D, Fernando RL, Dekkers JCM. The impact of genetic relationship information on genome-assisted breeding values. Genetics. 2007;177:2389–97.
3. de los Campos G, Hickey JM, Pong-Wong R, Daetwyler HD, Calus MP. Whole-genome regression and prediction methods applied to plant and animal breeding. Genetics. 2013;193:327–45.
4. Gianola D, van Kaam JB. Reproducing kernel Hilbert spaces regression methods for genomic assisted prediction of quantitative traits. Genetics. 2008;178:2289–303.
5. González-Recio O, Rosa GJ, Gianola D. Machine learning methods and predictive ability metrics for genome-wide prediction of complex traits. Livest Sci. 2014;166:217–31.
6. Long N, Gianola D, Rosa GJ, Weigel KA, Kranis A, Gonzalez-Recio O. Radial basis function regression methods for predicting quantitative traits using SNP markers. Genet Res (Camb). 2010;92:209–25.
7. de Haas Y, Pryce JE, Calus MP, Wall E, Berry DP, Løvendahl P, et al. Genomic prediction of dry matter intake in dairy cattle from an international data set consisting of research herds in Europe, North America, and Australasia. J Dairy Sci. 2015;98:6522–34.
8. Berry DP, Coffey MP, Pryce JE, De Haas Y, Løvendahl P, Krattenmacher N, et al. International genetic evaluations for feed intake in dairy cattle through the collation of data from multiple sources. J Dairy Sci. 2014;97:3894–905.
9. Zhu X, Goldberg AB. Introduction to semi-supervised learning. In: Brachman RJ, Dietterich T, editors. Synthesis lectures on artificial intelligence and machine learning, vol. 3. Williston: Morgan and Claypool Publishers; 2009. p. 1–130.
10. Drucker H, Burges CJC, Kaufman L, Smola A, Vapnik V. Support vector regression machines. Adv Neural Inform Process Syst. 1997;9:155–61.
11. Gunn SR. Support vector machines for classification and regression. Technical report. University of Southampton. 1998.
12. Yao C, Armentano LE, VandeHaar MJ, Weigel KA. Short communication: use of single nucleotide polymorphism genotypes and health history to predict future phenotypes for milk production, dry matter intake, body weight, and residual feed intake in dairy cattle. J Dairy Sci. 2015;98:2027–32.
13. Rosenberg C, Hebert M, Schneiderman H. Semi-supervised self-training of object detection models. Williston: Morgan and Claypool Publishers; 2005.
14. McClosky D, Charniak E, Johnson M. Effective self-training for parsing. In: Proceedings of the main conference on human language technology conference of the North American Chapter of the Association of Computational Linguistics; 2006. p. 152–9.
15. Tang D, Yu TH, Kim TK. Real-time articulated hand pose estimation using semi-supervised transductive regression forests. In: Proceedings of the IEEE international conference on computer vision, 1–8 Dec 2013, Sydney. 2013.

16. Besemer J, Lomsadze A, Borodovsky M. GeneMarkS: a self-training method for prediction of gene starts in microbial genomes. Implications for finding sequence motifs in regulatory regions. Nucleic Acids Res. 2001;29:2607–18.

17. Lomsadze A, Ter-Hovhannisyan V, Chernoff YO, Borodovsky M. Gene identification in novel eukaryotic genomes by self-training algorithm. Nucleic Acids Res. 2005;33:6494–506.

18. Dimitriadou E, Hornik K, Leisch F, Meyer D, Weingessel A, Leisch MF. e1071: misc functions of the department of statistics (e1071), TU Wien. R package version 1.5-7. 2005. http://CRAN.R-project.org/.

19. Tempelman RJ, Spurlock DM, Coffey M, Veerkamp RF, Armentano LE, Weigel KA, et al. Heterogeneity in genetic and nongenetic variation and energy sink relationships for residual feed intake across research stations and countries. J Dairy Sci. 2015;98:2013–26.

20. VanRaden PM, Null DJ, Sargolzaei M, Wiggans GR, Tooker ME, Cole JB, et al. Genomic imputation and evaluation using high-density Holstein genotypes. J Dairy Sci. 2013;96:668–78.

21. Wiggans GR, VanRaden PM, Cooper TA. Technical note: rapid calculation of genomic evaluations for new animals. J Dairy Sci. 2015;98:2039–42.

22. VanRaden PM, Van Tassell CP, Wiggans GR, Sonstegard TS, Schnabel RD, Taylor JF, et al. Invited review: reliability of genomic predictions for North American Holstein bulls. J Dairy Sci. 2009;92:16–24.

23. Pryce JE, Arias J, Bowman PJ, Davis SR, Macdonald KA, Waghorn GC, et al. Accuracy of genomic predictions of residual feed intake and 250-day body weight in growing heifers using 625,000 single nucleotide polymorphism markers. J Dairy Sci. 2012;95:2108–19.

24. Filipovych R, Davatzikos C, Alzheimer's Disease Neuroimaging Initiative. Semi-supervised pattern classification of medical images: application to mild cognitive impairment (MCI). Neuroimage. 2011;55:1109–19.

25. Cozman FG, Cohen I, Cirelo MC. Semi-supervised learning of mixture models. In: Proceedings of the twentieth international conference on machine learning, 21–24 Aug 2003, Washington. 2003.

26. Elworthy D. Does Baum-Welch re-estimation help taggers? In: Proceedings of the fourth conference on applied natural language processing. Association for Computational Linguistics, 13–15 Oct 1994, Stuttgart. 1994.

2

Single-step SNP-BLUP with on-the-fly imputed genotypes and residual polygenic effects

Matti Taskinen*⬤, Esa A. Mäntysaari and Ismo Strandén

Abstract

Background: Single-step genomic best linear unbiased prediction (BLUP) evaluation combines relationship information from pedigree and genomic marker data. The inclusion of the genomic information into mixed model equations requires the inverse of the combined relationship matrix **H**, which has a dense matrix block for genotyped animals.

Methods: To avoid inversion of dense matrices, single-step genomic BLUP can be transformed to single-step single nucleotide polymorphism BLUP (SNP-BLUP) which have observed and imputed marker coefficients. Simple block LDL type decompositions of the single-step relationship matrix **H** were derived to obtain different types of linearly equivalent single-step genomic mixed model equations with different sets of reparametrized random effects. For non-genotyped animals, the imputed marker coefficient terms in the single-step SNP-BLUP were calculated on-the-fly during the iterative solution using sparse matrix decompositions without storing the imputed genotypes. Residual polygenic effects were added to genotyped animals and transmitted to non-genotyped animals using relationship coefficients that are similar to imputed genotypes. The relationships were further orthogonalized to improve convergence of iterative methods.

Results: All presented single-step SNP-BLUP models can be solved efficiently using iterative methods that rely on iteration on data and sparse matrix approaches. The efficiency, accuracy and iteration convergence of the derived mixed model equations were tested with a small dataset that included 73,579 animals of which 2885 were genotyped with 37,526 SNPs.

Conclusions: Inversion of the large and dense genomic relationship matrix was avoided in single-step evaluation by using fully orthogonalized single-step SNP-BLUP formulations. The number of iterations until convergence was smaller in single-step SNP-BLUP formulations than in the original single-step GBLUP when heritability was low, but increased above that of the original single-step when heritability was high.

Background

The first model to simultaneously combine genomic information with non-genotyped animal information was single-step best linear unbiased prediction (BLUP) [1, 2] or ssGBLUP. When the number of genotyped animals is large, ssGBLUP may become computationally infeasible for practical purposes because it requires the inverses of dense matrices of size equal to the number of genotyped animals, particularly the inverse of the

genomic relationship matrix $\mathbf{G}_g^{-1}$. In addition, matrix $\mathbf{G}_g$ can be singular when the number of genotyped individuals exceeds the number of markers. Computational challenges may have been a reason for the slow adoption of ssGBLUP instead of a multi-step approach. A computationally scalable alternative, the algorithm for proven and young (APY), has been suggested [3]. In APY, a sparse $\mathbf{G}_{APY}^{-1}$ approximation to the $\mathbf{G}_g^{-1}$ matrix is created by setting a diagonal matrix for a group of individuals. In practice, APY has been able to reduce computational costs significantly when the number of genotyped animals is very large [4, 5]. However, different sets of core animals

*Correspondence: matti.taskinen@luke.fi
Natural Resources Institute Finland (Luke), Myllytie 1, Jokioinen, Finland

in APY will give different evaluations, which may affect selection decisions.

An alternative formulation called hereinafter single-step single nucleotide polymorphism BLUP (ssSNP-BLUP) [6] overcomes some of the major computational challenges in ssGBLUP. In particular, there is no need to construct or invert the genomic relationship matrix $\mathbf{G}_g$. The original idea in ssSNP-BLUP circumvents the problems in ssGBLUP by predicting or imputing genotypes for non-genotyped animals, and relying on computationally less demanding SNP-based prediction instead of breeding value based prediction. An additional advantage is that the marker effect solutions are easier to use for interim predictions.

The ssSNP-BLUP has some computational challenges as well. A simple implementation for ssSNP-BLUP generates and stores genotypes of all SNPs for all animals. This will lead to very large disk storage and fast reading requirements that will prohibit use of the approach for large populations. An alternative is to make the required genotype imputations "on-the-fly" instead of storing the very large amount of imputed genotypes to file. For practical purposes, the on-the-fly imputation requires a fast computing approach for the imputation step and/or fast convergence of the iterative method.

The original description for ssSNP-BLUP approach presents a wider range of models than ssGBLUP such as the use of a number of different Bayesian SNP model formulations [6]. In ssGBLUP, in contrast to ssSNP-BLUP, it is typical to include residual polygenic (RPG) information to enhance genomic information by including pedigree-based relationships into the genomic relationship matrix. Thus, the genomic relationship matrix is usually "adjusted" with part of the pedigree relationship matrix either to supply more additive relationship information or simply to make the genomic relationship matrix invertible. In the original ssSNP-BLUP formulation, this information has not been included. The computational challenges of ssGBLUP has led to the introduction of several equivalent models (e.g., [7–9]). However, these alternative approaches have had poor convergence by iterative methods [7, 9]. One reason is that the covariance structures have a poorer condition number which is a ratio of the largest and smallest eigenvalues and is used to measure numerical stability [9]. Some of the alternative versions of ssGBLUP have had SNP effects. Because ssSNP-BLUP is equivalent to ssGBLUP and ssGBLUP has many equivalent forms, alternative formulations of mixed model equations (MME) can be derived for ssSNP-BLUP as well.

In this paper, simple block LDL type decompositions [10] of the ssGBLUP relationship matrix are derived to obtain several linearly equivalent MME. This allows

derivation and testing of several equivalent ssSNP-BLUP MME that avoid making and storing the imputed genotypes. In this paper, an explicit imputation of genotypes is not needed but instead we apply sparse matrix decompositions to attain pedigree-based regressions of evaluations of genotyped animals on non-genotyped animals using sparse matrix decompositions. Accuracy and iteration convergence of the derived equivalent MME are tested on a small Nordic dairy cattle dataset.

Methods

For any model, an infinite number of equivalent models exist. In the following, first we recall the concept of equivalent models and how equivalent models can be made by attaching covariance information to the model design matrix. As an example, equivalence of genomic BLUP (GBLUP) and SNP-BLUP is presented. Then, ssGBLUP is recalled, and its covariance structure formulated using LDL decomposition. Equivalent MME are derived where information from the genomic relationship matrix are attached to the model design matrix similarly as shown for GBLUP and SNP-BLUP, resulting in ssSNP-BLUP. Finally, MME having orthogonalized random effects or diagonal covariance structures are derived in order to improve the convergence in iterative methods. A small dataset is used to illustrate performance of the derived equivalent models.

Linearly equivalent models

Two mixed linear effects models, i.e.

$$\mathbf{y} = \mathbf{Xb} + \mathbf{Zu} + \mathbf{e}, \, Var(\mathbf{u}) = \mathbf{G}, \, Var(\mathbf{e}) = \mathbf{R} \qquad (1)$$

$$\mathbf{y} = \widetilde{\mathbf{X}}\widetilde{\mathbf{b}} + \widetilde{\mathbf{Z}}\widetilde{\mathbf{u}} + \widetilde{\mathbf{e}}, \, Var(\widetilde{\mathbf{u}}) = \widetilde{\mathbf{G}}, \, Var(\widetilde{\mathbf{e}}) = \widetilde{\mathbf{R}} \qquad (2)$$

with the same observations $\mathbf{y}$ but different fixed ($\mathbf{b}$ and $\widetilde{\mathbf{b}}$) and random effects ($\mathbf{u}$ and $\widetilde{\mathbf{u}}$), residual errors ($\mathbf{e}$ and $\widetilde{\mathbf{e}}$), model matrices ($\mathbf{X}$, $\mathbf{Z}$, $\widetilde{\mathbf{X}}$, and $\widetilde{\mathbf{Z}}$) and variance structures ($\mathbf{G}$, $\mathbf{R}$, $\widetilde{\mathbf{G}}$, and $\widetilde{\mathbf{R}}$), are said to be *linearly equivalent models* [11–13] if the expected values and the variances of the observations are equal. Thus, models (1) and (2) are equivalent if:

$$\begin{cases} \mathbf{Xb} = \widetilde{\mathbf{X}}\widetilde{\mathbf{b}}, \\ \mathbf{V} = \mathbf{ZGZ}' + \mathbf{R} = \widetilde{\mathbf{Z}}\widetilde{\mathbf{G}}\widetilde{\mathbf{Z}}' + \widetilde{\mathbf{R}} = \widetilde{\mathbf{V}}. \end{cases} \qquad (3)$$

Separate equations for fixed and random effects

Mixed model (1) can be solved from separate equations for fixed and random effects [14] as:

$$\begin{aligned} \widehat{\mathbf{b}} &= (\mathbf{X}'\mathbf{V}^{-1}\mathbf{X})^{-1}\mathbf{X}'\mathbf{V}^{-1}\mathbf{y} \\ \widehat{\mathbf{u}} &= \mathbf{GZ}'\mathbf{V}^{-1}(\mathbf{y} - \mathbf{X}\widehat{\mathbf{b}}), \end{aligned} \qquad (4)$$

where matrix $\mathbf{V}$ needs to be invertible. The size of matrix $\mathbf{V}$ is the number of observations, which can be very large, and, therefore, solving the mixed model using this method is seldom feasible in practice.

Mixed model equations

In practice, Eq. (4) can be solved by Henderson's MME [14] as follows:

$$\begin{bmatrix} \mathbf{X'R^{-1}X} & \mathbf{X'R^{-1}Z} \\ \mathbf{Z'R^{-1}X} & \mathbf{Z'R^{-1}Z + G^{-1}} \end{bmatrix} \begin{bmatrix} \widehat{\mathbf{b}} \\ \widehat{\mathbf{u}} \end{bmatrix} = \begin{bmatrix} \mathbf{X'R^{-1}y} \\ \mathbf{Z'R^{-1}y} \end{bmatrix}, \quad (5)$$

where the variance matrix of the random effects $\mathbf{G}$ and the residual variance matrix $\mathbf{R}$ need to be invertible. MME (5) usually lead to more sparse matrix systems than Eq. (4).

Equivalent models by splitting the variance matrix

Suppose the variance matrix $\mathbf{G}$ can be expressed as a matrix product as follows:

$$\mathbf{G} = \mathbf{M}\widetilde{\mathbf{G}}\mathbf{M}', \quad (6)$$

where $\mathbf{M}$ is rectangular and $\widetilde{\mathbf{G}}$ is an invertible square matrix. Here, the matrix $\widetilde{\mathbf{G}}$ could be, for example, an identity matrix and could have different dimensions than the $\mathbf{G}$ matrix.

Matrices $\mathbf{G}$ and $\mathbf{Z}$ are always together in Eq. (4). This allows us to re-parametrize the model as:

$$\begin{aligned} \mathbf{V} &= \mathbf{ZGZ'} + \mathbf{R} \\ &= \mathbf{ZM}\widetilde{\mathbf{G}}\mathbf{M'Z'} + \mathbf{R} \quad (7) \\ &= \widetilde{\mathbf{Z}}\widetilde{\mathbf{G}}\widetilde{\mathbf{Z}}' + \widetilde{\mathbf{R}} = \widetilde{\mathbf{V}}, \end{aligned}$$

and thereafter:

$$\begin{aligned} \widehat{\mathbf{u}} &= \mathbf{M}\widetilde{\mathbf{G}}\mathbf{M'Z'V^{-1}(y-X\widehat{b})} \\ &= \mathbf{M}\widetilde{\mathbf{G}}\widetilde{\mathbf{Z}}'\widetilde{\mathbf{V}}^{-1}(\mathbf{y}-\mathbf{X}\widehat{\mathbf{b}}) = \mathbf{M}\widetilde{\mathbf{u}}, \end{aligned} \quad (8)$$

where the equivalent model has the same residual variance matrix ($\widetilde{\mathbf{R}} = \mathbf{R}$), the new model matrix $\widetilde{\mathbf{Z}} = \mathbf{ZM}$, and the random effects $\widetilde{\mathbf{u}}$ are defined as:

$$\widetilde{\mathbf{u}} = \widetilde{\mathbf{G}}\widetilde{\mathbf{Z}}'\widetilde{\mathbf{V}}^{-1}(\mathbf{y} - \mathbf{X}\widehat{\mathbf{b}}). \quad (9)$$

Now, according to Eq. (3), the quantities with a tilde together with the same observation vector $\mathbf{y}$, the original fixed effects ($\widetilde{\mathbf{b}} = \widehat{\mathbf{b}}$), and design matrix ($\widetilde{\mathbf{X}} = \mathbf{X}$) form a linearly equivalent model (2).

Linearly equivalent MME

Original fixed effects $\widehat{\mathbf{b}}$ and the new random effects $\widetilde{\mathbf{u}}$ of the linearly equivalent model can be solved, similarly as in Eq. (4), from:

$$\begin{aligned} \widehat{\mathbf{b}} &= (\mathbf{X'}\widetilde{\mathbf{V}}^{-1}\mathbf{X})^{-1}\mathbf{X'}\widetilde{\mathbf{V}}^{-1}\mathbf{y} \\ \widetilde{\mathbf{u}} &= \widetilde{\mathbf{G}}\widetilde{\mathbf{Z}}'\widetilde{\mathbf{V}}^{-1}(\mathbf{y} - \mathbf{X}\widehat{\mathbf{b}}), \end{aligned} \quad (10)$$

or from the corresponding MME (5):

$$\begin{bmatrix} \mathbf{X'R^{-1}X} & \mathbf{X'R^{-1}\widetilde{Z}} \\ \widetilde{\mathbf{Z}}'\mathbf{R^{-1}X} & \widetilde{\mathbf{Z}}'\mathbf{R^{-1}\widetilde{Z} + \widetilde{G}^{-1}} \end{bmatrix} \begin{bmatrix} \widehat{\mathbf{b}} \\ \widetilde{\mathbf{u}} \end{bmatrix} = \begin{bmatrix} \mathbf{X'R^{-1}y} \\ \widetilde{\mathbf{Z}}'\mathbf{R^{-1}y} \end{bmatrix}. \quad (11)$$

Because of the equivalence $\widehat{\mathbf{u}} = \mathbf{M}\widetilde{\mathbf{u}}$ in Eq. (8), the original random effects $\widehat{\mathbf{u}}$ can be obtained from the solution of the *linearly equivalent MME* (11) by pre-multiplying the new random effects $\widetilde{\mathbf{u}}$ with matrix $\mathbf{M}$, i.e.

$$\begin{bmatrix} \widehat{\mathbf{b}} \\ \widehat{\mathbf{u}} \end{bmatrix} = \begin{bmatrix} \mathbf{I}_b & 0 \\ 0 & \mathbf{M} \end{bmatrix} \begin{bmatrix} \mathbf{X'R^{-1}X} & \mathbf{X'R^{-1}\widetilde{X}} \\ \widetilde{\mathbf{Z}}'\mathbf{R^{-1}X} & \widetilde{\mathbf{Z}}'\mathbf{R^{-1}\widetilde{Z} + \widetilde{G}^{-1}} \end{bmatrix}^{-1} \begin{bmatrix} \mathbf{X'R^{-1}y} \\ \widetilde{\mathbf{Z}}'\mathbf{R^{-1}y} \end{bmatrix},$$
$$(12)$$

where identity matrix $\mathbf{I}_b$ has dimension of $\widehat{\mathbf{b}}$. Note that the inverse of the MME matrix in Eq. (12) is usually not evaluated explicitly, but rather, the corresponding linear matrix equation is solved using either direct or iterative solution methods.

The original MME (5) can, thus, be solved from a modified linearly equivalent MME (11) where the number of random effects in $\widetilde{\mathbf{u}}$ could be smaller or larger than in $\widehat{\mathbf{u}}$, the variance structure $\widetilde{\mathbf{G}}$ could be easier to obtain or invert than the original $\mathbf{G}$, or the new matrix system could be otherwise numerically more efficient.

Presentation for GBLUP and SNP-BLUP

As an example, consider single-trait GBLUP MME [15]. The variance matrix of random effects $\mathbf{u}$ is based on a genomic relationship matrix ($\mathbf{G}_g$), which describes the genomic relationships between individuals, i.e. $Var(\mathbf{u}) = \sigma_u^2 \mathbf{G}_g$. The genomic relationship matrix is usually fully dense and increases in order as the number of genotyped animals increases. The inverted genomic relationship matrix $\mathbf{G}_g^{-1}$ is needed in the solution of the GBLUP MME:

$$\begin{bmatrix} \widehat{\mathbf{b}} \\ \widehat{\mathbf{u}} \end{bmatrix} = \begin{bmatrix} \mathbf{X'X} & \mathbf{X'Z} \\ \mathbf{Z'X} & \mathbf{Z'Z} + \lambda\mathbf{G}_g^{-1} \end{bmatrix}^{-1} \begin{bmatrix} \mathbf{X'y} \\ \mathbf{Z'y} \end{bmatrix}, \quad (13)$$

where a single trait case is assumed for simplicity, $\mathbf{R} = \sigma_e^2\mathbf{I}$, and $\lambda = \frac{\sigma_e^2}{\sigma_u^2}$.

There are many ways to construct $\mathbf{G}_g$. Assume the genomic relationship matrix $\mathbf{G}_g$ can be expressed, in simplified form, using (centered and scaled) marker matrix $\mathbf{Z}_m$ [15] so that:

$$\mathbf{G}_g = \mathbf{Z}_m\mathbf{Z}_m' = \mathbf{M}\widetilde{\mathbf{G}}\mathbf{M}', \quad (14)$$

where

$$\mathbf{M} = \mathbf{Z}_m \quad \text{and} \quad \widetilde{\mathbf{G}} = \mathbf{I}_m, \quad (15)$$

and $\mathbf{I}_m$ is an identity matrix of size equal to the number of markers. Now, a linearly equivalent MME (11), alternative to GBLUP MME (13), can be derived and original effects solved similarly as in (12) so that:

$$\begin{bmatrix} \hat{\mathbf{b}} \\ \hat{\mathbf{u}} \end{bmatrix} = \begin{bmatrix} \mathbf{I}_b & 0 \\ 0 & \mathbf{Z}_m \end{bmatrix} \begin{bmatrix} \mathbf{X}'\mathbf{X} & \mathbf{X}'\tilde{\mathbf{Z}} \\ \tilde{\mathbf{Z}}'\mathbf{X} & \tilde{\mathbf{Z}}'\tilde{\mathbf{Z}} + \lambda\mathbf{I}_m \end{bmatrix}^{-1} \begin{bmatrix} \mathbf{X}'\mathbf{y} \\ \tilde{\mathbf{Z}}'\mathbf{y} \end{bmatrix},$$

where $\tilde{\mathbf{Z}} = \mathbf{Z}\mathbf{Z}_m$ and λ is the same variance ratio as in Eq. (13). This equivalent MME system, known as the SNP-BLUP [16], has markers as random effects instead of individuals. Random effects are also "orthogonalized", and, thus, inversion of the dense genomic relationship matrix $\mathbf{G}_g$ is avoided.

Note that, if the marker effects have unequal variances, the relationship matrix can be build as:

$$\mathbf{G}_g = \mathbf{Z}_m\mathbf{B}\mathbf{Z}'_m = \mathbf{M}\tilde{\mathbf{G}}\mathbf{M}', \tag{16}$$

where

$$\mathbf{M} = \mathbf{Z}_m \quad \text{and} \quad \tilde{\mathbf{G}} = \mathbf{B}, \tag{17}$$

and the matrix $\mathbf{B}$ is a diagonal covariance matrix describing the variances of different marker effects. Now the solution of SNP-BLUP becomes:

$$\begin{bmatrix} \hat{\mathbf{b}} \\ \hat{\mathbf{u}} \end{bmatrix} = \begin{bmatrix} \mathbf{I}_b & 0 \\ 0 & \mathbf{Z}_m \end{bmatrix} \begin{bmatrix} \mathbf{X}'\mathbf{X} & \mathbf{X}'\tilde{\mathbf{Z}} \\ \tilde{\mathbf{Z}}'\mathbf{X} & \tilde{\mathbf{Z}}'\tilde{\mathbf{Z}} + \lambda\mathbf{B}^{-1} \end{bmatrix}^{-1} \begin{bmatrix} \mathbf{X}'\mathbf{y} \\ \tilde{\mathbf{Z}}'\mathbf{y} \end{bmatrix}.$$

Single-step SNP-BLUP

In ssGBLUP [1, 2], some individuals have genomic information while some have only pedigree information. The model for ssGBLUP is a special case of mixed effect models, where the between-animal relationships are modeled via the aggregated relationship matrix $\mathbf{H}$ [1, 2]. The relationships in $\mathbf{H}$ are described by the pedigree-based relationship matrix $\mathbf{A}$, and the genomic relationship matrix among genotyped animals by $\mathbf{G}_g$. Relationships among non-genotyped individuals are constructed from the pedigree but modified according to the relationships among genotyped animals.

Assuming that the non-genotyped individuals are denoted with sub- and super-scripts 1 and the genotyped individuals by sub- and super-scripts 2, the pedigree relationship matrix and its inverse are the following:

$$\mathbf{A} = \begin{bmatrix} \mathbf{A}_{11} & \mathbf{A}_{12} \\ \mathbf{A}_{21} & \mathbf{A}_{22} \end{bmatrix} \quad \text{and} \quad \mathbf{A}^{-1} = \begin{bmatrix} \mathbf{A}^{11} & \mathbf{A}^{12} \\ \mathbf{A}^{21} & \mathbf{A}^{22} \end{bmatrix}. \tag{18}$$

Assume, as before, that the genomic relationship matrix has the form $\mathbf{G}_g = \mathbf{Z}_m\mathbf{Z}'_m$. If the genotyped population contains identical twins, i.e. clones, or if there are more individuals than markers, the genomic relationship matrix $\mathbf{G}_g$ becomes singular and the usual MME (5) cannot be constructed. Hence, $\mathbf{G}_g$ is commonly adjusted by regressing it towards the pedigree relationship matrix $\mathbf{A}_{22}$ with:

$$\mathbf{G}_w = w\mathbf{A}_{22} + (1 - w)\mathbf{G}_g, \tag{19}$$

where w is a scalar weight between 0 and 1 and can be interpreted as the relative weight on the polygenic effect [2, 15].

Single-step relationship matrix

The inverse of the ssGBLUP variance matrix $\mathbf{H}$ is [1, 2]:

$$\mathbf{H}^{-1} = \mathbf{A}^{-1} + \begin{bmatrix} 0 & 0 \\ 0 & \mathbf{G}_w^{-1} - (\mathbf{A}_{22})^{-1} \end{bmatrix} \tag{20}$$

$$= \begin{bmatrix} \mathbf{A}^{11} & \mathbf{A}^{12} \\ \mathbf{A}^{21} & \mathbf{A}^{22} + \mathbf{G}_w^{-1} - (\mathbf{A}_{22})^{-1} \end{bmatrix}. \tag{21}$$

Using block LDL decomposition, it is equal to:

$$\mathbf{H}^{-1} = \begin{bmatrix} \mathbf{I}_1 & 0 \\ -\mathbf{A}'_{imp} & \mathbf{I}_2 \end{bmatrix} \begin{bmatrix} \mathbf{A}^{11} & 0 \\ 0 & \mathbf{G}_w^{-1} \end{bmatrix} \begin{bmatrix} \mathbf{I}_1 & -\mathbf{A}_{imp} \\ 0 & \mathbf{I}_2 \end{bmatrix}, \tag{22}$$

where $\mathbf{I}_1$ and $\mathbf{I}_2$ are identity matrices of size equal to the number of non-genotyped and genotyped animals, respectively. For imputation of genotypes:

$$\mathbf{A}_{imp} = \mathbf{A}_{12}(\mathbf{A}_{22})^{-1} = -(\mathbf{A}^{11})^{-1}\mathbf{A}^{12} \tag{23}$$

is a regression prediction or an *imputation operator* that expands the genomic relationship information from the genotyped to the non-genotyped individuals [2, 6, 17]. By inverting the LDL decomposition of Eq. (22), the variance matrix $\mathbf{H}$ has a similar decomposition:

$$\mathbf{H} = \begin{bmatrix} \mathbf{I}_1 & \mathbf{A}_{imp} \\ 0 & \mathbf{I}_2 \end{bmatrix} \begin{bmatrix} (\mathbf{A}^{11})^{-1} & 0 \\ 0 & \mathbf{G}_w \end{bmatrix} \begin{bmatrix} \mathbf{I}_1 & 0 \\ \mathbf{A}'_{imp} & \mathbf{I}_2 \end{bmatrix}. \tag{24}$$

By using block matrix inversion identities (23) and

$$(\mathbf{A}^{11})^{-1} = \mathbf{A}_{11} - \mathbf{A}_{12}(\mathbf{A}_{22})^{-1}\mathbf{A}_{21} \tag{25}$$

to the "imputed" $\mathbf{A}_{22}$ matrix of $\mathbf{G}_w$ (19)

$$\begin{bmatrix} \mathbf{A}_{imp} \\ \mathbf{I}_2 \end{bmatrix} \mathbf{A}_{22} \begin{bmatrix} \mathbf{A}'_{imp} & \mathbf{I}_2 \end{bmatrix} = \mathbf{A} - \begin{bmatrix} (\mathbf{A}^{11})^{-1} & 0 \\ 0 & 0 \end{bmatrix}, \tag{26}$$

the variance matrix $\mathbf{H}$ (24) can be alternatively expressed as:

$$\mathbf{H} = (1 - w)\begin{bmatrix} (\mathbf{A}^{11})^{-1} & 0 \\ 0 & 0 \end{bmatrix} + w\mathbf{A} + (1 - w)\mathbf{G}_{imp}, \tag{27}$$

where $\mathbf{G}_{imp}$ is an imputed genomic relationship matrix as follows:

$$\mathbf{G}_{imp} = \begin{bmatrix} \mathbf{A}_{imp} \\ \mathbf{I}_2 \end{bmatrix} \mathbf{G}_g \begin{bmatrix} \mathbf{A}'_{imp} & \mathbf{I}_2 \end{bmatrix}. \tag{28}$$

Note that this operates on $\mathbf{G}_g$ instead of $\mathbf{G}_w$. Also, note that $\mathbf{G}_{imp}$ has a size equal to the number of all animals. Genotyped animals have observed marker data but non-genotyped animals have imputed marker data.

Equivalent single-step MME

In the following, the single-step relationship matrix $\mathbf{H}$ will be expressed as six different decompositions equivalent to Eq. (6):

$$\mathbf{H} = \mathbf{M}_i \widetilde{\mathbf{G}}_i \mathbf{M}'_i, \quad i = 1, \ldots, 6, \tag{29}$$

for different matrices $\mathbf{M}_i$ and $\widetilde{\mathbf{G}}_i$. All of these lead to a linearly equivalent ssGBLUP MME system of new sets of random effects with, potentially, different numerical properties. The linearly equivalent MME of these modified sets of random effects are similar to Eq. (11) and the original effects can be solved similarly as in Eq. (12):

$$\begin{bmatrix} \widehat{\mathbf{b}} \\ \widehat{\mathbf{u}} \end{bmatrix} = \begin{bmatrix} \mathbf{I}_b & 0 \\ 0 & \mathbf{M}_i \end{bmatrix} \begin{bmatrix} \mathbf{X}'\mathbf{X} & \mathbf{X}'\widetilde{\mathbf{Z}}_i \\ \widetilde{\mathbf{Z}}'_i\mathbf{X} & \widetilde{\mathbf{Z}}'_i\widetilde{\mathbf{Z}}_i + \lambda\widetilde{\mathbf{G}}_i^{-1} \end{bmatrix}^{-1} \begin{bmatrix} \mathbf{X}'\mathbf{y} \\ \widetilde{\mathbf{Z}}'_i\mathbf{y} \end{bmatrix},$$

where $\widetilde{\mathbf{Z}}_i = \mathbf{Z}\mathbf{M}_i$ and a single trait case is assumed.

Note that in these equivalent MME, square matrix $\widetilde{\mathbf{G}}_i$ represents the covariance structure for the reparametrized random effects, $\mathbf{M}_i$ has a row for each original random effect in $\mathbf{u}$ to change the model matrix $\mathbf{Z}$, and $\widetilde{\mathbf{Z}}_i$ is the redefined model matrix.

In order to derive linearly equivalent MME for multiple trait cases:

$$\mathbf{G} = \mathbf{G}_0 \otimes \mathbf{H}, \tag{30}$$

where $\otimes$ is the Kronecker product, the genetic (co)variance matrix $\mathbf{G}_0$ of size number of traits is assumed to have a decomposition:

$$\mathbf{G}_0 = \mathbf{M}_0 \widetilde{\mathbf{G}}_0 \mathbf{M}'_0. \tag{31}$$

For example, a simple case would have $\mathbf{M}_0$ as identity matrix and $\widetilde{\mathbf{G}}_0$ as $\mathbf{G}_0$. Now the variance matrix $\mathbf{G}$ can be expressed using the decompositions of the single-step relationship matrix (29) similarly as in Eq. (6):

$$\mathbf{G} = \mathbf{G}_0 \otimes \mathbf{H} = (\mathbf{M}_0 \widetilde{\mathbf{G}}_0 \mathbf{M}'_0) \otimes (\mathbf{M}_i \widetilde{\mathbf{G}}_i \mathbf{M}'_i) \tag{32}$$

$$= (\mathbf{M}_0 \otimes \mathbf{M}_i)(\widetilde{\mathbf{G}}_0 \otimes \widetilde{\mathbf{G}}_i)(\mathbf{M}_0 \otimes \mathbf{M}_i)' \tag{33}$$

$$= \mathbf{M}\widetilde{\mathbf{G}}\mathbf{M}', \tag{34}$$

where

$$\mathbf{M} = \mathbf{M}_0 \otimes \mathbf{M}_i \quad \text{and} \quad \widetilde{\mathbf{G}} = \widetilde{\mathbf{G}}_0 \otimes \widetilde{\mathbf{G}}_i. \tag{35}$$

Effects can then be solved from linearly equivalent multiple trait MME (12):

$$\begin{bmatrix} \widehat{\mathbf{b}} \\ \widehat{\mathbf{u}} \end{bmatrix} = \begin{bmatrix} \mathbf{I}_b & 0 \\ 0 & \mathbf{M}_0 \otimes \mathbf{M}_i \end{bmatrix}$$
$$\times \begin{bmatrix} \mathbf{X}'\mathbf{R}^{-1}\mathbf{X} & \mathbf{X}'\mathbf{R}^{-1}\widetilde{\mathbf{Z}}_i \\ \widetilde{\mathbf{Z}}'_i\mathbf{R}^{-1}\mathbf{X} & \widetilde{\mathbf{Z}}'_i\mathbf{R}^{-1}\widetilde{\mathbf{Z}}_i + \widetilde{\mathbf{G}}_0^{-1} \otimes \widetilde{\mathbf{G}}_i^{-1} \end{bmatrix}^{-1} \begin{bmatrix} \mathbf{X}'\mathbf{R}^{-1}\mathbf{y} \\ \widetilde{\mathbf{Z}}'_i\mathbf{R}^{-1}\mathbf{y} \end{bmatrix},$$

where $\widetilde{\mathbf{Z}}_i = \mathbf{Z}(\mathbf{M}_0 \otimes \mathbf{M}_i)$.

Basic equivalent ssGBLUP MME   The LDL decomposition (24) can be used directly to build the first linearly equivalent ssGBLUP MME of this paper using $\mathbf{H} = \mathbf{M}_1 \widetilde{\mathbf{G}}_1 \mathbf{M}'_1$ where:

$$\mathbf{M}_1 = \begin{bmatrix} \mathbf{I}_1 & \mathbf{A}_{imp} \\ 0 & \mathbf{I}_2 \end{bmatrix} \quad \text{and} \quad \widetilde{\mathbf{G}}_1 = \begin{bmatrix} (\mathbf{A}^{11})^{-1} & 0 \\ 0 & \mathbf{G}_w \end{bmatrix}. \tag{36}$$

From the modified relationship matrix $\widetilde{\mathbf{G}}_1$ (36), it can be seen that this *basic equivalent ssGBLUP* MME has random effects for non-genotyped animals with variances $(\mathbf{A}^{11})^{-1}$ and for genotyped animals with variances of the adjusted genomic relationship matrix $\mathbf{G}_w$. The number of effects in the system is, thus, the same as in the original ssGBLUP.

Basic RPG ssSNP-BLUP MME   Other linearly equivalent ssGBLUP MME of the form (29) can be derived as well. Note that the adjusted genomic relationship matrix $\mathbf{G}_w$ in Eq. (19) can be expressed by matrix products as follows:

$$\mathbf{G}_w = \begin{bmatrix} \mathbf{I}_2 & \mathbf{I}_2 \end{bmatrix} \begin{bmatrix} w\mathbf{A}_{22} & 0 \\ 0 & (1-w)\mathbf{G}_g \end{bmatrix} \begin{bmatrix} \mathbf{I}_2 \\ \mathbf{I}_2 \end{bmatrix} \tag{37}$$

$$= \begin{bmatrix} \mathbf{I}_2 & \mathbf{Z}_m \end{bmatrix} \begin{bmatrix} w\mathbf{A}_{22} & 0 \\ 0 & (1-w)\mathbf{I}_m \end{bmatrix} \begin{bmatrix} \mathbf{I}_2 \\ \mathbf{Z}'_m \end{bmatrix}, \tag{38}$$

where $\mathbf{G}_g = \mathbf{Z}_m\mathbf{Z}'_m$. The second linearly equivalent ssGBLUP MME can be built by substituting $\mathbf{G}_w$ in Eq. (38) to Eq. (36):

$$\mathbf{M}_2 = \begin{bmatrix} \mathbf{I}_1 & \sqrt{w}\mathbf{A}_{imp} & \sqrt{1-w}\mathbf{A}_{imp}\mathbf{Z}_m \\ 0 & \sqrt{w}\mathbf{I}_2 & \sqrt{1-w}\mathbf{Z}_m \end{bmatrix}$$
$$\widetilde{\mathbf{G}}_2 = \begin{bmatrix} (\mathbf{A}^{11})^{-1} & 0 & 0 \\ 0 & \mathbf{A}_{22} & 0 \\ 0 & 0 & \mathbf{I}_m \end{bmatrix}. \tag{39}$$

In this form, we avoid the inverse of $\mathbf{G}_g$ in the MME (11). The coefficients w and $(1 - w)$ were also split using square roots to matrix $\mathbf{M}_2$ so that the new variance matrix $\widetilde{\mathbf{G}}_2$ can be inverted even when w is 0 or 1. The first group of new random effects in Eq. (39), for the non-genotyped animals, is the same as in the first, basic equivalent ssGBLUP in Eq. (36). However, the genotyped animals now have random effects related through the variance matrix $\mathbf{A}_{22}$. Effects in this second effect group can be seen as *residual polygenic effects* that can describe effects that the marker effects are unable to model [8]. The third group of random effects are the marker effects as in SNP-BLUP (15) and so, this decomposition (39) can be called *basic RPG ssSNP-BLUP* MME. Compared to the original ssGBLUP, the second equivalent MME has marker effects in addition to the animal effects.

Expanded RPG ssSNP-BLUP MME A third linearly equivalent MME of form (29) can be derived from the alternative expression of matrix $\mathbf{H}$ in Eq. (27) and by splitting $\mathbf{G}_g = \mathbf{Z}_m\mathbf{Z}'_m$ in Eq. (28) as:

$$
\mathbf{M}_3 = \begin{bmatrix} \sqrt{1-w}\mathbf{I}_1 & \sqrt{w}\mathbf{E}_1 & \sqrt{1-w}\mathbf{A}_{imp}\mathbf{Z}_m \\ \mathbf{0} & \sqrt{w}\mathbf{E}_2 & \sqrt{1-w}\mathbf{Z}_m \end{bmatrix}
$$
$$
\widetilde{\mathbf{G}}_3 = \begin{bmatrix} (\mathbf{A}^{11})^{-1} & \mathbf{0} & \mathbf{0} \\ \mathbf{0} & \mathbf{A} & \mathbf{0} \\ \mathbf{0} & \mathbf{0} & \mathbf{I}_m \end{bmatrix}. \tag{40}
$$

Here, matrices $\mathbf{E}_1$ and $\mathbf{E}_2$ are rectangular sparse incidence matrices that select the subsets of non-genotyped and genotyped animals, respectively, from the $\mathbf{A}$ matrix. Both $\mathbf{E}_1$ and $\mathbf{E}_2$ have the same number of columns, i.e. number of all animals. Matrix $\mathbf{E}_1$ has a row for each non-genotyped and matrix $\mathbf{E}_2$ for each genotyped animal corresponding to animal's column in matrices $\mathbf{Z}_1$ and $\mathbf{Z}_2$ of

$$
\mathbf{Z} = [\mathbf{Z}_1 \;\; \mathbf{Z}_2]. \tag{41}
$$

Each row of both $\mathbf{E}_1$ and $\mathbf{E}_2$ has only one non-zero element, a value one at the column corresponding to that animal's location among all of the animals. Hence, when rows and columns of the matrices of all animals are in the same order as in matrix $\mathbf{A}$ in Eq. (18), matrix $\begin{bmatrix} \mathbf{E}_1 \\ \mathbf{E}_2 \end{bmatrix}$ is an identity matrix of the size of all animals.

The third equivalent MME (40) has three groups of effects similar to the second MME (39). The third effect group has, again, the orthogonal marker effects, and so this formulation is a ssSNP-BLUP as well. The first effect group, for the non-genotyped animals has, however, a constant multiplier $\sqrt{1-w}$. Also, the second group, related through the pedigree relationship matrix $\mathbf{A}$, has now effects for all animals, and not just for the genotyped animals. Thus, in this third *expanded RPG ssSNP-BLUP* MME, the non-genotyped animals have two sets of random effects.

Special cases of equivalent ssGBLUP MME These three equivalent MME, (36), (39) and (40), will approach the usual animal model when $w \to 1$. At the limit ($w = 1$), the expanded RPG ssSNP-BLUP MME 3 (40) has clearly the recognizable covariance structure of $\mathbf{A}$. The basic equivalent ssGBLUP MME 1 (36) and the basic RPG ssSNP-BLUP MME 2 (39) are models where the genotyped animals act as base animals and the non-genotyped animals are regressed on them.

For the other direction of $w \to 0$, the basic equivalent ssGBLUP MME 1 (36) converges to an alternative presentation of the standard ssGBLUP. However, it divides the breeding values of non-genotyped animals into regressions on genotyped animals and into non-imputed breeding values that are not conditional on them. Similarly, at the limit $w = 0$ the basic and the expanded RPG ssSNP-BLUP MME, 2 (39) and 3 (40), coincide with the simple ssSNP-BLUP without residual polygenic effects. For example, in the single trait case, the MME coefficient matrix of the basic RPG ssSNP-BLUP MME 2 (39) is

$$
\begin{bmatrix} \mathbf{X}'\mathbf{X} & \mathbf{X}'\mathbf{Z}_1 & \mathbf{0} & \mathbf{X}'\mathbf{W} \\ \mathbf{Z}'_1\mathbf{X} & \mathbf{Z}'_1\mathbf{Z}_1+\lambda\mathbf{A}^{11} & \mathbf{0} & \mathbf{Z}'_1\mathbf{W} \\ \mathbf{0} & \mathbf{0} & \lambda\mathbf{A}_{22}^{-1} & \mathbf{0} \\ \mathbf{W}'\mathbf{X} & \mathbf{W}'\mathbf{Z}_1 & \mathbf{0} & \mathbf{W}'\mathbf{W}+\lambda\mathbf{I}_m \end{bmatrix}, \tag{42}
$$

where $\mathbf{W} = (\mathbf{Z}_1\mathbf{A}_{imp} + \mathbf{Z}_2)\mathbf{Z}_m$.

In the case where $w = 0$, i.e. there is no adjustment of the genomic relationship matrix and, therefore, no residual polygenic effects, the basic and the expanded RPG ssSNP-BLUP MME, 2 (39) and 3 (40), are essentially the same MME as was derived by Fernando et al. [6]. The main differences are that they have moved the centering term of the marker matrix $\mathbf{Z}_m$ into an additional fixed effect, and they proposed to solve the MME using Bayesian regression.

Efficient implementation

The three linearly equivalent MME based on Eqs. (36), (39), and (40) contain inverted and non-inverted terms of the pedigree relationship matrix $\mathbf{A}$. In an efficient set up to solve these MME, all these terms can be expressed, or modified into a form that can be expressed, with sparse matrices or sparse decompositions of sparse matrices. This is expected to give three efficient implementations of these MME. In practice, matrix equations of these MME are assumed to be solved iteratively by the preconditioned conjugate gradient (PCG) algorithm. Then, only a matrix-vector product of the MME coefficient matrix times a vector is performed once every iteration.

Sparse matrices and decompositions
The inverse of the pedigree relationship matrix $\mathbf{A}^{-1}$ can be expressed efficiently [18] as:

$$
\mathbf{A}^{-1} = \mathbf{Q}\left(\mathbf{I} - \tfrac{1}{2}\mathbf{P}\right)'\mathbf{D}\left(\mathbf{I} - \tfrac{1}{2}\mathbf{P}\right)\mathbf{Q}' = \mathbf{Q}\mathbf{L}\mathbf{L}'\mathbf{Q}', \tag{43}
$$

where animals are sorted in (reversed) age order from the youngest to the oldest using sparse permutation matrix $\mathbf{Q}'$, so that matrix $\mathbf{L} = (\mathbf{I} - \tfrac{1}{2}\mathbf{P})'\mathbf{D}^{\frac{1}{2}}$ becomes a lower triangular matrix in $\mathbf{Q}'\mathbf{A}^{-1}\mathbf{Q} = \mathbf{L}\mathbf{L}'$. The diagonal matrix $\mathbf{D}$ has values $4/(4 - k - F_s)$ where k is the number of known parents and F_s is the sum of parent inbreeding coefficients. In the "parental matrix" $\mathbf{P}$ on row i, there are 1s in columns corresponding to parents of animal i. The parental matrix can be interpreted, together with identity matrix $\mathbf{I}$, as a very sparse lower triangular "Cholesky" matrix ($\mathbf{L}$) [18].

The pedigree relationship matrix $\mathbf{A}$ can be expressed as the inverse of its inverse,

$$\mathbf{A} = \left(\mathbf{A}^{-1}\right)^{-1} = \mathbf{Q}(\mathbf{L}')^{-1}\mathbf{L}^{-1}\mathbf{Q}', \tag{44}$$

and so the submatrices of the pedigree relationship matrix and its inverse (18) can be obtained by selecting the appropriate rows and columns as follows:

$$\mathbf{A}_{ij} = \mathbf{E}_i\mathbf{Q}(\mathbf{L}')^{-1}\mathbf{L}^{-1}\mathbf{Q}'\mathbf{E}_j' \tag{45}$$

$$\mathbf{A}^{ij} = \mathbf{E}_i\mathbf{Q}\mathbf{L}\mathbf{L}'\mathbf{Q}'\mathbf{E}_j', \tag{46}$$

where $i, j = 1, 2$. Matrix-vector products $\mathbf{A}^{ij}\mathbf{x}$ and $\mathbf{A}_{ij}\mathbf{x}$ can be efficiently computed using these decompositions [19, 20]. The submatrices $\mathbf{A}^{ij}$ are very sparse, so they could alternatively be expressed as separate sparse matrices.

The inverse of $\mathbf{A}^{-1}$ or particular parts of it (e.g. $(\mathbf{A}^{11})^{-1}$) are, however, in general non-sparse and, thus, these inverse matrix terms should never be computed explicitly. The sparse submatrix $\mathbf{A}^{11}$ can be expressed using *sparsity preserving Cholesky factorization* so that:

$$\mathbf{A}^{11} = \mathbf{Q}_1\mathbf{L}_1\mathbf{L}_1'\mathbf{Q}_1', \tag{47}$$

where matrix $\mathbf{L}_1$ is sparse lower triangular and $\mathbf{Q}_1$ sparse permutation matrix. Note that matrix $\mathbf{L}_1$ has to be computed explicitly, as opposed to matrix $\mathbf{L}$ in Eqs. (43) to (46). Matrix $\mathbf{L}_1$ has some more fill-ins compared to $\mathbf{A}^{11}$ but is still very sparse and efficient in use. In [4], it was demonstrated that the computations remain affordable even when the dataset size grows.

Computations involving matrix inversions of $\mathbf{A}^{-1}$ or parts of it can be transformed into solutions of sparse matrix equation systems [20]:

$$\begin{aligned}\mathbf{A}\mathbf{v} &= \mathbf{Q}(\mathbf{L}')^{-1}\mathbf{L}^{-1}\mathbf{Q}'\mathbf{v} \\ &= \mathbf{Q}\big(\mathbf{L}'\backslash(\mathbf{L}\backslash(\mathbf{Q}'\mathbf{v}))\big)\end{aligned} \tag{48}$$

$$\left(\mathbf{A}^{11}\right)^{-1}\mathbf{v}_1 = \mathbf{Q}_1\big(\mathbf{L}_1'\backslash(\mathbf{L}_1\backslash(\mathbf{Q}_1'\mathbf{v}_1))\big), \tag{49}$$

where $\mathbf{v}$ and $\mathbf{v}_1$ are vectors of appropriate sizes into which the inverse matrix operations are performed. Here the backslash ($\backslash$) is an operator indicating *forward or backward substitutions* and emphasizes the importance of avoiding inverting matrices. In other words, $\mathbf{L}\backslash\mathbf{y}$ is the solution $\mathbf{x}$ of equation $\mathbf{L}\mathbf{x} = \mathbf{y}$ or can be expressed as solving ($\mathbf{L}, \mathbf{y}$). Note that the matrix products are carefully

nested with parenthesis so that only matrix-vector operations are performed.

Furthermore, following [4, 9] the inverse of the matrix $\mathbf{A}_{22}$, needed in the inversion of the second modified relationship matrix $\widetilde{\mathbf{G}}_2$ in Eq. (39), can be expressed efficiently using block matrix inversion identity similar to Eq. (25) as:

$$(\mathbf{A}_{22})^{-1} = \mathbf{A}^{22} - \mathbf{A}^{21}(\mathbf{A}^{11})^{-1}\mathbf{A}^{12}, \tag{50}$$

where all terms can be computed using Eqs. (45) to (49).

On-the-fly imputation operation

The derived equivalent formulations in Eqs. (36), (39), and (40) contain imputation operator $\mathbf{A}_{imp} = -(\mathbf{A}^{11})^{-1}\mathbf{A}^{12}$ (23) in matrices $\mathbf{M}_i$ that are needed when operating with the modified model matrix $\widetilde{\mathbf{Z}}_i = \mathbf{Z}\mathbf{M}_i$ and its transpose $\widetilde{\mathbf{Z}}_i' = \mathbf{M}_i'\mathbf{Z}'$, and when calculating the original random effects in Eq. (12). When the MME are solved by the PCG iteration algorithm, the core of the algorithm is a multiplication of the so-called direction vector $\mathbf{v}$ by the left hand side of the MME (11). In this multiplication, the imputation operator, as part of the MME coefficient matrix, operates either with a part of the vector pertaining to random effects of the genotyped animals (i.e. $\mathbf{A}_{imp}\mathbf{v}_2$) or to a vector of the marker effects $\mathbf{v}_m$ through the marker matrix (i.e. $\mathbf{A}_{imp}\mathbf{Z}_m\mathbf{v}_m$). Thus, in the transpose $\widetilde{\mathbf{Z}}_i'$ side, the imputation term operates on a vector of size equal to the number of non-genotyped animals (i.e. $\mathbf{A}_{imp}'\mathbf{v}_1$).

In all cases, the size of the vector term that operates on $(\mathbf{A}^{11})^{-1}$ equals the number of non-genotyped animals, i.e. size of $\mathbf{v}_1$. For example, the *imputed genomic marker data* term, $-(\mathbf{A}^{11})^{-1}\mathbf{A}^{12}\mathbf{Z}_m\mathbf{v}_m$, that expands the genomic information from genotyped to non-genotyped animals, can be calculated using:

$$\widetilde{\mathbf{v}}_2 = \mathbf{Z}_m\mathbf{v}_m \tag{51}$$

$$\mathbf{v}_1 = \mathbf{A}^{12}\widetilde{\mathbf{v}}_2 \tag{52}$$

and Eq. (49) so that:

$$-\left(\mathbf{A}^{11}\right)^{-1}\mathbf{A}^{12}\mathbf{Z}_m\mathbf{v}_m = -\mathbf{Q}_1\big(\mathbf{L}_1'\backslash(\mathbf{L}_1\backslash(\mathbf{Q}_1'\mathbf{v}_1))\big). \tag{53}$$

Vector $\mathbf{v}_1$ is calculated from Eq. (46), or without constructing any of the matrices by using rules for $\mathbf{A}^{-1}$ by pedigree information [18], or, alternatively, as a sparse matrix-vector product of separate sparse matrix $\mathbf{A}^{12}$.

Note that the actual imputation of the genomic marker information is not needed. The imputation operation is performed only implicitly, "on-the-fly" during the iterative solution without the need to use, for example, disk storage. In the normal imputation process [6], the marker information needs to be calculated for thousands, or even hundreds of thousands marker vectors of genotyped animals, i.e. columns of marker matrix $\mathbf{Z}_m$. The predicted marker data matrix contains real numbers and can be very large, and, thus, takes a lot of time and disk space to generate and use.

In the on-the-fly imputation process of genetic effects, however, imputation is an operation on a "projection vector" of the genotyped animals, i.e. a linear combination of the marker vectors. It needs to be performed only twice within each iteration round for each trait. Once for matrix $\widetilde{\mathbf{Z}}_i$ and another time for the transpose $\widetilde{\mathbf{Z}}_i'$ in matrix multiplication of MME coefficient matrix of Eq. (11). The imputation operation is also needed once before the iteration when calculating the right-hand-side for the new random effects ($\widetilde{\mathbf{Z}}_i'\mathbf{R}^{-1}\mathbf{y}$) in Eq. (11) and once at the end of the iteration in order to retrieve the original random effects ($\widehat{\mathbf{u}} = \mathbf{M}_i\widetilde{\mathbf{u}}$) in Eq. (12).

Orthogonalization of random effects
In the SNP-BLUP versions of the derived equivalent ssGBLUP, in Eqs. (39) and (40), the marker effects are orthogonal, i.e. their covariance matrix is diagonal. It turns out that the PCG iteration numbers of these two equivalent ssSNP-BLUP MME are considerably larger than the original ssGBLUP. In Eq. (39), the RPG effects and genomic values predicted by SNPs have colinearity, and in Eq. (40), the RPG and the animal effects for non-genotyped animals are difficult to separate.

The key for maintaining good numerical properties of the original ssGBLUP seems to be to "orthogonalize" the remaining new random effects, too. The remaining variance structures can be orthogonalized by splitting the variance matrices and attaching the two "halves" into the coefficient matrices $\mathbf{M}$ as in Eqs. (6) and (29).

The term $(\mathbf{A}^{11})^{-1}$ in Eqs. (39) and (40) can be orthogonalized by using the sparse Cholesky factorization in Eq. (47) as follows:

$$(\mathbf{A}^{11})^{-1} = \mathbf{M}_{11}\widetilde{\mathbf{G}}_{11}\mathbf{M}_{11}', \tag{54}$$

where

$$\mathbf{M}_{11} = \mathbf{Q}_1(\mathbf{L}_1')^{-1} \text{ and } \widetilde{\mathbf{G}}_{11} = \mathbf{I}_1. \tag{55}$$

Note that the permutation operator $\mathbf{Q}_1$ can be performed outside the inverse operator. However, the term $\mathbf{A}_{22}$ in Eq. (39) seems to be much more difficult to decompose. Still, it can be expressed using the sparse decomposition of the full matrix $\mathbf{A}$ in Eq. (44) as:

$$\mathbf{A}_{22} = \mathbf{E}_2\mathbf{A}\mathbf{E}_2' = \mathbf{M}_{22}\widetilde{\mathbf{G}}_{22}\mathbf{M}_{22}', \tag{56}$$

where

$$\mathbf{M}_{22} = \widetilde{\mathbf{A}}_2^{\frac{1}{2}} \text{ and } \widetilde{\mathbf{G}}_{22} = \mathbf{I}, \tag{57}$$

and

$$\widetilde{\mathbf{A}}_k^{\frac{1}{2}} = \mathbf{E}_k\mathbf{Q}(\mathbf{L}')^{-1}, \quad k = 1, 2. \tag{58}$$

The rectangular matrix $\widetilde{\mathbf{A}}_2^{\frac{1}{2}}$ has dimensions number of genotyped individuals times total number of individuals, hence the trade-off here is that Eq. (56) will expand the second random effect group of Eq. (39) from genotyped to all individuals (size of $\mathbf{I}$).

Using Eqs. (54), (56), and (58), the linearly equivalent MME (39) and (40) can be "orthogonalized" into fourth:

$$\mathbf{M}_4 = \begin{bmatrix} \mathbf{M}_{11} & \sqrt{w}\mathbf{A}_{imp}\widetilde{\mathbf{A}}_2^{\frac{1}{2}} & \sqrt{1-w}\mathbf{A}_{imp}\mathbf{Z}_m \\ \mathbf{0} & \sqrt{w}\widetilde{\mathbf{A}}_2^{\frac{1}{2}} & \sqrt{1-w}\mathbf{Z}_m \end{bmatrix}, \tag{59}$$

and fifth

$$\mathbf{M}_5 = \begin{bmatrix} \sqrt{1-w}\mathbf{M}_{11} & \sqrt{w}\widetilde{\mathbf{A}}_1^{\frac{1}{2}} & \sqrt{1-w}\mathbf{A}_{imp}\mathbf{Z}_m \\ \mathbf{0} & \sqrt{w}\widetilde{\mathbf{A}}_2^{\frac{1}{2}} & \sqrt{1-w}\mathbf{Z}_m \end{bmatrix}, \tag{60}$$

equivalent MME. Both of these linearly equivalent (29) ssSNP-BLUPs share the same orthogonal variance structure:

$$\widetilde{\mathbf{G}}_4 = \widetilde{\mathbf{G}}_5 = \begin{bmatrix} \mathbf{I}_1 & \mathbf{0} & \mathbf{0} \\ \mathbf{0} & \mathbf{I} & \mathbf{0} \\ \mathbf{0} & \mathbf{0} & \mathbf{I}_m \end{bmatrix}, \tag{61}$$

and, thus, both also have the same number of new random effects: random effects for the genotyped individuals, two sets of random effects for the non-genotyped individuals, and random effects for the markers. The difference in equivalent MME 4 (59) and 5 (60) is on how they divide the RPG on non-genotyped animals.

The fourth equivalent MME (59) can be called *orthogonal ssSNP-BLUP* MME, and the fifth MME (60), originating from the expanded RPG ssSNP-BLUP (40), *orthogonal expanded ssSNP-BLUP* MME.

Reduction of the number of effects by using ancestors of genotyped animals
Matrix $\mathbf{A}_{22}$, as the covariance structure for the genotyped animals, was reparametrized in Eq. (56) using the full pedigree relationship matrix $\mathbf{A}$. This reparametrization increases the number of corresponding new random effects from genotyped animals to all animals in the pedigree. However, computations involving $\mathbf{A}_{22}$ require only the genotyped individuals and their ancestors. Thus, to reduce the number of extra new effects, $\mathbf{A}_{22}$ can be expressed using a smaller pedigree and relationship

matrix $\widehat{\mathbf{A}}$ containing the genotyped animals and their ancestors [4].

Let the inverse of the pedigree relationship matrix (43) of this smaller pedigree be:

$$\widehat{\mathbf{A}}^{-1} = \widehat{\mathbf{Q}}\widehat{\mathbf{L}}\widehat{\mathbf{L}}'\widehat{\mathbf{Q}}', \tag{62}$$

where $\widehat{\mathbf{Q}}$ and $\widehat{\mathbf{L}}$ are as before in Eq. (44) but involve genotyped animals and their ancestors only. Matrix $\mathbf{A}_{22}$ in Eq. (56) can then be represented using the smaller pedigree as:

$$\mathbf{A}_{22} = \widehat{\mathbf{E}}_2\widehat{\mathbf{A}}\widehat{\mathbf{E}}_2' = \widehat{\mathbf{M}}_{22}\widehat{\mathbf{G}}_{22}\widehat{\mathbf{M}}_{22}', \tag{63}$$

where

$$\widehat{\mathbf{M}}_{22} = \widehat{\mathbf{E}}_2\widehat{\mathbf{Q}}(\widehat{\mathbf{L}}')^{-1} \text{ and } \widehat{\mathbf{G}}_{22} = \mathbf{I}_{ganc}, \tag{64}$$

$\widehat{\mathbf{E}}_2$ selects the genotyped individuals from the smaller pedigree, and the size of identity matrix $\mathbf{I}_{ganc}$ is the number of genotyped animals and their ancestors.

The sixth linearly equivalent, *reduced orthogonal ssSNP-BLUP* MME, can be derived from Eqs. (59) and (61) as:

$$\mathbf{M}_6 = \begin{bmatrix} \mathbf{M}_{11} & \sqrt{w}\mathbf{A}_{imp}\widehat{\mathbf{M}}_{22} & \sqrt{1-w}\mathbf{A}_{imp}\mathbf{Z}_m \\ \mathbf{0} & \sqrt{w}\widehat{\mathbf{M}}_{22} & \sqrt{1-w}\mathbf{Z}_m \end{bmatrix}$$
$$\widetilde{\mathbf{G}}_6 = \begin{bmatrix} \mathbf{I}_1 & \mathbf{0} & \mathbf{0} \\ \mathbf{0} & \mathbf{I}_{ganc} & \mathbf{0} \\ \mathbf{0} & \mathbf{0} & \mathbf{I}_m \end{bmatrix}. \tag{65}$$

Here only the non-genotyped ancestors of the genotyped have two sets of random effects, all the other non-genotyped and all genotyped animals have single sets of effects, in addition to the marker effects.

Data

The derived MME were tested using a small Nordic Red dairy cattle dataset and a simple model. The small dataset and the model were partially chosen in order to be able to use direct sparse matrix solutions of the original ssGBLUP to obtain accurate "correct solutions". The data were deregressed proofs of milk yield that were based on estimated breeding values from the Nordic production trait evaluations by NAV (Nordic Evaluations, Denmark). There were 73,579 animals in the pedigree of which 2885 were genotyped. Genotyped animals together with their ancestors form a smaller pedigree of 6833 animals. The animals had been genotyped with the Illumina Bovine SNP50 Bead Chip (Illumina, San Diego, USA). The analysis used 37,526 SNPs that passed quality control. There were 66,426 non-genotyped and 1222 genotyped animals with phenotypes. Hence, 1663 animals had a genotype but no phenotype. We considered a single trait model

and assumed a heritability of 0.5. The genomic data contained one pair of animals with identical genomic marker data and a couple of more near identical pairs that led to problems for the inversion of the genomic relationship matrix $\mathbf{G}_g$ without $\mathbf{A}_{22}$ adjustment, i.e. in the case $w = 0$.

Comparison statistics

The original ssGBLUP with inverse variance matrix $\mathbf{H}^{-1}$ of Eq. (20) and the six linearly equivalent formulations of the form (29), from Eqs. (36), (39), (40), (59), (60), (61), and (65), were implemented and tested in an Octave [21] environment. Sparse matrix factorizations were based on CHOLMOD routines [22]. Six different weights w were tested: 0.00, 0.01, 0.10, 0.20, 0.30, and 1.00. Because of the singularity in the inverse of the genomic relationship matrix $\mathbf{G}_g^{-1}$ with the test data, the original ssGBLUP matrix (20) and the first equivalent formulation (36) were not calculated when $w = 0$. The derived new formulations were compared against the original ssGBLUP, mainly focusing on efficiency, accuracy, and number of iterations.

Efficiency of the derived equivalent ssGBLUP formulations relies on the sparsity of the pedigree relationship matrices and their decompositions. Inverse matrix operations of these sparse matrices were transformed into solving sparse lower triangular matrix systems. The efficiency of these solving operations depend on the sparsity structure of the matrices, i.e. number of non-zero elements.

Accuracy of the formulations was tested by solving the MME with the PCG method using Octave's PCG routine (pcg) with the diagonal of the MME coefficient matrix as the preconditioner, or without preconditioning. Convergence tolerance in pcg was relative residual norm. The tolerance was chosen to be small (10^{-12}) so that all solved effects, without doubt, converged. Accuracies, or rather the differences from the "exact solution", were calculated as relative residual errors ($\widetilde{\mathbf{e}}_i$) between iteratively obtained MME solutions ($\mathbf{s}_i$) and the direct solution ($\mathbf{s}_{direct}$) of the original ssGBLUP:

$$\widetilde{\mathbf{e}}_i = \frac{\|\mathbf{s}_{direct} - \mathbf{s}_i\|}{\|\mathbf{s}_{direct}\|}, \tag{66}$$

where subscript $i = 1, \ldots, 6$ is the formulation number.

Implementations of the derived equivalent ssGBLUP formulation were not yet streamlined for speed and, thus, the execution times were neither optimal, nor comparable. The performance of the formulations is, therefore, tested by comparing the number of iterations of the iterative solution. The purpose was to demonstrate that the iteration counts are comparable to those obtained by the original ssGBLUP. With a larger number of genotyped individuals, the inversion of the genomic relationship matrix in the original ssGBLUP becomes a bottleneck and ssSNP-BLUP formulations, avoiding the inverse, become relatively faster.

Two versions of the genomic marker matrix encodings were tested. The first was VanRaden method 1 matrix ($\mathbf{Z}_m^{vR1}$) where the marker information is centered around the mean of the observed genotyped animals, and scaled [15]. The second was "$-1,0,1$ encoding" ($\mathbf{Z}_m^{-1,0,1}$) where the 0,1,2 genotypes were assigned values of $-1,0,1$, then scaled. In both cases, the centered $\mathbf{Z}_m$ was scaled by dividing by $\sqrt{\sum_{i=1}^{m} 2p_i(1-p_i)}$ where m is the number of markers, and p_i is the allele frequency of marker i. In case of $-1,0,1$ coding, the allele frequencies were all $p_i = 0.5$, and the scaling factor was $\sqrt{\frac{m}{2}}$. In VanRaden 1, the allele frequencies were those of the observed genotypes.

Results and discussion
Efficiency
In general, all sparse matrices in this study were very sparse. Table 1 shows the sizes and sparsity of the various sparse matrices and their decomposition in the test case. The most important matrix is $\mathbf{L}_1$ which is used in the imputation process of Eq. (23). Compared to the matrix $\mathbf{A}^{11}$, to which the Cholesky matrix $\mathbf{L}_1$ belongs, there is only a minor additional fill-in. Both matrices have less than three non-zero elements on average on each row or column. Note that the number of non-zeros in $\mathbf{A}^{-1}$ equals the sum of those in $\mathbf{A}^{11}$, $\mathbf{A}^{22}$, and twice in $\mathbf{A}^{12}$. On average, matrix $\mathbf{A}^{12}$ has less than one non-zero element on a row, but almost 22 non-zero elements on a column. This matrix has elements due to non-genotyped animals being offspring, parents and/or mates to a genotyped animal.

Table 1 Number of rows (N_r), columns (N_c), non-zeros (N_z), and mean number of non-zeros on row or column (M_z) by matrix used in MME coefficient matrices in the test case with 73,579 animals

Matrix	N_r	N_c	N_z	M_z
$\mathbf{A}^{-1}$	73,579	73,579	235,669[a]	3.20[a]
$\mathbf{A}^{11}$	70,694	70,694	168,818[a]	2.39[a]
$\mathbf{A}^{12}$	70,694	2885	62,489	0.88/21.66
$\mathbf{A}^{22}$	2885	2885	4362[a]	1.51[a]
$\mathbf{L}$	73,579	73,579	191,026	2.60
$\mathbf{L}_1$	70,694	70,694	181,536	2.57
$\widehat{\mathbf{A}}^{-1}$	6833	6833	22,612[a]	3.31[a]
$\widehat{\mathbf{L}}$	6833	6833	18,173	2.66

$\mathbf{L}$ and $\mathbf{L}_1$ are Cholesky decomposition matrices of $\mathbf{A}^{-1}$ (inverse of pedigree relationship matrix) and $\mathbf{A}^{11}$ (submatrix of $\mathbf{A}^{-1}$), respectively. $\widehat{\mathbf{A}}$ and $\widehat{\mathbf{L}}$ are the corresponding matrices for smaller pedigree of genotyped animals and their ancestors

[a] Non-zeros of symmetric matrices counted from the lower/upper triangular region only

In this study, an implicit "on-the-fly" imputation process was used. Fernando et al. [6] suggested imputing the genotypes for the non-genotyped animals, i.e. computing the predicted values of genotypes based on pedigree. Their approach for Bayesian estimation of SNP effects requires, at least the diagonal elements of, the block that pertains to SNP effects:

$$\mathbf{Z}'_{imp}\mathbf{Z}'_1\mathbf{R}^{-1}\mathbf{Z}_1\mathbf{Z}_{imp} + \mathbf{Z}'_m\mathbf{Z}'_2\mathbf{R}^{-1}\mathbf{Z}_2\mathbf{Z}_m,$$

in equivalent MME 2 or 3 (basic and expanded RPG ssSNP-BLUP) with $w = 0$ and where $\mathbf{Z}_{imp} = \mathbf{A}_{imp}\mathbf{Z}_m$ contains the imputed genotypes. If genotypes in $\mathbf{Z}_{imp}$ had been predicted for the non-genotyped animals in our data and stored using single precision accuracy, then about 11 gigabytes would have been read from the file or kept in memory. Note that the imputed genotypes for the non-genotyped animals are real numbers, so they cannot be stored as integers while retaining full accuracy. Also, the marker matrix is a dense matrix of size equal to the number of animals times markers. For this small example, an 11 GB file is quite a large extra file to be read when all the other files would take only some tens of megabytes. Our implicit on-the-fly implementation process, however, works with sparse matrices. For our example case, for the largest MME size, this means storing 372,562 non-zeros due to sparse matrices $\mathbf{L}$, and $\mathbf{L}_1$, i.e., about 3 megabytes using double precision.

PCG iteration was implemented such that all operations were matrix by vector products. Thus, there was no need to build matrix $\mathbf{Z}'_{imp}\mathbf{Z}'_1\mathbf{R}^{-1}\mathbf{Z}_1\mathbf{Z}_{imp}$ but instead the required computations were performed stepwise from right to left in $\mathbf{Z}'_{imp}(\mathbf{Z}'_1(\mathbf{R}^{-1}(\mathbf{Z}_1(\mathbf{Z}_{imp}\mathbf{v}))))$ where $\mathbf{v}$ is a vector. This approach saves memory and allows fast computations [19].

Because of the very sparse pedigree relationship ($\mathbf{A}^{-1}$) and factorization ($\mathbf{L}$) matrices, the operations on each PCG iteration step that involve inverses of the sparse matrices, e.g. the imputation operations, can be calculated in linear time with respect to the number of individuals. The matrix multiplication of the marker matrix $\mathbf{Z}_m$ is also linear if the number of markers is assumed to be constant. Hence, the cubic complexity of inverting the genomic relationship matrix can be replaced by linear computational complexity of ssSNP-BLUP formulations. This holds if the iteration counts remain low.

Accuracy
All the derived ssGBLUP MME formulations in this paper were linearly equivalent. Consequently, the final iterative solutions by all formulations were numerically equal and dictated only by the convergence tolerance. All formulations had "real" relative residual errors $\widetilde{\mathbf{e}}_i$ in Eq. (66) of

10^{-10} scale when using the residual convergence tolerance 10^{-12} in pcg. Thus, all formulations indicated convergence to the same solutions, and no divergence of the iterative method was observed.

Speed of iterative convergence
Genetic relationship: VanRaden 1
Without preconditioning, the original ssGBLUP achieved relative convergence of 10^{-12} in about 360 iterations when VanRaden 1 marker matrix encodings ($\mathbf{Z}_m^{vR1}$) and assumed heritability 0.5 were used (Table 2). The iteration counts of the first three equivalent formulations 1 to 3 were higher than with the original ssGBLUP. In particular, the third formulation (40), i.e. expanded RPG ssSNP-BLUP, had clearly the worst iteration counts although the formulation is very similar to the second formulation (39), basic RPG ssSNP-BLUP. In the third formulation, the full $\mathbf{A}$ matrix was used instead of $\mathbf{A}_{22}$ matrix having the genotyped relationships. This increased the number of unknowns by the number of non-genotyped animals, in our case c. 64%.

When $w = 1$, all equivalent MME coincide with the traditional animal model with no genomic information and the numbers of iterations are smaller, even for the badly behaving third formulation (40). When $w = 0$, the original ssGBLUP and the first equivalent MME (36), basic equivalent ssGBLUP, cannot be calculated because of the singularity in the inverse of the genomic relationship matrix $\mathbf{G}_g^{-1}$ in the test case. The numbers of iterations of the second (39) and third (40) MME are much lower in this case, which implies that the higher iteration counts are due to the RPG terms.

All fully orthogonalized equivalent ssSNP-BLUP MME 4 to 6 needed about half the number of iterations of the original ssGBLUP in all cases of w. Note that the fifth formulation (60), i.e. orthogonal expanded ssSNP-BLUP, is an orthogonalized version of the badly behaving third formulation (40) while the fourth (59), i.e. orthogonal ssSNP-BLUP, and the sixth (65), i.e. reduced orthogonal ssSNP-BLUP, are orthogonalized versions of the second MME (39). The applied orthogonalization clearly reduced the number of iterations. Of the three orthogonalized ssSNP-BLUP formulations 4 to 6, the last, number 6 (65) is preferred because it has the smallest number of unknowns (115,054).

It should be noted that the convergence results apply only on the data used in the example. The equivalent MME formulation 2 (39), i.e. basic RPG ssSNP-BLUP, had 37,526 equations more than the MME formulation 1 (36), i.e. basic equivalent ssSNP-BLUP. These extra equations were for the SNP solutions. Furthermore, equivalent MME 3 (40), i.e. expanded RPG ssSNP-BLUP, had again 70,694 new equations associated with RPG of non-genotyped animals. It remains to be tested whether MME 2 and 3 are more competitive when the number of genotyped animals is either close to or larger than the number of SNPs.

When diagonal preconditioning was applied, the original ssGBLUP achieved relative convergence of 10^{-12} much faster than without preconditioning, in about 60 iterations (vs. 360 iterations) (Table 3). Similarly, the first equivalent MME formulation gained from the preconditioning, whereas the convergence speed of the formulations 2 and 3 was about the same as without preconditioning.

However, all fully orthogonalized ssSNP-BLUP formulations 4 to 6 converged much more slowly with diagonal preconditioning. For these formulations, the inverse of the diagonal of the MME matrix is not a good approximation of the inverse MME coefficient matrix. This could mean that the inverse MME coefficient matrix is not diagonally dominant or that the off-diagonal parts of the MME matrix contribute to the diagonal of the inverse MME matrix.

Table 2 Number of iterations in PCG of linearly equivalent ssGBLUP MME using marker matrix Z_m^{vR1} (VanRaden 1), convergence tolerance 10^{-12}, heritability 0.5, and no preconditioning under different polygenic proportions w

MME	Size	Weight w					
		0.00	0.01	0.10	0.20	0.30	1.00
Orig.	73,580	–	362	358	358	355	357
1	73,580	–	536	512	536	523	536
2	111,106	646	1203	1085	987	886	536
3	181,800	646	4023	3660	3307	3040	355
4	181,800	193	196	193	191	190	182
5	181,800	193	197	194	192	190	181
6	115,054	193	196	193	191	190	182

MME, original ssGBLUP; 1, basic equivalent ssGBLUP; 2, basic RPG ssSNP-BLUP; 3, expanded RPG ssSNP-BLUP; 4, orthogonal ssSNP-BLUP; 5, orthogonal expanded ssSNP-BLUP; 6, reduced orthogonal ssSNP-BLUP

Table 3 Number of iterations in PCG of linearly equivalent ssGBLUP MME using marker matrix Z_m^{vR1} (VanRaden 1), convergence tolerance 10^{-12}, heritability 0.5, and diagonal preconditioning under different polygenic proportions w

MME	Size	Weight w					
		0.00	0.01	0.10	0.20	0.30	1.00
Orig.	73,580	–	93	62	59	57	57
1	73,580	–	152	153	158	158	171
2	111,106	847	1176	1099	1007	950	171
3	181,800	847	4058	3658	3195	2873	57
4	181,800	442	443	702	853	920	283
5	181,800	442	455	720	868	917	124
6	115,054	442	443	702	853	920	283

MME, original ssGBLUP; 1, basic equivalent ssGBLUP; 2, basic RPG ssSNP-BLUP; 3, expanded RPG ssSNP-BLUP; 4, orthogonal ssSNP-BLUP; 5, orthogonal expanded ssSNP-BLUP; 6, reduced orthogonal ssSNP-BLUP

The same dataset was analyzed using lower heritability values of 0.2 and 0.1 as well. This change in heritability had a large impact on convergence. Lower heritability leads to an increased relative weight on the variance matrix $\mathbf{H}^{-1}$ in MME of the original ssGBLUP. Consequently, the number of PCG iterations until convergence is expected to increase. However, in ssSNP-BLUP versions 4 to 6 the number of iterations decreased when heritability decreased. For these, the relative weight multiplies the orthogonalized variance matrix, i.e. the identity matrix, which grows dominant. In a single trait case

$$\widetilde{\mathbf{Z}}_i'\widetilde{\mathbf{Z}}_i + \lambda\mathbf{I} \xrightarrow[h^2 \to 0]{} \lambda\mathbf{I}, \tag{67}$$

because λ increases when heritability h^2 is small:

$$\lambda = \frac{1-h^2}{h^2} \xrightarrow[h^2 \to 0]{} \infty. \tag{68}$$

With a lower heritability of 0.1, the orthogonalized equivalent ssSNP-BLUP formulations 4 to 6 achieved a relative convergence of 10^{-12} more quickly, in about 70 iterations without preconditioning (Table 4) whereas

the original ssGBLUP needed 130 iterations with diagonal preconditioning (Table 5). Equivalent formulations 1 to 3 gained from the diagonal preconditioning but the orthogonalized formulations 4 to 6, again, did not.

When the heritability was equal to 0.2, the diagonally preconditioned original ssGBLUP and non-preconditioned orthogonalized ssSNP-BLUP formulations all achieved relative convergence of 10^{-12} in about the same 100 iterations (results not shown).

Genetic relationship: −1,0,1 encoding
Tables 6 and 7 show the numbers of pcg iterations needed for convergence using marker matrix $\mathbf{Z}_m^{-1,0,1}$ (−1,0,1 encoding) and a heritability of 0.5, without and with diagonal preconditioning, respectively. The results were similar to the $\mathbf{Z}_m^{vR1}$ (VanRaden 1) case (Tables 2, 3) but the number of required iterations was overall a little smaller, at least in the preconditioned case. In the pure SNP-BLUP type of computations, it is expected that observed genotype centering will lead to faster convergence, at least in Gibbs sampling or Gauss–Seidel type of iterations [23]. One reason for the poorer convergence may be that base

Table 4 Number of iterations in PCG of linearly equivalent ssGBLUP MME using marker matrix Z_m^{vR1} (VanRaden 1), convergence tolerance 10^{-12}, heritability 0.1, and no preconditioning under different polygenic proportions w

MME	Size	Weight w					
		0.00	0.01	0.10	0.20	0.30	1.00
Orig.	73,580	–	619	622	624	624	623
1	73,580	–	758	733	701	728	744
2	111,106	736	1005	970	907	836	748
3	181,800	736	3422	3315	3154	2934	623
4	181,800	74	74	72	72	71	71
5	181,800	74	73	72	70	71	70
6	115,054	74	74	72	72	71	71

MME, original ssGBLUP; 1, basic equivalent ssGBLUP; 2, basic RPG ssSNP-BLUP; 3, expanded RPG ssSNP-BLUP; 4, orthogonal ssSNP-BLUP; 5, orthogonal expanded ssSNP-BLUP; 6, reduced orthogonal ssSNP-BLUP

Table 5 Number of iterations in PCG of linearly equivalent ssGBLUP MME using marker matrix Z_m^{vR1} (VanRaden 1), convergence tolerance 10^{-12}, heritability 0.1, and diagonal preconditioning under different polygenic proportions w

MME	Size	Weight w					
		0.00	0.01	0.10	0.20	0.30	1.00
Orig.	73,580	–	178	131	126	122	119
1	73,580	–	191	156	148	145	139
2	111,106	438	491	459	429	398	139
3	181,800	438	1732	1592	1416	1247	119
4	181,800	107	105	130	151	160	82
5	181,800	107	107	132	151	162	49
6	115,054	107	105	130	151	160	82

MME, original ssGBLUP; 1, basic equivalent ssGBLUP; 2, basic RPG ssSNP-BLUP; 3, expanded RPG ssSNP-BLUP; 4, orthogonal ssSNP-BLUP; 5, orthogonal expanded ssSNP-BLUP; 6, reduced orthogonal ssSNP-BLUP

Table 6 Number of iterations in PCG of linearly equivalent MME using marker matrix $Z_m^{-1,0,1}$ ($-1,0,1$ encoding), convergence tolerance 10^{-12}, heritability 0.5, and no preconditioning under different polygenic proportions w

MME	Size	Weight w					
		0.00	0.01	0.10	0.20	0.30	1.00
Orig.	73,580	–	372	366	362	364	357
1	73,580	–	518	512	512	515	536
2	111,106	620	1141	1082	996	896	536
3	181,800	620	3794	3586	3390	3096	355
4	181,800	189	193	192	190	190	182
5	181,800	189	193	191	190	192	181
6	115,054	189	193	192	190	190	182

MME, original ssGBLUP; 1, basic equivalent ssGBLUP; 2, basic RPG ssSNP-BLUP; 3, expanded RPG ssSNP-BLUP; 4, orthogonal ssSNP-BLUP; 5, orthogonal expanded ssSNP-BLUP; 6, reduced orthogonal ssSNP-BLUP

Table 7 Number of iterations in PCG of linearly equivalent MME using marker matrix $Z_m^{-1,0,1}$ ($-1,0,1$ encoding), convergence tolerance 10^{-12}, heritability 0.5, and diagonal preconditioning under different polygenic proportions w

MME	Size	Weight w					
		0.00	0.01	0.10	0.20	0.30	1.00
Orig.	73,580	–	96	64	60	58	57
1	73,580	–	144	144	147	152	171
2	111,106	785	1059	1068	1010	953	171
3	181,800	785	3570	3411	3080	2826	57
4	181,800	418	413	636	762	817	283
5	181,800	418	423	673	805	857	124
6	115,054	418	413	636	762	817	283

MME, original ssGBLUP; 1, basic equivalent ssGBLUP; 2, basic RPG ssSNP-BLUP; 3, expanded RPG ssSNP-BLUP; 4, orthogonal ssSNP-BLUP; 5, orthogonal expanded ssSNP-BLUP; 6, reduced orthogonal ssSNP-BLUP

population allele frequencies were not used in VanRaden 1 as advocated in [15]. Use of base population allele frequencies might give a genomic relationship matrix that is more appropriate in ssGBLUP, and deviations from this matrix may lead to poorer convergence.

Compatibility of the genomic relationship matrix G_w

Convergence properties of the PCG method depend on the model used, data, and parameters. The model in our statistical analysis was very simple but we used different genomic relationship matrices. When genomic data is involved, several approaches are available to construct the genomic relationship matrix and the marker matrix $\mathbf{Z}_m$. Previously, Strandén and Christensen [23] had shown that differences in $\mathbf{Z}_m$ marker matrix in SNP-BLUP type models can give different mixing properties in Markov chain Monte Carlo computations. In ssGBLUP, the genomic and pedigree relationship matrices need to be constructed properly in order to avoid bias in the breeding values. We used different genomic relationship matrices by changing the w parameter without trying to maximize prediction ability in our data. Our choice for the family of genomic relationship matrices showed differences in convergence that may be partly due to, a potentially suboptimal, $\mathbf{H}^{-1}$ matrix.

In practice, the genomic relationship matrix in ssG-BLUP or ssSNP-BLUP can be built such that it is "compatible" with the pedigree relationship matrix. There are several strategies for this e.g., [24, 25]. For each strategy an equivalent ssSNP-BLUP can be derived similarly as done for the family of relationship matrices in our study. For example, when the genomic relationship matrix has the form $a\mathbf{11}' + \mathbf{G}_g$ instead of $\mathbf{G}_w$, there will be one effect due to $a\mathbf{11}'$ instead of the residual polygenic effects. The equations for the marker effects remain the same.

Some studies have indicated that the $(\mathbf{A}_{22})^{-1}$ matrix in ssGBLUP should be scaled by a factor less than 1, e.g., [26, 27]. This suggests that not only the genomic relationship matrix should be carefully constructed but also the pedigree relationship matrix should be adjusted. This has been properly formulated in the metafounders approach [28] where the pedigree relationship matrix is modified.

Comparison to other approaches

The model by Fernando et al. [6] did not include RPG effects. The existence of RPG effects can be justified because not all the additive genetic variation can be explained by marker genotypes [2, 29]. Moreover Goddard et al. [30] suggested that with a finite number of markers, estimates of the genomic relationships are subject to error. The error can be due to sampling variation or inaccuracies in the analysis, and is inversely related to the number of markers in the analysis. In practice, the RPG has been included in most genomic evaluations because a moderate w is known to reduce the prediction bias in young selection candidates [27]. However, w might not have notable effects in single-step models [27].

The RPG effect could be included in the models of Fernando et al. [6] as a general random effect with $Var(\mathbf{u}) \sim N(\mathbf{0}, w\mathbf{A})$. However, when the same observations of non-genotyped animals in [6] are modelled by RPG, the iterative approaches might face problems for separating the RPG and the "imputation residual" [6] (i.e. $\mathbf{a}_1$) effects from each other. This was clearly visible in our

equivalent MME 3 (40), i.e. expanded RPG ssSNP-BLUP, which showed very poor convergence.

When RPG was not included ($w = 0$) in equivalent MME 2 and 3, basic and expanded RPG ssSNP-BLUP, they converged much faster. However, all the other equivalent MME alternatives reached convergence with a smaller number of iterations.

Liu et al. [8] proposed a different approach for the use of marker effects in single-step models. Their model for the observations did not include the SNP effects, but instead the SNP effects were introduced into the MME as augmented effects correlated with the aggregated genomic breeding values, i.e. the sum of the genomic breeding value and the RPG effect. In this way, the marker matrix generated the dependencies among genotyped animals similar to genomic relationships in the $\mathbf{H}$ matrix. However, the MME by Liu et al. [8] was reported to have problematic convergence properties [8] (Liu Z: personal communication). This may have been due to poor condition number of MME coefficient matrix which resulted from large off-diagonal elements in blocks connecting marker effects and aggregated genomic values.

Conclusions

A procedure was presented to derive linearly equivalent MME formulations for ssGBLUP. Six ssGBLUP based MME were derived, of which five were ssSNP-BLUP. In ssSNP-BLUP, inversion of the genomic relationship matrix is avoided. Three of the derived formulations were fully orthogonalized such that all random effects had diagonal covariance matrices.

All matrix operations and matrices, except the marker matrix $\mathbf{Z}_m$, were expressed using sparse matrices and sparse decompositions. During the iteration, the on-the-fly imputation from the genotyped to the non-genotyped animals was used on the genomic breeding values and residual polygenic effects without any need to explicitly predict and store genotypes of relatives of genotyped animals. All implementations used efficient matrix times vector operations where very sparse matrices were saved in memory. This enables efficient iteration on data-based implementations for large datasets and models.

All the derived MME gave exactly the same breeding value estimates at convergence with the small test data. Using the expected heritability of 0.5, the fully orthogonalized non-preconditioned ssSNP-BLUP formulations needed more iterations than the diagonally preconditioned original ssGBLUP. However, the number of iterations depended on the heritability value used. With a smaller heritability (0.1), the non-preconditioned ssSNP-BLUP formulations needed less iterations. The ssSNP-BLUP formulations did not benefit from diagonal preconditioner in PCG iteration.

The blending of the genomic relationship matrix $\mathbf{G}_g$ with the pedigree relationship matrix $\mathbf{A}_{22}$ was transformed into an additional residual polygenic effect in MME. The number of estimated additional random effects from all animals was reduced to include genotyped and their non-genotyped ancestors only. However, this did not improve convergence, although the number of unknowns to solve was smaller. When no residual polygenic effect was included, the ssSNP-BLUP models converged with a smaller number of iterations.

In conclusion, inversion of the large and dense genomic relationship matrix in the ssGBLUP can be avoided by using fully orthogonalized ssSNP-BLUP formulations. Although the new algorithms are more complicated than the original ssGBLUP, numerical efficiency is better when the number of genotyped individuals is large. The number of iterations until convergence by PCG was smaller in orthogonalized ssSNP-BLUP than in the original ssGBLUP when the heritability was low, but increased above that of the original ssGBLUP when heritability was higher.

The performance of the new MME should be further tested by analyzing data with more genotyped and non-genotyped animals.

Authors' contributions
MT derived the formulae together with IS and EAM. MT did the main data analysis with IS supplying the data and performing additional comparisons. MT wrote the first drafts of the manuscript, and EAM and IS helped to revise and finalize it. All authors read and approved the final manuscript.

Acknowledgements
This work was a part of the Genomics in Herds project which is a joint effort of Luke and Aarhus University. Breeding organizations Viking Genetics, Faba, and Breed4Food, the MAKERA foundation (Ministry of Agriculture and Forestry) and Valio Ltd were all participating funding of the work.

Competing interests
The authors declare that they have no competing interests.

References
1. Aguilar I, Misztal I, Johnson DL, Legarra A, Tsuruta S, Lawlor TJ. Hot topic: a unified approach to utilize phenotypic, full pedigree, and genomic information for genetic evaluation of Holstein final score. J Dairy Sci. 2010;93:743–52.
2. Christensen OF, Lund MS. Genomic prediction when some animals are not genotyped. Genet Sel Evol. 2010;42:2.
3. Misztal I, Legarra A, Aguilar I. Using recursion to compute the inverse of the genomic relationship matrix. J Dairy Sci. 2014;97:3943–52.
4. Masuda Y, Misztal I, Tsuruta S, Legarra A, Aguilar I, Lourenco DAL, et al. Implementation of genomic recursions in single-step genomic best linear unbiased predictor for US Holsteins with a large number of genotyped animals. J Dairy Sci. 2016;99:1968–74.
5. Masuda Y, Misztal I, VanRaden PM. Single-step GBLUP using APY inverse for protein yield in U.S. Holstein with a large number of genotyped animals. In: Proceedings of the 2016 ASAS-ADSA-CSAS-WSASAS joint annual meeting; Salt Lake City. 2016.
6. Fernando RL, Dekkers JCM, Garrick DJ. A class of Bayesian methods to combine large numbers of genotyped and non-genotyped animals for whole-genome analyses. Genet Sel Evol. 2014;46:50.
7. Legarra A, Ducrocq V. Computational strategies for national integration of phenotypic, genomic, and pedigree data in a single-step best linear unbiased prediction. J Dairy Sci. 2012;95:4629–45.
8. Liu Z, Goddard ME, Reinhardt F, Reents R. A single-step genomic model with direct estimation of marker effects. J Dairy Sci. 2014;97:5833–50.
9. Strandén I, Mäntysaari EA. Comparison of some equivalent equations to solve single-step GBLUP. In: Proceedings of the 10th World Congress on genetics applied to Livestock production. Vancouver; 2014. p. 22.
10. Golub GH, Van Loan CF. Matrix computations. Baltimore: Johns Hopkins University Press; 1985.
11. Henderson CR. Applications of linear models in animal breeding. Guelph: University of Guelph Press; 1984.
12. Mrode R, Thompson R. An alternative algorithm for incorporating the relationships between animals in estimating variance components. J Anim Breed Genet. 1989;106:89–95.
13. Quaas RL. Linear prediction. In: BLUP School Handbook. Armidale: A.G.B.U., University of New England; 1984. https://www.cabdirect.org/cabdirect/abstract/19850186676.
14. Henderson CR. Sire evaluation and genetic trends. In: Proceedings of the animal breeding and genetics symposium in honor of Dr. Jay L. Lush: 29 July 1972. Blacksburg; 1973. p. 10–41.
15. VanRaden PM. Efficient methods to compute genomic predictions. J Dairy Sci. 2008;91:4414–23.
16. Strandén I, Garrick DJ. Technical note: Derivation of equivalent computing algorithms for genomic predictions and reliabilities of animal merit. J Dairy Sci. 2009;92:2971–5.
17. Legarra A, Aguilar I, Misztal I. A relationship matrix including full pedigree and genomic information. J Dairy Sci. 2009;92:4656–63.
18. Henderson CR. A Simple method for computing the inverse of a numerator relationship matrix used in prediction of breeding values. Biometrics. 1976;32:69–83.
19. Strandén I, Lidauer M. Solving large mixed linear models using preconditioned conjugate gradient iteration. J Dairy Sci. 1999;82:2779–87.
20. Colleau JJ. An indirect approach to the extensive calculation of relationship coefficients. Genet Sel Evol. 2002;34:409–21.
21. Eaton JW, et al. GNU Octave. www.gnu.org/software/octave. Accessed 15 Mar 2017.
22. Chen Y, Davis TA, Hager W, Rajamanickam S. Algorithm 887: CHOLMOD, supernodal sparse Cholesky factorization and update/downdate. ACM Trans Math Softw. 2008;35:22.
23. Strandén I, Christensen OF. Allele coding in genomic evaluation. Genet Sel Evol. 2011;43:25.
24. Vitezica ZG, Aguilar I, Misztal I, Legarra A. Bias in genomic predictions for populations under selection. Genet Res (Camb). 2011;93:357–66.
25. Gao H, Christensen OF, Madsen P, Nielsen US, Zhang Y, Lund MS, et al. Comparison on genomic predictions using three GBLUP methods and two single-step blending methods in the Nordic Holstein population. Genet Sel Evol. 2012;44:8.
26. Tsuruta S, Misztal I, Aguilar I, Lawlor T. Multiple-trait genomic evaluation of linear type traits using genomic and phenotypic data in US Holsteins. J Dairy Sci. 2011;94:4198–204.
27. Koivula M, Strandén I, Pösö J, Aamand GP, Mäntysaari EA. Single-step genomic evaluation using multitrait random regression model and test-day data. J Dairy Sci. 2015;98:2775–84.
28. Legarra A, Christensen OF, Vitezica ZG, Aguilar I, Misztal I. Ancestral relationships using metafounders: finite ancestral populations and across population relationships. Genetics. 2015;200:455–68.
29. Erbe M, Gredler B, Seefried FR, Bapst B, Simianer H. A function accounting for training set size and marker density to model the average accuracy of genomic prediction. PLoS One. 2013;8:e81046.
30. Goddard ME, Hayes BJ, Meuwissen THE. Using the genomic relationship matrix to predict the accuracy of genomic selection. J Anim Breed Genet. 2011;128:409–21.

3

Genomic prediction using preselected DNA variants from a GWAS with whole-genome sequence data in Holstein–Friesian cattle

Roel F. Veerkamp[1,2]* , Aniek C. Bouwman[1], Chris Schrooten[3] and Mario P. L. Calus[1]

Abstract

Background: Whole-genome sequence data is expected to capture genetic variation more completely than common genotyping panels. Our objective was to compare the proportion of variance explained and the accuracy of genomic prediction by using imputed sequence data or preselected SNPs from a genome-wide association study (GWAS) with imputed whole-genome sequence data.

Methods: Phenotypes were available for 5503 Holstein–Friesian bulls. Genotypes were imputed up to whole-genome sequence (13,789,029 segregating DNA variants) by using run 4 of the 1000 bull genomes project. The program GCTA was used to perform GWAS for protein yield (PY), somatic cell score (SCS) and interval from first to last insemination (IFL). From the GWAS, subsets of variants were selected and genomic relationship matrices (GRM) were used to estimate the variance explained in 2087 validation animals and to evaluate the genomic prediction ability. Finally, two GRM were fitted together in several models to evaluate the effect of selected variants that were in competition with all the other variants.

Results: The GRM based on full sequence data explained only marginally more genetic variation than that based on common SNP panels: for PY, SCS and IFL, genomic heritability improved from 0.81 to 0.83, 0.83 to 0.87 and 0.69 to 0.72, respectively. Sequence data also helped to identify more variants linked to quantitative trait loci and resulted in clearer GWAS peaks across the genome. The proportion of total variance explained by the selected variants combined in a GRM was considerably smaller than that explained by all variants (less than 0.31 for all traits). When selected variants were used, accuracy of genomic predictions decreased and bias increased.

Conclusions: Although 35 to 42 variants were detected that together explained 13 to 19% of the total variance (18 to 23% of the genetic variance) when fitted alone, there was no advantage in using dense sequence information for genomic prediction in the Holstein data used in our study. Detection and selection of variants within a single breed are difficult due to long-range linkage disequilibrium. Stringent selection of variants resulted in more biased genomic predictions, although this might be due to the training population being the same dataset from which the selected variants were identified.

Background

Genomic selection is increasingly applied in breeding programs for livestock species, e.g. [1, 2], and has led to dramatic increases in genetic progress [3], especially in dairy cattle. However until now, accuracies of genomic prediction are still not close to 1, although one of the expectations was that, compared to the currently used common single nucleotide polymorphism (SNP) panels, whole-genome sequence data would increase accuracies of genomic prediction. Because most of the causal mutations that underlie quantitative trait loci (QTL) are expected to be included as genetic markers in the sequence data, it is expected that causal mutations will be identified more precisely than with the common lower

---

*Correspondence: Roel.Veerkamp@wur.nl
[1] Animal Breeding and Genomics Centre, Wageningen UR Livestock Research, P.O. Box 338, 6700 AH Wageningen, The Netherlands
Full list of author information is available at the end of the article

density SNP chips [4] and that the reliability of genomic predictions and its persistency across generations and even across breeds [5, 6] will improve. This was confirmed on simulated data [7], but in practice, the use of cattle and chicken sequence data has not increased the reliability of genomic predictions [8, 9].

Several reasons may explain why the accuracy of genomic predictions does not increase when sequence data is used: (1) if the number of training individuals is small, the effects of QTL may be estimated with too large errors and thus, little advantage is gained by using sequence data [10]; (2) if training is performed within a breed or line, long-range linkage disequilibrium (LD) may prevent the precise localisation of quantitative trait nucleotides (QTN) when all sequence variants are fitted simultaneously [8]; and (3) many different linear combinations of variants (that are in high LD) may occur and result in equally accurate genomic predictions for the same set of phenotypes. Therefore, it is not possible to construct a unique prediction equation and no benefit can be expected from using more precise measures at the DNA level (i.e. more variants). In fact, it might be better to use fewer variants that are located closer to the QTN, than to rely on the complex LD structure between variants for the prediction of selection candidates. This was also found in a simulation study for across-breed prediction by Wientjes et al. [11].

These previous studies raise several questions i.e. how much of the total genetic variation is tagged by using different sets of variants, from commercial SNP chips up to whole-genome sequence data and to variants selected from a genome-wide association study (GWAS) using (imputed) sequence data, and how is accuracy of genomic prediction affected. Our objective was to compare the proportion of variance explained and the accuracy of genomic prediction based on imputed sequence data, lower density SNP panels, and preselected variants from a GWAS based on imputed whole-genome sequence.

Methods

Phenotypes

De-regressed proofs (DRP) were available for somatic cell score (SCS), interval between first and last insemination (IFL), and protein yield (PY) for 5503 Holstein–Friesian bulls provided by CRV (Arnhem, the Netherlands). DRP were calculated according to [12]:

$$DRP = PA + (EBV - PA) * \left(\frac{EDC_{EBV}}{EDC_{prog}} \right),$$

where EBV is the estimated breeding value of a bull for a trait available from the national evaluations, and PA is the parent average of the bull for that trait. Effective daughter contribution, EDC_{EBV}, represents the effective number

of daughters with phenotypes that contributed to the EBV of a bull [13] and was calculated according to [12] as $\alpha * REL_{EBV}/(1 - REL_{EBV})$, where REL_{EBV} is the published reliability for EBV and $\alpha = (4 - h^2)/h^2$, where h^2 is the heritability of the trait. $EDC_{prog} = EDC_{EBV} - EDC_{PA}$, where $EDC_{PA} = \alpha REL_{PA}/(1 - REL_{PA})$ and $REL_{PA} = (REL_{sire} + REL_{dam})/4$ [14]. As the number of daughters with phenotypic information for a trait increases, the reliability of the EBV of a bull and EDC_{EBV} increase. The average EDC_{EBV} (and its range) for animals in the training set was equal to 266 (24 to 971) for SCS, 643 (47 to 4851) for IFL, and 245 (24 to 693) for PY.

Following van Binsbergen et al. [8], the bulls were assigned either to the population used for variant detection (discovery population) in the GWAS (and training for genomic prediction) or to the validation population. Assignment was based on year of birth, bulls born before 2001 (3416 bulls) were assigned to the discovery population and bulls born between 2001 and 2008 (2087 bulls) to the validation population.

Genotypes

In total, 551 of the bulls in this study were genotyped with the Illumina BovineHD BeadChip (Illumina Inc., San Diego) and the other 4952 bulls were genotyped with a 50k SNP panel and imputed to BovineHD (734,403 SNPs). Imputation from the 50k panel to the BovineHD SNP panel was performed with BEAGLE 3.3.0 [15, 16], using additional Holstein bulls in a reference set of 1333 animals genotyped with the BovineHD SNP panel. For this first step, the error rate of imputation was low (with a slightly smaller reference population, it was equal to 0.41%) [17]. The HD genotypes of the bulls were imputed to whole-genome sequence using the sequenced population from the 1000 Bull Genomes Project Run 4 as reference population. This multi-breed reference population included 1147 sequenced animals with on average an 11-fold coverage, among which 311 Holstein bulls. All the individuals were used as reference because earlier studies showed that a multi-breed sequenced reference population can be beneficial for imputation accuracy, especially for SNPs with a low minor allele frequency (MAF) [4, 18, 19]. Polymorphic sites, including SNPs and short insertions and deletions (InDels), were identified for the 1147 individuals simultaneously using the multi-sample approach implemented in SAMtools' mpileup along with BCFtools as described in Daetwyler et al. [4]. Genotype calls for the 1000 Bull Genomes reference population were improved with BEAGLE [15] using genotype likelihoods from SAMtools and inferred haplotypes in the samples. The sequence data contained 36,916,855 bi-allelic variants of which 30,339,468 had four or more copies of the minor allele in the reference population and were used for imputation. Imputation of HD genotypes to whole-genome sequence was done using standard settings in MINIMAC2 [20] and the pre-phased reference genotypes that resulted from BEAGLE. MINIMAC2 gave empirical imputation reliabilities (squared correlations between imputed and true genotypes for typed SNPs only) of 0.99 on average per chromosome including only the SNPs with MAF higher than 0.01, except for chromosomes 2, 4, 5, 26, and 27 where the average per chromosome ranged between 0.63 and 0.66.

GWAS using sequence information

For the three traits analyzed, the bulls in the discovery set were used to perform a GWAS in which each variant was fitted separately and a genomic relationship matrix (GRM) based on the BovineHD SNPs was constructed to account for population structure. The mixed linear model based association analysis (MLMA) in the package GCTA [21] was used. All sequence variants (SNPs and biallelic InDels) with a MAF higher than 0.01 (n = 13,789,029) were tested for their association. The model was:

$$\mathbf{y} = \mathbf{1}\mu + \mathbf{Z}\mathbf{g} + \mathbf{b}\mathbf{x} + \mathbf{e},$$

where $\mathbf{y}$ is the vector of DRP of all individuals, μ is the overall mean, $\mathbf{1}$ is a vector of ones, $\mathbf{Z}$ is an incidence matrix that links records to bulls, $\mathbf{g}$ is a vector of the genomic breeding values of all individuals, b is the additive (fixed) effect of the candidate variants to be tested for association, $\mathbf{x}$ is a vector of the variants' genotype indicator variable coded as 0, 1 or 2, and $\mathbf{e}$ is a vector of random residuals. Genomic breeding values were assumed to be distributed as $\mathbf{g}|\mathbf{GRM}, \sigma_g^2 \sim N(\mathbf{0}, \mathbf{GRM}\sigma_g^2)$, where $\mathbf{GRM}$ is the genomic relationship matrix calculated from the variants present on the BovineHD chip, and σ_g^2 is the additive genetic variance picked up by the markers. For ease of computation, σ_g^2 is estimated based on the null model without variants and then fixed while testing for the association between each of the variants and the trait. Diagonal and off-diagonal values of the $\mathbf{GRM}$ were calculated following [22, 23] as:

$$GRM_{jk} = \frac{1}{N}\sum_i GRM_{ijk}$$

$$= \begin{cases} \frac{1}{N}\sum_i \frac{(x_{ij}-2p_i)(x_{ik}-2p_i)}{2p_i(1-p_i)}, & j \neq k \\ 1 + \frac{1}{N}\sum_i \frac{x_{ij}^2-(1+2p_i)x_{ij}+2p_i^2}{2p_i(1-p_i)}, & j = k \end{cases}$$

where GRM_{ijk} is the estimated relationship between individuals j and k at locus i, and N is the number of variants. The genotypes of the variants (x_i) were coded as 0, 1 or 2, and p_i is the allele frequency of the allele for which the homozygous genotype was coded as 2. Residual effects

were assumed to be distributed as $\mathbf{e}|\sigma_e^2 \sim N(\mathbf{0}, \mathbf{I}\sigma_e^2)$, where σ_e^2 is the residual variance. This is not the usual estimate of the residual variance associated with an individual phenotype, but the residual of the DRP. Ideally the DRP should have been weighted according to the EDC but this was not feasible in GCTA.

Manhattan plots were created using the R package qqman [24] excluding all variants with a $-\log_{10}(p)$ less than 1 for computational ease.

Selection of variants

From the full set of 13,789,029 imputed sequence variants (ISQ), SNPs that were present on the two commonly used SNP panels (50k or Bovine HD) were selected as subsets. Then, the GWAS results for the discovery population were used to select 10 subsets of variants within ISQ, HD and 50k variants, which totalled 33 sets of variants. Selection was "p value based" using arbitrary cutoff levels of 3 and 5 for the $-\log_{10}(p)$. A disadvantage is that selecting variants purely on a $-\log10(p)$ threshold results in many variants in one region being selected for genomic prediction, due to LD between variants and to running regression on each variant separately. Therefore, we also carried out a conditional and joint GWAS (COJO) using the results from the single-variant GWAS model [25]. In the COJO analysis, variants were added to the model one by one, starting with the variants that had the most significant effect, on the basis of joint and conditional significance level from the GWAS. The joint and conditional significant level is the significance level from the GWAS results conditional on the LD with the selected variants already in the model and the joint significance level of these variants. Variants were added to the model only when more variance was explained compared to that obtained with the other variants already in the model. By performing the COJO, the large number of variants led to computing limitations for the calculation of LD and selection from all variants, while the large family structures of the dataset led to over-fitting due to high collinearity between the variants. Collinearity resulted in grossly overestimated conditional variant effects and inflated p values. In order to circumvent these two issues, four different COJO analyses were performed. For the first two analyses, all variants with a $-\log_{10}(p)$ less than 3 were a priori removed and variants that were in LD (defined as r^2) with the variants already in the model with an r^2 higher than 0.8 were not added in the forward selection step. Then, variants were selected based on a conditional and joint significance level $-\log_{10}(p)$ greater than 3 (COJO3) or 5 (COJO5). For the third and fourth COJO analyses, all variants were considered a priori, but it was assumed that variants that were more than 100 Mb apart were in complete linkage equilibrium. Thus, estimated effects were not adjusted for loci that were more than 100 Mb apart since they are assumed to be independent, and the LD threshold was only applied for loci that were less than 100 Mb apart. Also, variants that were in LD with the variants already in the model with an r^2 higher than 0.5 were not added. Then, variants were selected based on a conditional and joint significance level $-\log_{10}(p)$ higher than 5 (COJO5LD) or the 100 variants with the largest effect were selected (COJO#100).

Variance explained by the selected variants

The first method to evaluate the value of the selected variants consisted in estimating the variance of the DRP that can be explained by the variants for the validation animals. The estimated genetic variance was expressed as a proportion of the total variance i.e. the so-called genomic heritability (h^2) [26] as relevant for the DRP. This heritability is not directly comparable to the usual heritability of a single phenotypic record since the estimated residual variance is not directly comparable with the residual variance of a single phenotypic record. Using the 33 sets of variants (Tables 1 and 2), the 33 **GRM** were calculated following [22] as described above, and variance components were estimated using GREML in GCTA. Variances were not only estimated using the **GRM** for the subsets of selected variants, but also by using a complementary GRM (**GRMc**) based on the remaining variants that were not selected for inclusion in the **GRM** for the subsets of selected variants. For example, the 50k panel contained 49,580 variants, thus the remaining 13,739,449 (=13,789,029 − 49,580) variants were used to create the complementary **GRMc**. For the scenarios with variant selection based on the 50k SNP or Bovine HD panels only, no additional pruning on LD was performed for the **GRMc**. For the "p value based variant selection" (Table 1), a GREML analysis with these **GRMc** matrices reflected the variance explained by variants without an association with the trait. For the subsets selected with the COJO analysis (Table 2), many variants in high LD with the selected variants were still present in the

Table 1 Number of variants in each of the subsets of variants selected from the SNP panels and selection criteria

Trait	Selection criteria	Imputed sequence (ISQ)	HD	50k
	All variants	13,789,029	656,044	49,580
PY	$-\log10(p) > 3$	24,387	1238	120
	$-\log10(p) > 5$	2,194	159	27
SCS	$-\log10(p) > 3$	23,346	1203	98
	$-\log10(p) > 5$	1539	90	7
IFL	$-\log10(p) > 3$	22,833	987	61
	$-\log10(p) > 5$	853	27	4

Table 2 Number of variants in each of the subsets of variants selected using COJO, and number of variants in linkage disequilibrium (LD) with the selected variants, which were ignored in the GRMc

Trait	Selection criteria	Number of variants in subset of selected variants	Number of variants in LD with selected variants
PY	COJO3	90	1,650,152
	COJO5	64	1,154,416
	COJO5LD	35	615,586
	COJO#100	100	1,688,270
SCS	COJO3	195	3,241,932
	COJO5	215	3,449,212
	COJO5LD	42	757,095
	COJO#100	100	1,652,678
IFL	COJO3	264	3,835,730
	COJO5	209	3,151,538
	COJO5LD	35	607,631
	COJO#100	100	1,675,727

remaining set. Therefore, an additional step was performed to exclude from the **GRMc** not only the selected variants but also the variants that were in significant LD ($p < 0.01$) with the selected variants. GCTA was used to search for variants in significant LD with the selected variants [21], and the search was limited to a 2-Mb window on either side of each selected variant.

Finally, each **GRM** was fitted together with its **GRMc** to obtain a more conservative and probably better estimate of the variance explained by the selected set of variants. When fitting multiple **GRM**, GREML will partition the variances according to the maximum likelihood.

Accuracy of genomic predictions with selected variants

The second method to evaluate the value of the selected variants consisted in calculating genomic predictions for the validation animals (GEBV) and correlating these with the phenotypes of the same animals. Since GCTA excluded by default the animals without phenotypes from the **GRM**, several steps were required. First, using GREML in GCTA, each of the 33 **GRM** was fitted separately for the discovery (training) animals. Secondly, BLUP solutions for the effects of variants were back-solved from the GEBV for the discovery animals. Finally, using the package PLINK (v1.90b3c 64-bit; 2 Feb 2015; http://pngu.mgh.harvard.edu/purcell/plink/; [27]), the BLUP solutions for the effects of variants were used to calculate the GEBV for the validation animals. Similar to the estimation of the variance, GEBV for the validation animals were also computed using both the **GRM** and the complementary **GRMc** simultaneously in the GREML model, followed by back-solving the effects of variants and calculating the breeding values with the combined solutions.

Accuracy of genomic prediction was calculated for the validation animals as the correlation between the DRP and GEBV for the different traits, assuming that the DRP was based on very many progeny. Furthermore, the regression coefficient of the DRP on the GEBV was calculated to evaluate the bias of predictions.

Results
GWAS
The GWAS results for PY, SCS and IFL are in the Manhattan plots in Figs. 1, 2 and 3 (Q–Q plots are in Additional file 1: Figure S1, Additional file 2: Figure S2, and Additional file 3: Figure S3). Compared to SNP data, when sequence data was used, the peaks became higher and sharper, suggesting a more precise detection of the QTL. For PY, a strong association was found with the *diacylglycerol O-acyltransferase 1* (*DGAT1*) gene, and each of the three traits, were associated with several additional variants ($-\log_{10}(p) > 5$) when using the imputed sequence data. The total number of variants with a $-\log_{10}(p)$ value higher than 3 or 5 differed only slightly between traits when using the sequence data (Table 1), and was larger than expected by chance (13,789 and 138 for $-\log_{10}(p) > 3$ and $-\log_{10}(p) > 5$ respectively). If only the SNPs on the 50k and HD panels were considered, more SNPs with a $-\log_{10}(p)$ higher than 3 and 5 were found for PY than for SCS and IFL.

In the COJO analysis, variants were selected only when they explained more variance than the other variants already added in the model (starting with the most significant variant). When performing the COJO3 analysis (preselection of variants with a $-\log_{10}(p) > 3$), 195 and 264 variants were retained for IFL and SCS, respectively, while for PY only 90 variants were selected (Table 2). However, when performing the COJO5LD analysis (using the more stringent LD criteria of 0.5, i.e. assuming no LD between variants that were more than 100 Mb apart and $-\log_{10}(p) > 5$), between 35 and 42 variants were selected and their number for each trait varied little. Many of the remaining variants within the 2-Mb window on either side of the selected variants were in significant LD with the selected variants (as shown in Additional file 4: Figure S4), and up to 3,449,212 variants were excluded from the GRMc (Table 2).

Variance explained by the selected variants
The GRM of all the variants in the full sequence data resulted in genomic heritabilities (h^2) of 0.83, 0.87 and 0.72 for PY, SCS and IFL for the validation animals (Table 3), respectively. Compared to these values, the decrease in h^2 when the HD or 50k SNP panels were

used was only marginal (less than 0.04), which indicates that little additional genetic variance is picked up by the sequence data.

Selection of variants based on the $-\log_{10}(p)$ value resulted in fewer variants being used for the GRM and the proportion of variance explained by the GRM was smaller. Exceptions were found for variants selected with a $-\log_{10}(p) > 5$ from the full sequence data for PY and SCS; in this case, h^2 increased with fewer variants compared to when the variants were selected with a $-\log_{10}(p) > 3$. However, estimated phenotypic variances were highly inflated for this scenario (see Additional file 5: Table S1): 621 kg^2, 55 SCS^2, and 28 d^2 compared with 308 kg^2, 19 SCS^2 and 16 d^2, for PY, SCS and IFL, respectively. Also, when the lower density SNP panels were used and the variants were strongly selected, and when variants from sequence data were selected with a $-\log_{10}(p)$ higher than 3, the estimated phenotypic variances were inflated but to a much lesser extent. This inflation of the h^2 was probably due to the properties of the GRM when it was calculated from a few variants in high LD with each other. Comparing the GRM from HD, 50k, and ISQ $-\log_{10}(p) > 5$ variants with the GRM elements from ISQ variants in Additional file 6: Figure S5 and Additional file 7: Table S2, it is clear that the ISQ $-\log_{10}(p) > 5$ GRM contained many off-diagonal elements that were equal to the size of the diagonal elements, and therefore, in the analysis, the GRM had to adjust for positive definiteness. When the few variants selected from the COJO analysis were used, h^2 were not inflated, for example the GRM from the 100 most informative variants in the discovery population resulted in h^2 that ranged from 0.17 to 0.23 in the validation population. Still, it was clear that even the variants selected from GWAS with (imputed) sequence data could not compete in terms of variance explained with a GRM based on a larger number of variants (e.g. 50k).

Another way of testing the importance of selecting variants was to investigate how much h^2 was lost when the selected variants were discarded from the GRM, i.e. the complementary variants in the GRMc. In the scenarios that applied a simple SNP selection, fitting only the GRMc resulted in a drop in h^2 that was less than 0.01 compared to fitting the full sequence data. With the COJO scenario, the drop in h^2 compared to fitting the full sequence data was less than 0.04 (results not shown).

To judge the relative importance of the GRM and GRMc, both GRM and GRMc were fitted together in a single model (Table 4). For PY, SCS and IFL, in nearly all the scenarios with the p value-based selection, the sum of the two h^2 was close to the total genetic variance that was explained by the full sequence information (0.83 for PY, 0.87 for SCS, and 0.72 for IFL), except in the analysis

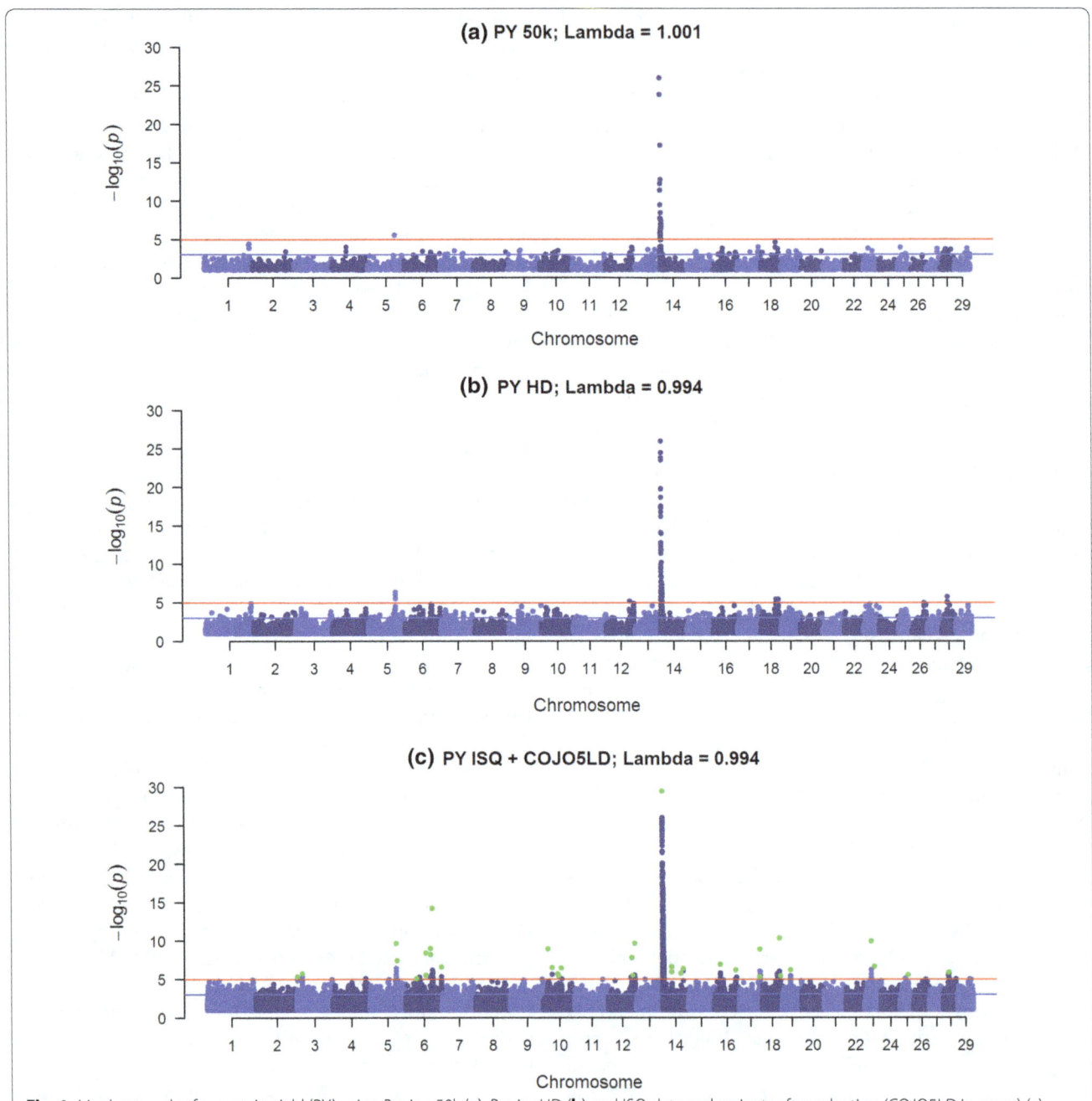

Fig. 1 Manhattan plot for protein yield (PY) using Bovine 50k (**a**), BovineHD (**b**) and ISQ data and variants after selection (COJO5LD in *green*) (**c**). Significance of variants effects (−log10(p)) based on the GCTA single variant analyses for protein yield (PY) using Bovine 50k (**a**), BovineHD (**b**), and full sequence data (ISQ) and the variants selected after the COJO5LD analysis (*green*) (**c**)

with the HD **GRM** and its **GRMc**, which resulted in highly inflated estimates of h^2 for PY and IFL. Separately, the HD **GRM** and the **GRMc** can both fully explain the genetic variance and among the SNPs that were used to build the **GRMc**, some are probably in strong LD with variants on the HD chip. Consequently, estimation of the genetic variance for these two sets of data with redundant information is probably difficult. For the three traits, the combined effect of **GRM** and **GRMc** for −log10(p) > 5 selection from imputed sequence variants (ISQ), i.e. weighting the selected variants differently from the rest of the variants, resulted in a very small improvement of 0.01 for the combined h^2. In comparison with the p value-based selection, the COJO scenarios resulted in lower h^2 since many variants were removed from the **GRMc** on the basis of LD with the selected variants. The 50k panel

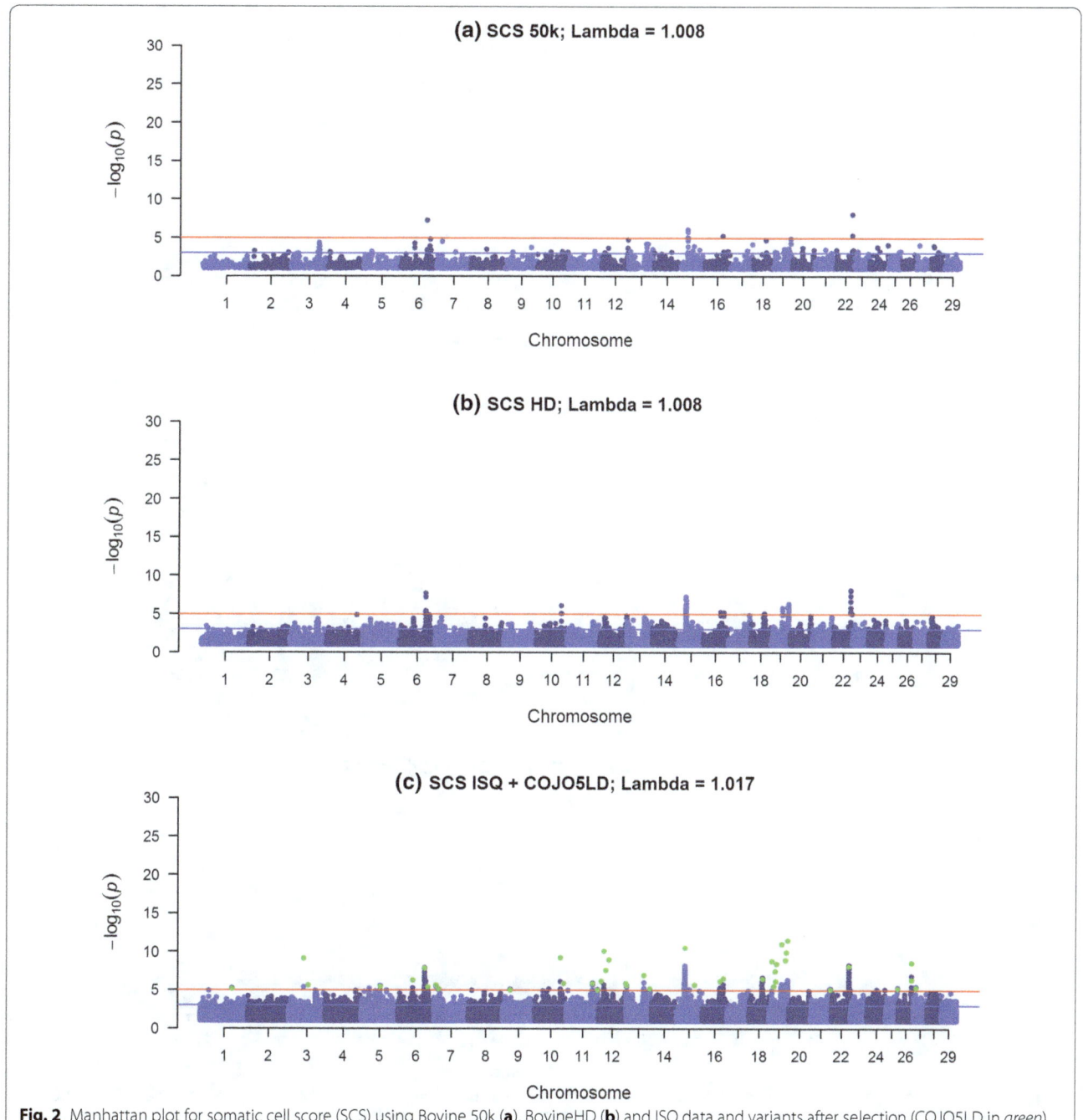

Fig. 2 Manhattan plot for somatic cell score (SCS) using Bovine 50k (**a**), BovineHD (**b**) and ISQ data and variants after selection (COJO5LD in *green*) (**c**). Significance of variants effects (−log10(p)) based on the GCTA single variant analyses for somatic cell score (SCS) using Bovine 50k (**a**), BovineHD (**b**), and full sequence data (ISQ) and the variants selected after the COJO5LD analysis (*green*) (**c**)

explained 85% (= 0.70/0.82) of the genetic variance for PY and only 15% was partitioned to the rest of the variants on the sequence, whereas the 50k panel explained 56 and 70% for SCS and IFL. For the COJO analyses, the sum of the two h^2 was smaller than the total genetic variance that was explained by the full sequence information, but the selected variants from the GWAS accounted for 6 to 18%

of the total genetic variance, when they were estimated conditional on the **GRMc** for the complementary variants.

Genomic prediction with selected variants

Using ISQ variants or any of the two SNP panels resulted in the same prediction accuracy for PY (0.68), SCS (0.70 to 0.71) and IFL (0.60) (Table 5). Compared to these

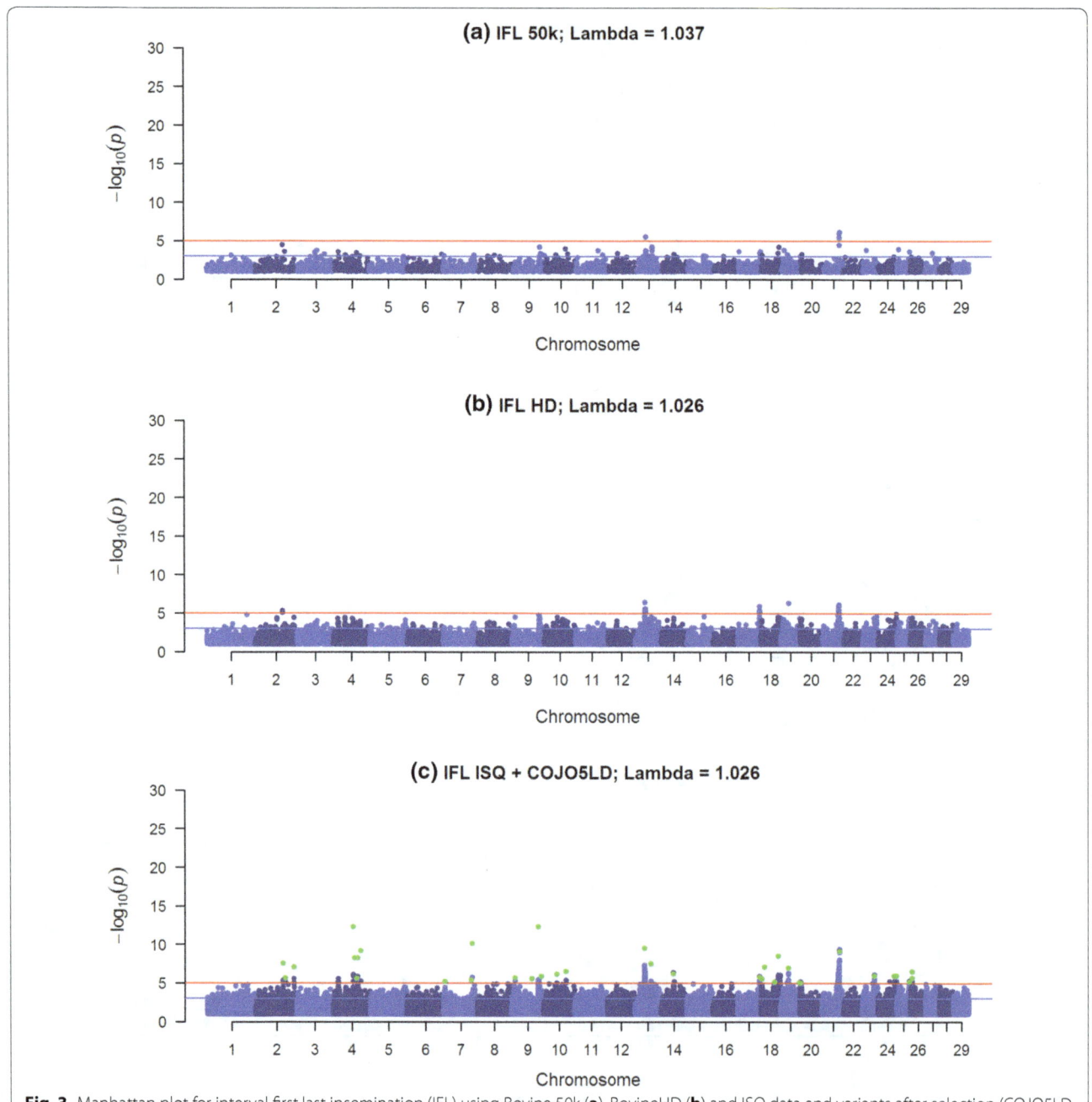

Fig. 3 Manhattan plot for interval first last insemination (IFL) using Bovine 50k (**a**), BovineHD (**b**) and ISQ data and variants after selection (COJO5LD in *green*) (**c**). Significance of variants effects (−log10(p)) based on the GCTA single variant analyses for interval between first and last lactation using Bovine 50k (**a**), BovineHD (**b**), and full sequence data (ISQ) and the variants selected after the COJO5LD analysis (*green*) (**c**)

values, the prediction accuracy for all scenarios decreased when the number of variants in the **GRM** decreased. However, compared to the simple selection of variants with a −log10(p) > 5, there was a clear advantage in the COJO analyses especially for IFL and to a lesser extent for SCS. For IFL, the prediction accuracy increased from 0.27 for the **GRM** based on ISQ −log10(p) > 5 to between 0.30 and 0.38 for the COJO scenarios while the number of variants decreased from 853 to between 35 and 264.

All variant selection scenarios showed a clear bias (slope <1.0) in the scale of the predictions (Table 5). In general, the bias increased as selection was more stringent and the number of selected variants decreased.

When both **GRM** and **GRMc** are fitted together (Table 6), in the simple variant selection scenarios, all the variants are used but accuracy of genomic prediction may differ between models, because a separate weight is given to the variants in the **GRM** and **GRMc**. Apart from two of

Table 3 Phenotypic variance (h^2) explained in 2287 validation animals fitting GRM based on the selected set of variants for protein yield (PY), somatic cell score (SCS) and interval first–last insemination (IFL)

Trait	Selection criteria	ISQ	HD	50k
		Selected set of variants (GRM)		
PY	All variants	0.83	0.82	0.81
	$-\log10(p) > 3$	0.53[a]	0.40	0.22
	$-\log10(p) > 5$	0.60[a]	0.43[a]	0.22[a]
	COJO3	0.21		
	COJO5	0.19		
	COJO5LD	0.19		
	COJO#100	0.23		
SCS	All variants	0.87	0.84	0.83
	$-\log10(p) > 3$	0.57[a]	0.45[a]	0.19
	$-\log10(p) > 5$	0.72[a]	0.25[a]	0.03[a]
	COJO3	0.31		
	COJO5	0.31		
	COJO5LD	0.16		
	COJO#100	0.22		
IFL	All variants	0.72	0.70	0.69
	$-\log10(p) > 3$	0.51[a]	0.32	0.14
	$-\log10(p) > 5$	0.50[a]	0.15[a]	0.03
	COJO3	0.25		
	COJO5	0.23		
	COJO5LD	0.13		
	COJO#100	0.17		

ISQ are all imputed sequence variants, and HD and 50k are the SNPs on the common HD and 50k panels. Variants were selected using GWAS results on 3469 discovery animals

[a] Inflated phenotypic variance (see Additional file 5: Table S1)

the variant selection scenarios, no increase in accuracy was observed in any scenario when fitting **GRM** and **GRMc** compared with fitting the ISQ **GRM** for all variants. Bias in the prediction was smaller than when each **GRM** was fitted separately. When variants were selected from HD with $-\log10(p) > 5$ and fitted in a **GRM** separately from the **GRMc** with the remaining ISQ variants, prediction accuracies for PY and SCS were 0.01 higher than when all ISQ variants were fitted through the **GRM**. This result is similar to that mentioned above for the h^2, and is in contrast to that of the scenarios fitting $-\log10(p) > 3$ separately, which resulted in lower accuracy and more bias.

Discussion

The objective of this study was to identify the usefulness of imputed sequence data, in particular regarding the proportion of variance explained by different sets of variants for three traits PY, SCS and IFL, and for the accuracy of genomic prediction. Full imputed sequence data,

lower density SNP panels, and preselected variants from GWAS that used imputed whole-genome sequence were considered. Using the **GRM** based on full sequence data explained marginally more variation than that based on the common SNP panels. Compared to SNP data, the use of sequence data allowed to identify more variants linked to QTL, and peaks across the genome were sharper, which is in line with other studies using the data of the 1000 Bull Genomes Project [4]. This study clearly showed that the 35 and 42 selected variants from the COJO analysis led to h^2 that ranged from 0.13 to 0.19 when fitted alone, and from 0.05 to 0.08 when the **GRM** is competing with a **GRM** based on the full ISQ information. Thus, such QTL information should be beneficial in genomic prediction. However, no clear benefit for genomic prediction was detected with our data where training and validation populations were both composed of Holstein animals.

Improving genomic prediction

The fact that sequence data did not improve genomic prediction was previously reported using the same data [8, 28]. In the study of van Binsbergen et al. [8], a Bayesian variable selection method was used with all ISQ variants fitted simultaneously, but the Manhattan plots in that study demonstrated the difficulty of precise QTL detection. QTL were detected, given the prediction accuracy achieved, but the effects were smeared across DNA variants that were in high LD with each other. Calus et al. [28] investigated the split-and-merge approach to alleviate the severe $n \ll p$ problem with sequence data. Neither of these two studies showed an advantage of using sequence data for genomic prediction. Both studies suggested and discussed several explanations for these results and some of these still hold in our study. One explanation concerns the imputed sequence data used, with imputation accuracy being low for some chromosomes. Poor imputation could be due to errors in the genomic map, which reduce accuracy of prediction and detection of causal mutations. Also the training set is relatively small with highly related animals in contrast with the large number of variants available from ISQ. Still, the prior expectation for our study was that, by pre-selecting the ISQ variants some of the limitations (e.g. extreme $p \gg n$ and strong LD between many SNPs) would be overcome [11, 29], and more precise QTL detection with ISQ variants would lead to higher accuracy of genomic prediction, especially since ISQ helps to identify more precisely the variants that are associated with the traits [4]. Our results also demonstrated that ISQ helped to identify the QTL, and a limited number of selected variants explained 11 to 14% of the genetic variance, even when fitted with the complementary **GRMc** at the same time. Hence, there is no

Table 4 Phenotypic variance explained (h^2) in 2287 validation animals for protein yield (PY), somatic cell score (SCS) and interval first –last insemination (IFL)

Trait	Selection criteria	ISQ	HD	50k	ISQ	HD	50k	ISQ	HD	50k
		Selected set of variants (GRM)			Complementary set of variants (GRMc)			Sum of GRM and GRMc		
PY	All variants	0.83	0.98	0.70		0.00	0.12	0.83	0.98	0.82
	−log10(p) > 3	0.19	0.15	0.09	0.61	0.65	0.73	0.80	0.80	0.82
	−log10(p) > 5	0.10	0.04	0.03	0.74	0.79	0.80	0.84	0.83	0.83
	COJO3	0.11			0.70			0.81		
	COJO5	0.10			0.71			0.81		
	COJO5LD	0.08			0.73			0.82		
	COJO#100	0.09			0.72			0.82		
SCS	All variants	0.87	0.87	0.48		0.00	0.38	0.87	0.87	0.86
	−log10(p) > 3	0.22	0.15	0.05	0.60	0.68	0.80	0.82	0.83	0.85
	−log10(p) > 5	0.24	0.03	0.01	0.64	0.84	0.85	0.88	0.87	0.86
	COJO3	0.14			0.68			0.81		
	COJO5	0.14			0.66			0.80		
	COJO5LD	0.05			0.79			0.84		
	COJO#100	0.08			0.76			0.83		
IFL	All variants	0.72	0.85	0.50		0.00	0.21	0.72	0.85	0.70
	−log10(p) > 3	0.20	0.12	0.05	0.51	0.57	0.64	0.70	0.69	0.69
	−log10(p) > 5	0.11	0.03	0.03	0.63	0.69	0.70	0.73	0.72	0.72
	COJO3	0.11			0.57			0.67		
	COJO5	0.12			0.57			0.69		
	COJO5LD	0.07			0.64			0.71		
	COJO#100	0.08			0.64			0.71		

COJO analysis with −log10(p) > 3 (COJO3) or −log10(p) > 5 (COJO5); ISQ are all imputed sequence variants, HD and 50k are the SNPs on the common HD and 50k panels

Variances are estimated fitting **GRM** and **GRMc** together in one model where **GRM** were based on the selected set of variants and **GRMc** on the complementary variants. Set of variants that were selected using GWAS results on 3469 discovery animals

doubt that associated regions were identified for all three traits. However, when weighting this prior information in a separate **GRM**, it was difficult to improve the accuracy of genomic prediction compared with the common SNP panels. This confirms the expectation that, within the Holstein population, it is probably difficult to increase the accuracy of prediction, due to the small size of the effective population and the long-range LD in the population, as was previously demonstrated in a simulation study by MacLeod [30]. Hence, using ISQ and selected variants might be especially beneficial for across-breed prediction in small populations [31] or when traits are used with some QTL having large effects, as for fat percentage [32].

Bias in genomic prediction
Our study showed that the bias in genomic prediction became stronger when variants were strongly preselected. Regressions of DRP on GEBV were expected to be 1, but we found that the stronger the selection of variants was, the stronger the bias was when comparing the predictions in the validation animals. When all ISQ variants

or the SNPs on the common panels were fitted in a single **GRM**, the bias in the slope of prediction was limited (slope > 0.86). Also, when **GRM** and **GRMc** were fitted together, the bias in the genomic prediction was more controlled. However, when strongly selected variants were used, the genomic predictions became more biased, with slopes even lower than 0.5. Szyda et al. [33] showed that genomic predictions for milk yield were biased when 3 k variants were selected for their effect on milk yield [33]. Brondum et al. [32] reported no extra bias when 1623 selected SNPs were added to the 54 k SNP panel, but when the 1623 SNPs were fitted with their own variance in a model with the 54 k SNPs, the bias increased for some traits.

GEBV could be biased because reported effects of SNPs on a trait tend to be larger in magnitude than the true effects of these SNPs. This phenomenon is well-known, as discussed by Goddard et al. [34]; it is known as the "Beavis effect" [35] and has been described as a form of the "winner's curse" [36]. The reason underlying the "Beavis effect" is that effects are estimates, and the

Table 5 Prediction accuracy in 2287 validation animals, and the intercept and slope for the regression of phenotype on the breeding value estimated using GRM with different selected sets of variants for protein yield (PY), somatic cell score (SCS) and interval first–last insemination (IFL)

Trait	Selection criteria	ISQ	HD	50k	ISQ	HD	50k	ISQ	HD	50k
		Accuracy			Intercept			Slope		
PY	All variants	0.68	0.68	0.68	−0.6	−0.6	−0.7	0.90	0.90	0.89
	−log10(p) > 3	0.58	0.56	0.42	2.3	3.6	6.9	0.73	0.65	0.57
	−log10(p) > 5	0.39	0.30	0.28	7.2	8.7	9.4	0.54	0.51	0.71
	COJO3	0.40			7.2			0.45		
	COJO5	0.38			7.7			0.41		
	COJO5LD	0.33			8.1			0.51		
	COJO#100	0.34			7.2			0.47		
SCS	All variants	0.70	0.71	0.70	100	100	100	1.02	1.03	1.03
	−log10(p) > 3	0.63	0.55	0.36	100	100	101	0.82	0.79	0.70
	−log10(p) > 5	0.40	0.22	0.11	100	101	101	0.79	0.66	0.57
	COJO3	0.48			100			0.64		
	COJO5	0.48			100			0.60		
	COJO5LD	0.35			100			0.68		
	COJO#100	0.39			100			0.66		
IFL	All variants	0.60	0.60	0.60	99	99	99	0.88	0.87	0.86
	−log10(p) > 3	0.51	0.45	0.31	99	99	99	0.70	0.62	0.52
	−log10(p) > 5	0.27	0.16	0.10	99	98	98	0.47	0.51	0.77
	COJO3	0.38			99			0.45		
	COJO5	0.35			99			0.41		
	COJO5LD	0.30			99			0.52		
	COJO#100	0.32			99			0.45		

ISQ are all imputed sequence variants, HD and 50k are the SNPs on the common HD and 50k panels. Set of variants that were selected using GWAS and subsequently trained in 3469 discovery animals

uncertainty of these estimates is not taken into account. When selecting significant SNPs, we tend to select those for which the uncertainty of the estimate has a positive effect on the variant effect. As pointed out by Goddard et al. [34], when effects of variants are fitted as random effects, this form of the "Beavis effect" is expected to be minimised, since estimates are regressed towards the mean, at least when proper variances are used for each SNP. However, we selected the variants and subsequently trained them for genomic prediction in the same (discovery) population. Thus, the fact that the validation was biased, was a form of the "Beavis effect": the combined effect of a small set of preselected SNPs was overestimated since the SNPs were selected to have an effect in the same training population.

Another reason for the observed bias is that, rather than the estimates being biased, the bias comes from the overlap between discovery and validation data due to relationships between discovery and validation animals. Overlaps between the validation and discovery data cause bias due to the prediction error covariance between the phenotypes and predictions [37]. Initially, the effect of overlap in the validation and discovery data might be considered as very small here, since validation animals were excluded from both the GWAS and the derivation of the prediction equation, and bulls had highly accurate EBV. However, the validation population consisted of animals from subsequent generations of the training animals, e.g. 84% of the validation animals had their sire included in the discovery data [28]. Hence, DNA variants selected from the GWAS were validated within the same families from the discovery population. Also, the phenotypes used are DRP derived from the EBV from national genetic evaluations, in which all records are estimated simultaneously, and therefore the validation animals are strictly speaking not a completely external and independent population. The phenotypic records of the daughters of the young bulls might have also contributed to the breeding values of the sires of the young bulls, and thus result in erroneous correlations between the validation and training or discovery set [38]. The consequence would be that the estimates are not necessarily biased, but the validation was biased due to correlations between the residuals between the training and validation sets.

Which of these underlying reasons is the major cause of the bias observed in our study is not clear. Also, to what

Table 6 Prediction accuracy in 2287 validation animals, and the intercept and slope for the regression of phenotype on the breeding value estimated using the effects of variants from GRM and GRMc fitted together for different selected sets of variants for protein yield (PY), somatic cell score (SCS) and interval first –last insemination (IFL)

Trait	Selection criteria	ISQ	HD	50k	ISQ	HD	50k	ISQ	HD	50k
		Accuracy			Intercept			Slope		
PY	All variants	0.68	0.68	0.68	−0.6	−0.6	−0.7	0.90	0.90	0.90
	−log10(p) > 3	0.64	0.65	0.67	1.0	1.1	0.4	0.79	0.75	0.83
	−log10(p) > 5	0.67	0.69	0.69	0.2	−0.5	−0.6	0.84	0.90	0.91
	COJO3	0.64			1.4			0.72		
	COJO5	0.64			1.1			0.75		
	COJO5LD	0.67			0.2			0.84		
	COJO#100	0.63			1.2			0.79		
SCS	All variants	0.70	0.71	0.70	100	100	100	1.02	1.03	1.02
	−log10(p) > 3	0.67	0.66	0.66	100	100	100	0.85	0.83	0.87
	−log10(p) > 5	0.67	0.69	0.69	100	100	100	0.93	0.99	1.00
	COJO3	0.63			100			0.76		
	COJO5	0.62			100			0.73		
	COJO5LD	0.65			100			0.88		
	COJO#100	0.62			100			0.83		
IFL	All variants	0.60	0.60	0.60	99	99	99	0.88	0.87	0.87
	−log10(p) > 3	0.55	0.56	0.58	99	99	99	0.73	0.71	0.80
	−log10(p) > 5	0.58	0.61	0.60	99	99	99	0.80	0.88	0.88
	COJO3	0.51			99			0.60		
	COJO5	0.51			99			0.59		
	COJO5LD	0.57			99			0.76		
	COJO#100	0.54			99			0.70		

ISQ are all imputed sequence variants, HD and 50k are the SNPs on the common HD and 50k panels. Set of variants that were selected using GWAS and subsequently trained in 3469 discovery animals

extent the bias is controlled by fitting additional variants is not completely clear yet. Given the importance of validation results in practical breeding (i.e. used to assess the scale and reliability of published breeding values), more thought should be given on the validation of genomic breeding values within populations. For example, what are the effects of removing the sires of the validation population on the bias and accuracy when selected SNPs are used, or using separate populations for discovery, training and validation.

Variant selection

To benefit from the use of sequence data, it needs to be combined with a careful variant selection to pinpoint the QTN [29, 39]. Detection of causal variants based on the data only proved to be difficult due to the large number of variants, and the high LD between variants due to the family relationships in our discovery population. Initially, variant selection was based purely on $-\log_{10}(p)$ values of the GWAS results. When a high $-\log_{10}(p)$ threshold was maintained, variants were selected from a few chromosomal regions, but the resulting **GRM** from these selected variants had poor properties (see Additional

file 6: Figure S5 and Additional file 7: Table S2), since the genotypes of too many animals within the population were not sufficiently different for these regions to estimate genetic relationships that differ from 1. Therefore, simply selecting all associated variants was not a good criterion for variant selection. To overcome the issue of selecting variants from the same regions, we used different options of GCTA to do a conditional and joint (COJO) analysis [22]. The first COJO application used only variants pre-selected based on $-\log_{10}(p)$ value (to reduce the number of variants) but calculated the conditional and joint significance considering LD between all the variants across the whole genome. This variant selection was hindered by collinearity in the data. In spite of excluding from the model variants that were in LD with a r^2 higher than 0.8, many variants were selected with large effects and $-\log_{10}(p)$ values, calculated conditional on the joint effects already included in the model. Sometimes the same variants had no effect or effects close to zero $-\log_{10}(p)$ in the first single variant analyses. Also, when comparing the LD between the variants, the COJO analysis selected few variants that were in moderate to high LD with each other and had opposite effects. Since the estimates were unrealistic, alternative approaches were tested by controlling the LD between variants more stringently. Fewer variants were selected with COJO5LD and only using these in the **GRM** resulted in lower h^2 and prediction accuracy, mainly because fewer variants were used. However, combining the COJO5LD together with the **GRM**c resulted in slightly higher h^2 and higher prediction accuracy and less bias for all three traits, than any of the other conditional and joint analyses. Thus, when selecting variants, the way that the variants are selected and LD is accounted for is important.

Ideally, Bayesian variable selection methods should be able to separate out the causal variants when all fitted together. However, using the same dataset as in our study, van Binsbergen et al. [8] did not succeed in detecting clear peaks and significance levels for variants in the Manhattan plots when they were fitted all together, and detection of causal variants became even less precise using ISQ in comparison with HD variants [8]. Other studies have combined the biological information available on the functional classes that the variants belong to with the Bayesian variable selection (BAYESRC) [40]. However, in the case of a population with animals as closely related as in our Holstein discovery population, it remains intrinsically difficult to identify the causal variants very precisely.

Brondum et al. [32] performed the GWAS in Nordic cattle for three separate breeds and for three different sets of traits. They selected QTL and three to five variants to tag each QTL and combined 1623 variants with the 50k SNP panel. In contrast to our study, they obtained improved accuracies within the breeds that were used for the GWAS, and the largest improvements in genomic prediction were observed for a French Holstein population that was not used for the GWAS. Also, bias was improved when tested in the independent population of French Holsteins. An extensive study using sequence data, and using across-breed QTL and genomic prediction was performed by van den Berg [41]. Using multibreed information, increases in reliability of up to 10% were found for all the breeds, but they were sensitive to the selection of variants and the model used. In both these studies, LD-pruning was used to select variants [32, 39]. Therefore, the use of sequence information should be accompanied by careful detection and selection of causal variants using concordance analysis or using biological information [29].

Conclusions

When only the Holstein breed is considered for the discovery of variants and prediction, there is little advantage in using dense sequence data for genomic prediction, although 35 to 42 variants were detected that explained 13 to 19% of the total variation when fitted alone, and 5 to 10% of the variance when they were in competition with other variants. With the within-breed approach, detection of variants and their selection were difficult due to LD. Selection of variants gave more biased genomic predictions. It is unclear if predictions were more biased due to estimating the effects of selected SNPs in the same training population as that from which SNPs were selected, or if the validation was biased due to common family structure or to the use of common data in the national analyses between the training and validation sets.

Additional files

Additional file 1: Figure S1. Q–Q plot for PY using the variants from the Bovine 50k (A), BovineHD (B) and the full imputed sequence data (C).

Additional file 2: Figure S2. Q–Q plot for SCS using the variants from the Bovine 50k (A), BovineHD (B) and the full imputed sequence data (C).

Additional file 3: Figure S3. Q–Q plot for IFL using the variants from the Bovine 50k (A), BovineHD (B) and the full imputed sequence data (C).

Additional file 4: Figure S4. Manhattan plot for three chromosomes and PY using ISQ variants and the variants excluded from **GRMc** based on LD within a 2-Mb window on either side of each selected variant (*green*).

Additional file 5: Table S1. Estimated variances, h^2 and log likelihood for PY, SCS and IFL using models with different single **GRM**, or **GRM** + **GRMc** combined in one model. Description: **GRM** were based on SNPs selected from GWAS. Standard errors are below the estimates.

Additional file 6: Figure S5. Plot of the elements of a **GRM** based on the 50k SNPs, $-\log10(p) > 5$ and COJO5LD versus the same elements using ISQ.

Additional file 7: Table S2. Summary statistics for the diagonal and off diagonal elements of the different **GRM**.

Authors' contributions
RFV designed the study, performed the statistical analyses, and drafted the manuscript. ACB performed the imputation, and together with MPLC, participated in the design of the study. ACB, MPLC and CS helped to draft the manuscript. All authors read and approved the final manuscript.

Author details
[1] Animal Breeding and Genomics Centre, Wageningen UR Livestock Research, P.O. Box 338, 6700 AH Wageningen, The Netherlands. [2] Department of Animal and Aquacultural Sciences, Norwegian University of Life Sciences, P.O. Box 5003, 1432 Ås, Norway. [3] CRV BV, P.O. Box 454, 6800 AL Arnhem, The Netherlands.

Acknowledgements
The authors acknowledge CRV BV (Arnhem, the Netherlands) for financial support and for providing the deregressed proofs and the HD genotype data, the 1000 Bull Genomes consortium for providing the sequence data, and also acknowledge financial support from the Dutch Ministry of Economic Affairs, Agriculture, and Innovation (Public–private partnership "Breed4Food" code BO-22.04-011-001-ASG-LR-3).

Competing interests
The authors declare that they have no competing interests.

References

1. Goddard ME, Hayes BJ, Meuwissen THE. Genomic selection in livestock populations. Genet Res (Camb). 2010;92:413–21.

2. Hayes BJ, Bowman PJ, Chamberlain AJ, Goddard ME. Invited review: genomic selection in dairy cattle: Progress and challenges. J Dairy Sci. 2009;92:433–43.

3. Bouamra-Mechemache Z, Jongeneel R, Réquillart V. Impact of a gradual increase in milk quotas on the EU dairy sector. Eur Rev Agric Econ. 2008;35:461–91.

4. Daetwyler HD, Capitan A, Pausch H, Stothard P, Van Binsbergen R, Brondum RF, et al. Whole-genome sequencing of 234 bulls facilitates mapping of monogenic and complex traits in cattle. Nat Genet. 2014;46:858–65.

5. Clark SA, Hickey JM, van der Werf JHJ. Different models of genetic variation and their effect on genomic evaluation. Genet Sel Evol. 2011;43:18.

6. MacLeod IM, Hayes BJ, Goddard ME. Will sequence SNP data improve the accuracy of genomic prediction in the presence of long term selection? Proc Assoc Advmt Anim Breed Genet. 2013;20:215–9.

7. Meuwissen T, Goddard M. Accurate prediction of genetic values for complex traits by Whole-genome resequencing. Genetics. 2010;185:623–31.

8. van Binsbergen R, Calus MPL, Bink MCAM, van Eeuwijk FA, Schrooten C, Veerkamp RF. Genomic prediction using imputed whole-genome sequence data in Holstein Friesian cattle. Genet Sel Evol. 2015;47:71.

9. Heidaritabar M, Calus MPL, Megens HJ, Vereijken A, Groenen MAM, Bastiaansen JWM. Accuracy of genomic prediction using imputed whole-genome sequence data in white layers. J Anim Breed Genet. 2016;133:167–79.

10. Druet T, Macleod IM, Hayes BJ. Toward genomic prediction from whole-genome sequence data: impact of sequencing design on genotype imputation and accuracy of predictions. Heredity (Edinb). 2014;112:39–47.

11. Wientjes YCJ, Veerkamp RF, Calus MPL. Using selection index theory to estimate consistency of multi-locus linkage disequilibrium across populations. BMC Genet. 2015;16:87.

12. VanRaden PM, Van Tassell CP, Wiggans GR, Sonstegard TS, Schnabel RD, Taylor JF, et al. Invited review: reliability of genomic predictions for North American Holstein bulls. J Dairy Sci. 2009;92:16–24.

13. Fikse WF, Banos G. Weighting factors of sire daughter information in international genetic evaluations. J Dairy Sci. 2001;84:1759–67.

14. VanRaden PM, Wiggans GR. Derivation, calculation, and use of national animal model information. J Dairy Sci. 1991;74:2737–46.

15. Browning BL, Browning SR. A unified approach to genotype imputation and haplotype-phase inference for large data sets of trios and unrelated individuals. Am J Hum Genet. 2009;84:210–23.

16. Browning SR, Browning BL. Rapid and accurate haplotype phasing and missing-data inference for whole-genome association studies by use of localized haplotype clustering. Am J Hum Genet. 2007;81:1084–97.

17. Schrooten C, Dassonneville R, Ducrocq V, Brondum RF, Lund MS, Chen J, et al. Error rate for imputation from the Illumina BovineSNP50 chip to the Illumina BovineHD chip. Genet Sel Evol. 2014;46:10.

18. Bouwman AC, Veerkamp RF. Consequences of splitting whole-genome sequencing effort over multiple breeds on imputation accuracy. BMC Genet. 2014;15:105.

19. Brondum RF, Guldbrandtsen B, Sahana G, Lund MS, Su GS. Strategies for imputation to whole genome sequence using a single or multi-breed reference population in cattle. BMC Genomics. 2014;15:728.

20. Fuchsberger C, Abecasis GR, Hinds DA. minimac2: faster genotype imputation. Bioinformatics. 2015;31:782–4.

21. Yang J, Lee SH, Goddard ME, Visscher PM. GCTA: a tool for genome-wide complex trait analysis. Am J Hum Genet. 2011;88:76–82.

22. Yang J, Benyamin B, McEvoy BP, Gordon S, Henders AK, Nyholt DR, et al. Common SNPs explain a large proportion of the heritability for human height. Nat Genet. 2010;42:565–9.

23. VanRaden PM. Efficient methods to compute genomic predictions. J Dairy Sci. 2008;91:4414–23.

24. Turner SD. qqman: an R package for visualizing GWAS results using Q–Q and manhattan plots. bioRxiv. 2014. doi:10.1101/005165.

25. Yang J, Ferreira T, Morris AP, Medland SE, Madden PAF, Heath AC, et al. Conditional and joint multiple-SNP analysis of GWAS summary statistics identifies additional variants influencing complex traits. Nat Genet. 2012;44:369–75.

26. de los Campos g, Sorensen D, Gianola D. Genomic heritability: what is it? PLoS Genet. 2015;11:e1005048.

27. Purcell S, Neale B, Todd-Brown K, Thomas L, Ferreira MAR, Bender D, et al. PLINK: a tool set for whole-genome association and population-based linkage analyses. Am J Hum Genet. 2007;81:559–75.

28. Calus MPL, Bouwman AC, Schrooten C, Veerkamp RF. Efficient genomic prediction based on whole genome sequence data using split-and-merge Bayesian variable selection. Genet Sel Evol. 2016;48:49.

29. Perez-Enciso M, Rincon JC, Legarra A. Sequence- vs. chip-assisted genomic selection: accurate biological information is advised. Genet Sel Evol. 2015;47:43.

30. MacLeod IM, Hayes BJ, Goddard ME. The effects of demography and long-term selection on the accuracy of genomic prediction with sequence data. Genetics. 2014;198:1671–84.

31. Lund MS, van den Berg I, Ma P, Brondum RF, Su G. Review: how to improve genomic predictions in small dairy cattle populations. Animal. 2016;10:1042–9.

32. Brondum RF, Su G, Janss L, Sahana G, Guldbrandtsen B, Boichard D, et al. Quantitative trait loci markers derived from whole genome sequence data increases the reliability of genomic prediction. J Dairy Sci. 2015;98:4107–16.

33. Szyda J, Zukowski K, Kaminski S, Zarnecki A. Testing different single nucleotide polymorphism selection strategies for prediction of genomic breeding values in dairy cattle based on low density panels. Czech J Anim Sci. 2013;58:136–45.

34. Goddard ME, Wray NR, Verbyla K, Visscher PM. Estimating effects and making predictions from genome-wide marker data. Stat Sci. 2009;24:517–29.

35. Xu SZ. Theoretical basis of the Beavis effect. Genetics. 2003;165:2259–68.

36. Zollner S, Pritchard JK. Overcoming the winner's curse: estimating penetrance parameters from case-control data. Am J Hum Genet. 2007;80:605–15.

37. Wray NR, Yang J, Hayes BJ, Price AL, Goddard ME, Visscher PM. Pitfalls of predicting complex traits from SNPs. Nat Rev Genet. 2013;14:507–15.

38. Amer PR, Banos G. Implications of avoiding overlap between training and testing data sets when evaluating genomic predictions of genetic merit. J Dairy Sci. 2010;93:3320–30.

39. van den Berg I, Boichard D, Guldbrandtsen B, Lund MS. Using sequence variants in linkage disequilibrium with causative mutations to improve across breed prediction in dairy cattle: A simulation study. 2016;G3 (Bethesda)(6):2553–61.

40. MacLeod IM, Bowman PJ, Vander Jagt CJ, Haile-Mariam M, Kemper KE, Chamberlain AJ, et al. Exploiting biological priors and sequence variants enhances QTL discovery and genomic prediction of complex traits. BMC Genomics. 2016;17:144.

41. van den Berg I, Boichard D, Lund MS. Sequence variants selected from a multi-breed GWAS can improve the reliability of genomic prediction. Genet Sel Evol. 2016;48:83.

4

Estimating the genetic merit of sires by using pooled DNA from progeny of undetermined pedigree

Amy M. Bell[1*], John M. Henshall[1], Laercio R. Porto-Neto[2], Sonja Dominik[1], Russell McCulloch[2], James Kijas[2] and Sigrid A. Lehnert[2]

Abstract

Background: DNA-based predictions for hard-to-measure production traits hold great promise for selective breeding programs. DNA pooling might provide a cheap genomic approach to use phenotype data from commercial flocks which are commonly group-mated with parentage unknown. This study on sheep explores if genomic breeding values for stud sires can be estimated from genomic relationships that were obtained from pooled DNA in combination with phenotypes from commercial progeny.

Methods: Phenotypes used in this study were categorical data. Blood was pooled strategically aiming at even pool sizes and within sex and phenotype category. A hybrid genomic relationship matrix was constructed relating pools to sires. This matrix was used to determine the contribution of sires to each of the pools and therefore phenotype category by using a simple regression approach. Genomic breeding values were also estimated using the hybrid genomic relationship matrix.

Results: We demonstrated that, using pooled DNA, the genetic performance of sires can be illustrated as their contribution to phenotype categories and can be expressed as a regression coefficient. Genomic estimated breeding values for sires were equivalent to the regression coefficients and are a commonly used industry tool.

Conclusions: Genotyping of DNA from pooled biological samples offers a cheap method to link phenotypic information from commercial production animals to the breeding population and can be turned into information on the genetic value of stud sires for traits that cannot be measured in the stud environment.

Background

Genomic predictions have had a significant impact on livestock breeding systems for which large reference populations with genotypic and phenotypic information exist [1]. The opportunity to develop genomic predictions has been addressed by forming specialized nucleus herds or flocks that are extensively phenotyped for the beef and sheep industries [2, 3]. Commercial flocks provide an unmined resource of abundant phenotypes that are assessed or measured during routine commercial husbandry procedures. Using commercial phenotypes for genetic evaluation has been hindered by the fact that performance records are not usually captured, animals are often not individually identified and/or no parentage information exists because flocks or herds are group-mated. However, in combination with affordable genotyping, commercial phenotypes could add genetic information on sire performance under commercial conditions. In spite of the decreasing cost of genotyping, it would still be a substantial expense to assess the performance of sires in a commercial environment, based on individual genotypes. Commercial phenotypes can be exploited in a cost-effective manner without needing to capture individual records by strategically pooling DNA and using it in a genetic evaluation approach [4].

*Correspondence: Amy.Bell@csiro.au
[1] CSIRO Agriculture, F D McMaster Laboratory Chiswick, Armidale, NSW 2350, Australia
Full list of author information is available at the end of the article

Allele frequencies can be estimated from pooled genotype data and subsequently estimated effects of single nucleotide polymorphisms (SNPs) from a genome-wide association study (GWAS) have been demonstrated to be equivalent to effects of SNPs from individual genotyping [4, 5]. This approach reduces the cost of GWAS [6–8]. It has also been demonstrated that the genetic merit of sires can be estimated from pooled DNA in combination with phenotype information collected on commercial properties during routine husbandry procedures [5, 9].

The objective of this study was to determine whether, in the absence of individual genotypes, pooled DNA genotypes can be used in combination with commercial progeny records on a categorical phenotype to estimate genomic breeding values and to illustrate these in a regression approach as a sire's genetic contribution to a particular phenotype. This approach could be a cost-effective commercial progeny test to inform stud breeders and commercial producers on the genetic suitability of sires for specific environments.

Methods
Animals
Approval was granted (AEC approval number 1582) to use the animals in this study by the Animal Ethics Committee of the Australian Animal Health Laboratory, Victoria. Two thousand six hundred 13 to 14 months old Merino sheep were available for the trial. The sires of the sheep in the study were obtained from a stud in southern New South Wales which had been the sole provider of rams to the commercial property for many years. For management purposes, the sheep were maintained in two groups according to sex, ewes (female) and wethers (castrated males).

The phenotype of interest in this study is called "dag score" and describes the amount of faecal soiling in the breech area of the sheep. Breech soiling devalues the wool harvested from the sheep, increases time and management costs of routine husbandry practices and can predispose the animal to increased risk of flystrike. Dag score is a heritable trait with a heritability of about 0.35, depending on

the age of the animal at the time of phenotype assessment [10], but is not expressed in all environments. Dags were a problem for this specific commercial property, but the stud from which this commercial property sourced rams was located in an environment where dags do not occur and no information existed for the sires' propensity for dag formation. The dag score phenotype was assessed on a scale of 1 (no soiling) to 5 (heavy soiling) based on Visual Sheep Scores, a commercial guide for visually assessed traits developed by Australian Wool Innovation Limited (AWI) and Meat and Livestock Australia (MLA) [11]. Dag score is a visual assessment and a large number of animals can be phenotyped in a short period of time. All sheep were moved through the sampling race for scoring and bleeding until a maximum of 80 individuals per sex and dag score was reached, resulting in a subset of 400 males and 386 females as outlined in Table 1.

Pooling design
Pool formation within contemporary groups or fixed effects has been suggested as the most effective pooling design [12]. Generally no fixed effects or contemporary group information is recorded on commercial properties. For this property, sex was the only known fixed effect. Within the two sexes and five dag scores, with 80 individuals each, samples were randomly split into two replicates, with 40 individuals per pool, with the exception of the pools of females with dag score 5, for which only 66 samples were available, and which formed two pools of 33 samples each. This resulted in a total of 20 pools. Although parentage of individual sheep was unknown, 33 of the 45 sires used to produce the flock of sheep sampled were still present for DNA sample collection.

Once samples were assigned to pools, samples of 20 µL of whole blood from each individual sample within each pool were combined to create a pooled blood sample. 200 µL of the pooled blood was then used for genomic DNA extraction following manufacturer's instructions (Qiagen DNeasy® Blood and Tissue Kit).

For genotyping, each of the pooled DNA samples and the 33 individual sires were assayed with the Illumina

Table 1 Description of phenotypic values for dag scores [11] and pool sizes (number of pools × number of individuals in the pool)

Dag score	Description	Male pools	Female pools
1	No dags	2 × 40	2 × 40
2	Some dags around the breech area	2 × 40	2 × 40
3	Dags around the breech area, some dags reaching down the inner hind leg to above the hock	2 × 40	2 × 40
4	Dags around the breech area, reaching down the inner hind legs to the hock and extend out	2 × 40	2 × 40
5	Extensive dags around breech and extending down the hind legs to the pasterns, covering extensive amount of the hind legs	2 × 40	2 × 33

Ovine SNP 50 chip [13]. To obtain the relevant data, the Illumina GenomeStudio™ software was formatted to export a variable called "B-allele frequency" [14, 15]. These are quantitative estimates of the proportion of the alternative SNP allele. For an individual genotype, the B-allele frequency is 0 or 1 for homozygous individuals and 0.5 for heterozygous individuals. For a pooled sample, the B-allele frequency for a SNP can range from 0 to 1. Genotypes for pooled DNA were generated based on the diploid clustering algorithm [14]. Pooled DNA presents like polyploidy data, which consequently, renders some of the routine quality control parameters, such as GenCall and HetExcess [15], which are not meaningful since they aim to eliminate rare alleles, whereas they are informative for this study. Other classic quality control steps such as thresholds for minor allele frequencies are not applicable either. The aim of the approach presented here is to relate allele frequencies from the pooled progeny data to the individual sire data and rare alleles provide useful information to this process.

Statistical analysis

Hybrid genomic relationship matrix based on pooled DNA

Sire relationships with pools were estimated through a genomic relationship matrix. The method described here has previously been termed "hybrid genomic relationship matrix" (h-GRM) because it consists of three blocks of relationships, i.e. (1) between pools, (2) between individual sires, and (3) between pools and sires [5]. The first method of VanRaden was applied [16], but instead of discrete genotype calls, B-allele frequencies were used which describe the allele frequency of the second allele at each locus.

VanRaden uses matrix $\mathbf{M}$ which specifies which SNP alleles each individual inherited, and the dimensions of $\mathbf{M}$ are the number of individuals (n) by the number of loci (i), containing values -1 and 1 for individuals that are homozygous for the respective allele of the locus and 0 for heterozygous individuals. For this study, matrix $\mathbf{M}^*$ was used, which is equivalent to $\mathbf{M}$. Let $\mathbf{M}^* = (\mathbf{Bfreq} - 0.5) * 2$, with $\mathbf{Bfreq}$ being a matrix of the dimension of number of sires (s) plus the number of pools (p) by the number of loci (i), containing B-allele frequencies. The B-allele frequencies for sires were 0.0, 0.5, and 1.0 for the homozygote, heterozygote and other homozygote, respectively, and for pools these were expressed as a real number between 0 and 1. For vector $\mathbf{P}^*$ of size $(1 \times (s + p))$, the same formula is used as for $\mathbf{P}$ by VanRaden, but $\mathbf{P}$ is of size I [16]. Let vector $\mathbf{P}^*$ be $\mathbf{P}^* = (\mathbf{freq} - 0.5) * 2$ with $\mathbf{freq}$ being a vector of B-allele frequencies for sires and pools.

Let matrix $\mathbf{Z}^*$ be the difference between $\mathbf{M}^*$ and $\mathbf{P}^*$, equivalent to $\mathbf{Z} = \mathbf{M} - \mathbf{P}$ [16].

Matrix $\mathbf{G}^*$ was calculated in the same way as $\mathbf{G}$ by VanRaden with $\mathbf{G}^* = \frac{Z^* Z^*}{2 \sum p_i (1 - p_i)}$, with p_i the frequency at locus i [16]. For this study, we re-scaled the B-allele frequencies as described above for $\mathbf{P}^*$ to obtain p, but with missing values set to 0.5.

Then, the distribution of pool phenotypes is not necessarily a scaled equivalent of the distribution of phenotypes in the population. In our sheep data, pool sizes were fairly even. Although not necessary in this case, matrix $\mathbf{H}^*$ was used to scale h-GRM elements to account for potential differences in pool sizes. Therefore, to account for differences in pool sizes, we scaled the elements of $\mathbf{G}^*$ by the square roots of the product of the diagonals to produce a matrix $\mathbf{H}$ with elements $H_{ij} = \frac{G_{ij}^*}{\sqrt{G_{ii}^* \times G_{ij}^*}}$. This is similar to multiplying the relationships by the number of individuals (n) in the pool. The problem is that n is not known with certainty, because the "effective n" depends on the variations in the concentration of DNA in the blood samples and on the accuracy of mixing the samples. Since this is impossible to determine, the scaling of $\mathbf{G}^*$ into $\mathbf{H}$ provides an analytical solution to the technical problem.

Regression analysis of sire relationship with pool on dag score

The relationship of the sires with pools was regressed on the dag score. The DNA pooling strategy was based on phenotype category, therefore, the linear relationship between genetic contribution of a sire and phenotype categories is expressed in the regression coefficient. In this study, a positive regression slope indicates a higher degree of relatedness of the sire to the pools with higher dag scores. Conversely, a negative slope indicates higher relatedness of the sire to the pools with low dag score. Therefore, the latter would characterize sires that are genetically favorable for dag score.

For the regression approach, we fitted the following model:

$$\mathbf{Y}_i = \beta_0 + \beta_1 \mathbf{X}_{i1} + \beta_2 \mathbf{X}_{i2} + \varepsilon_i,$$

where $\mathbf{Y}_i$ is the vector of the GRM relationships of sire i with the pools, β_0 is the intercept, β_1 and β_2 are regression coefficients, $\mathbf{X}_{i1}$ is a vector of the fixed effect of sex of contributors to the pools, to account for any stratification due to sex, $\mathbf{X}_{i2}$ is a vector of the fixed effect of dag phenotype of contributors to the pools, and ε_i is a random error term.

P values of the regression coefficient were empirically validated through permutation testing. Sires' phenotype data were permuted 100 times within sex. The distribution of counts for the real data compared to the distribution of counts for the permuted data using a Pearson's Chi squared test with simulation was used to derive the significance level. Results were tabulated, and means were calculated for each sire's genomic relationship to a pool and for the slope of the relationship between each sire and each pool calculated.

Genomic breeding values from pooled data

Genomic breeding values were estimated using h-GRM in a genomic best linear unbiased prediction (gBLUP) approach in ASReml [17]. The following model was fitted:

$$\mathbf{y} = \mathbf{Xb} + \mathbf{Zg} + \mathbf{e},$$

where $\mathbf{y}$ is a vector of dag phenotypes for pools and missing values for sires, $\mathbf{X}$ is a design matrix relating the fixed effect of sex to each pool and sire, $\mathbf{b}$ is a vector of sex for each pool and sire, $\mathbf{Z}$ is a design matrix allocating records to genetic values to each pool and sire, $\mathbf{g}$ is a vector of genetic effects for each pool and sire, $\mathbf{e}$ is a vector of random normal deviates with variance σ_e^2.

It was assumed that $\text{var}(\mathbf{g}) = \mathbf{G} * \sigma_g^2$, where g is the h-GRM and σ_g^2 is the genetic variance in this model. As outlined above, the gBLUP model fits the dag phenotype of the pool as the dependent variable and includes sex as the only known fixed effect. The previously constructed h-GRM was used in the model instead of the numerator relationship matrix.

Results and discussion

Pooling strategy

An appropriate pooling strategy strikes a balance between cost effectiveness and accuracy. Here, we were not in a position to assess our pooling strategy on accuracy, but previous studies suggested that 64 pools of 46 individuals each estimated SNP effects equally well as individual genotypes [12]. We used pools of 33 to 40 individuals each. Although cost and accuracy are considerations, the numbers and sizes of pools are mainly determined by the total number of animals, phenotype distribution and contemporary group structure. Here, pools were formed within fixed effects, as suggested by [12], with sex being the only known fixed effect. Pooling strategies based on contemporary group information and phenotype are likely to have uneven contributions of sires to each of the pools, in particular if it is a moderately heritable trait, such as dag score in this study. Since a larger number of smaller pools would estimate allele frequencies more accurately [12], in this study, groups of animals of the same sex and phenotype category were randomly split into smaller pools of 40 because this was demonstrated to be an appropriate pool size [12]. In a study on beef cattle, 15 to 28 individuals were pooled, but again, the number of pools and resulting pool sizes were determined by the contemporary group structure and phenotype categories [5]. More comprehensive knowledge on contemporary group effects, e.g. year

of birth, might have added more objective information to the pooling strategy, but in a commercial setting, individual records are not kept and ear tags only indicate year of birth. Therefore, pooling strategies for commercial data might often have to take a pragmatic approach. However, one of the attractive characteristics of a pooling approach is the ease of the logistics of phenotype collection, which should slot into commercial husbandry procedures without major additional workload for the producer.

Genomic relationships

The interpretation of the genomic relationships between sires provides some insights into the choice of sires for the commercial flock. Genomic relationships between sires, which are the off-diagonal values of the sire-by-sire block of the h-GRM, ranged between 0 and 0.5, with the majority around 0.1 (Fig. 1a). The commercial property is a pure-bred, self-replacing Merino flock where the replacement rams are sourced from one stud and have been for a number of years. The distribution of genomic relationships suggests that the sires of the commercial property, in spite of being from the same stud, had a low degree of relatedness. Only a small number of sires were highly related.

As a consequence of the low sire-by-sire relationships, we would expect the relationships between sires and animals that contributed to a pool and which are not progeny of the sire to be also low. Multiple sires contribute to a pool, therefore the sire-by-pool relationships can be expected to reflect a wider range of expected values than the sire-by-sire relationships. For a heritable trait, this may be enhanced through the pooling by phenotype strategy, if more related sires contribute more often to pools with the same phenotype. The frequencies of the genomic relationship estimates between sires and pools are plotted in Fig. 1b. The majority of the estimates ranged from −0.02 to 0.02. Within breed one might expect to see only positive relationship values, but since the relationships are estimated based on identity-by-state, the range of relationship values depends on the population of genotypes that are being used. Therefore, it is not unusual to see negative relationships for the lower relationship values between sires and pools. However, the variation in the genomic relationships between sires and pools indicates that sire contributions to pools vary and it was demonstrated that this variation can be exploited to obtain information on the genetic merit of sires.

Sire genetic merit from pooled DNA

To determine whether the relationships between sires and pools were associated with the phenotypes of the pools, for each sire we regressed the genomic relationships on the pool dag scores. Departure from the null

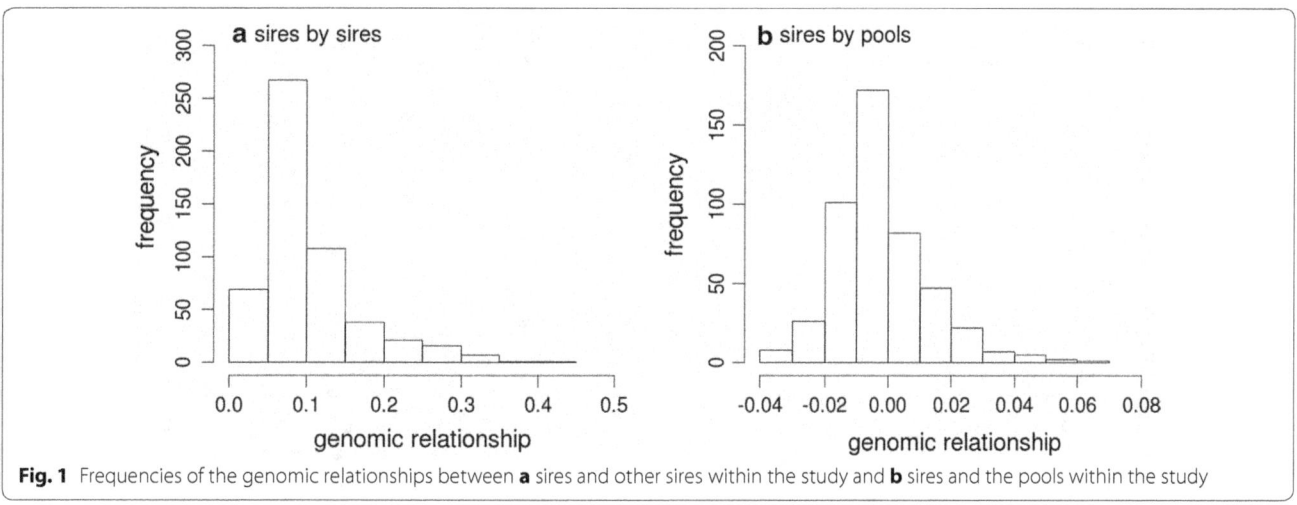

Fig. 1 Frequencies of the genomic relationships between **a** sires and other sires within the study and **b** sires and the pools within the study

hypothesis, assuming no association between sire-pool relationship and pool phenotype, was assessed by examining the distribution of the significance levels of the regressions. The regressions of sire relationship on dag score were more often significant than would be expected by chance. For example, 10 of 33 sires (30%) were significant at the 5% level (Table 2), far more than would be expected by chance, and this trend was also observed at other significance levels. To check that this result was not due to our small sample size, we performed the analyses again after permuting the pool phenotypes. When P values were allocated to significance level classes and the counts compared for the observed and permuted data, the Chi square test was significant ($P = 0.015$), which indicates that the variation observed between sires in the contributions to pools of different dag scores is likely to be real, as one would expect for a heritable trait.

The "best" and "worst" sires with respect to the regression coefficients for dag score are illustrated in Fig. 2a, b. The best sire had the strongest relationship with lower dag score phenotypes, and therefore the most significant negative slope of the regression line (Fig. 2a). The worst sire had the most significant positive slope of the regression line and therefore a stronger relationship with the

higher dag score phenotype. This suggests that the slope of the regression can be used to obtain information on genetic sire performance for the categorical phenotype of dag score.

The replicate pools for each phenotype category, i.e. two male and two female pools (Fig. 2) show that a random split of pools influenced the relationships of pools with sires. Figure 2 demonstrates that the random split resulted in the progeny from the same sire to be divided unevenly across the replicate pools. For example, the relationships of the replicates of female pools for the best and worst sire are in many cases different. As discussed earlier, more objective information on the formation of appropriate size pools might assist in devising a strategy that does not decrease the number of progeny of a sire to a particular pool.

The equivalence of the regression approach compared to genomic estimated breeding values (GEBV) obtained with a gBLUP approach is shown in Fig. 3. Not only did we demonstrate that the contribution of a sire to a phenotype category can be estimated in a regression approach, but this can be translated into a breeding value as it is commonly known and used in the stud industry.

Implications

A probability-based approach was suggested to estimate a numerator relationship matrix for multiple sire combinations [18], but genomic information provides not only a more rigorous approach to identify parentage of an individual but also the representation of a sire's genes to a pool of individuals [9]. There are likely to be tradeoffs in accuracy in genomic breeding values that are derived from pooling compared to individual genotypes, which could not be demonstrated from the data in this study.

Table 2 Proportions of analyses that were significant at various levels for the observed data and for the data with phenotypes permuted

	Significance level				
	0.05	0.01	0.005	0.001	0.0005
Observed	0.300	0.120	0.061	0.030*	0.030*
Permuted	0.049	0.011	0.005	0.001	0.001

* 0.0303 is one out of 33 sires

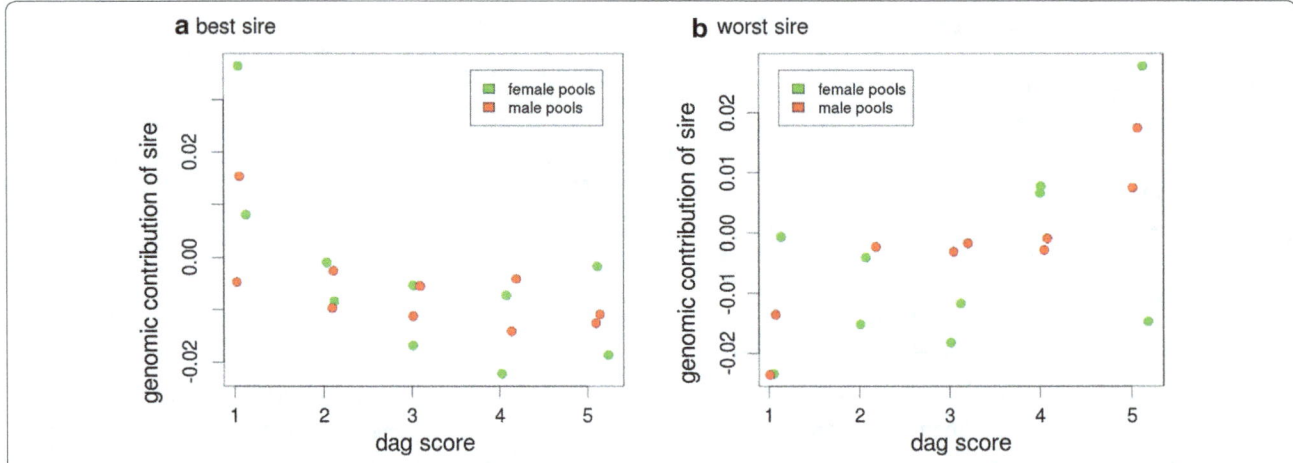

Fig. 2 An example of the best versus the worst sire when a sire's genomic contribution is regressed on the dag score phenotype. The best sire has the most negative slope, indicating a greater contribution to lower dag score phenotypes. The worst sire has the more positive slope, contributing more to higher dag score phenotypes

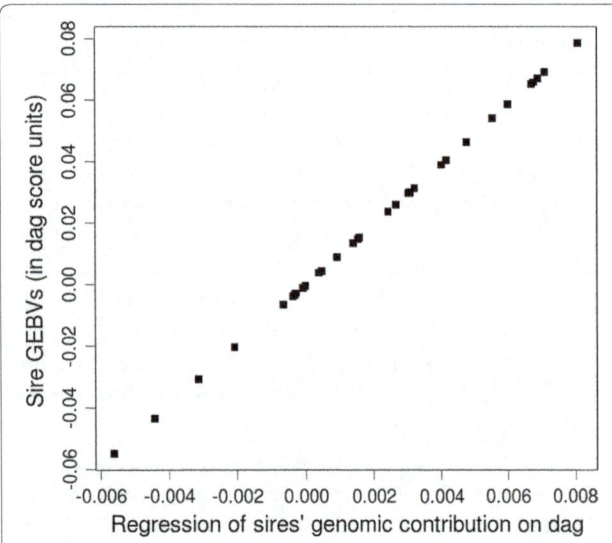

Fig. 3 Relationship between sires' genomic estimated breeding value (in dag score units) and the coefficient of the regression from sires' genomic contribution on dag score

However, assaying pooled DNA is cheap compared to individual genotypes and the resulting genomic breeding values provide a ranking for commercial performance of the sires under evaluation, which fills a gap for which there was previously no available information.

In the hierarchical structure of most livestock industries, where genetic improvement is undertaken in the stud breeding sector, and the genetic gains flow to the commercial sector through the sale of sires and semen for artificial insemination, no performance information from the commercial sector returns to the stud. This is a lost

opportunity to genetically characterize sires across environments. The approach demonstrated in this study has multiple benefits for the stud and commercial sector. It provides an opportunity to apply cost-effective genomic technologies to harvest commercial performance data, which is either routinely measured or assessed during general husbandry procedures or could be obtained with only small additional labour investment. The resulting information on the sires provides the commercial producer with the knowledge of which sires have contributed to particular phenotypes, which can inform future sire or stud selection. Although, in this study sires were evaluated retrospectively, individual genotypes of related current generation sires could be included in a pooling study to obtain information of their genetic merit in a commercial environment [5].

For studs, the proposed pooling approach offers genomic breeding values for their sires for traits that are impossible to obtain in the stud environment, e.g. disease or performance in a commercial environment. It has been demonstrated that significant genotype × environment (G × E) interactions exist in the Merino industry between the stud and commercial level [19] and the information generated from the DNA pooling approach could inform such G × E interactions.

The next step in defining the value proposition of DNA pooling for the livestock industries is to establish the loss in accuracy of pooling versus individual genotyping. Here, we demonstrated that the contribution of sires to phenotypes reflects their genetic merit and it can be translated into a breeding value which is a known industry tool. DNA pooling is a cheap approach that can inform a knowledge gap on commercial performance of sires which can be exploited by stud breeders and producers.

Conclusion

Estimates of the genetic merit of sires using pooled DNA from progeny in a commercial production system can be determined using this technique, and it can provide a cost effective option to inform on the performance of sires for traits that cannot be measured in the stud environment, but are important for commercial operations, and to ultimately increase the amount of data available to stud breeders to inform on the genetic value of sires for a range of traits.

Authors' contributions
JMH, SAL, AMB and RM conceived, designed and performed the experiments. JMH, SD, AMB analysed the data. JK and LPRN contributed SNP chips and additional data. AMB, JMH, SD, LRPN and SAL wrote the article. All authors read and approved the final manuscript.

Author details
[1] CSIRO Agriculture, F D McMaster Laboratory Chiswick, Armidale, NSW 2350, Australia. [2] CSIRO AgricultureQueensland Bioscience Precinct, Brisbane, QLD 4067, Australia.

Acknowledgements
The sheep sampling as part of this project was conducted on "Tramore", Woodside, VIC, and we thank Fergus and Rosemary Irving for access to their sheep and assistance in collecting the samples. Jim Litchfield "Hazeldean", Cooma, NSW, is thanked for his facilitation between the stud and commercial levels of the sheep project. Dr Brad Hine (CSIRO) and Dominic Niemeyer (CSIRO) are thanked for their proficient collection of sheep blood samples for DNA extraction. Rowan Bunch (CSIRO) provided expert technical assistance for the Ovine SNP50 chip genotyping. Dr Aaron Ingham is thanked for his discussion and comments on drafts of the paper.

Competing interests
The authors declare that they have no competing interests. J Henshall is currently an employee of Cobb-Vantress Inc., a commercial company which has funded research on the feasibility of using pooled DNA as a cost-effective genomics strategy.

References
1. Van Eenennaam AL, Weigel KA, Young AE, Cleveland MA, Dekkers JCM. Applied animal genomics: results from the field. Annu Rev Anim Biosci. 2014;2:105–39.
2. Bindon B. Genesis of the cooperative research centre for the cattle and beef industry: integration of resources for beef quality research (1993–2000). Aust J Exp Agric. 2001;41:843–53.
3. Fogarty NM, Banks RG, Van Der Werf JHJ, Ball AJ, Gibson JP. The information nucleus—a new concept to enhance sheep industry genetic improvement. Proc Assoc Advmt Anim Breed Genet. 2007;17:29–32.
4. Reverter A, Henshall JM, McCulloch R, Sasazaki S, Hawken R, Lehnert SA. Numerical analysis of intensity signals resulting from genotyping pooled DNA samples in beef cattle and broiler chicken. J Anim Sci. 2014;92:1874–85.
5. Reverter A, Porto-Neto LR, Fortes MRS, McCulloch R, Lyons RE, Moore S, et al. Genomic analyses of tropical beef cattle fertility based on genotyping pools of Brahman cows with unknown pedigree. J Anim Sci. 2016;94:4096–108.
6. Futschik A, Schlötterer C. The next generation of molecular markers from massively parallel sequencing of pooled DNA samples. Genetics. 2010;186:207–18.
7. Cutler DJ, Jensen JD. To pool, or not to pool? Genetics. 2010;186:41–3.
8. Craig JE, Hewitt AW, McMellon AE, Henders AK, Ma L, Wallace L, et al. Rapid inexpensive genome-wide association using pooled whole blood. Genome Res. 2009;19:2075–80.
9. Bell AM, Henshall JM, McCulloch R, Kijas J. Evaluating sires from commercial progeny data using pooled DNA. In Proceedings of the 10th World Congress of Genetics Applied to Livestock Production: 17–22 August 2014; Vancouver. 2014.
10. Greeff JCKL, Schlink AC. Identifying indicator traits for breech strike in Merino sheep in a Mediterranean environment. Anim Prod Sci. 2014;54:125–40.
11. Visual Sheep Scores—Researcher Version. Australian Wool Innovation Limited and Meat & Livestock Australia. Version 2—2013. 2013. http://www.wool.com/globalassets/start/on-farm-research-and-development/sheep-health-welfare-and-productivity/sheep-breeding/visual-sheep-scores/visual_sheep_scores_researcher_version_lr.pdf. Accessed on 30 March 2016.
12. Henshall JM, Hawken RJ, Dominik S, Barendse W. Estimating the effect of SNP genotype on quantitative traits from pooled DNA samples. Genet Sel Evol. 2012;44:12.
13. Illumina I. OvineSNP50 Genotyping BeadChip. 2015. http://www.illumina.com/documents/products/datasheets/datasheet_ovinesnp50.pdf. Accessed on 30 March 2016.
14. Illumina I. Infinium genotyping data analysis. 2014. http://www.illumina.com/Documents/products/technotes/technote_infinium_genotyping_data_analysis.pdf. Accessed 30 March 2016.
15. Illumina I. Interpreting Infinium assay data for whole-genome structural variation. 2010. http://www.illumina.com/Documents/products/technotes/technote_cytoanalysis.pdf. Accessed 30 March 2016.
16. VanRaden PM. Efficient methods to compute genomic predictions. J Dairy Sci. 2008;91:4414–23.
17. Gilmour AR, Gogel BJ, Cullis BR, Thompson R. ASReml user guide release 3.0. Hemel Hempstead: VSN International Ltd. 2009.
18. Henderson CR. Use of an average numerator relationship matrix for multiple-sire joining. J Anim Sci. 1988;66:1614–21.
19. Dominik S, Crook BJ, Kinghorn BP. Genotype x management interaction on wool production traits and body weight in Western Australian merino sheep. Proc Assoc Advmt Anim Breed Genet. 1999;13:98–101.

5

Metafounders are related to F_{st} fixation indices and reduce bias in single-step genomic evaluations

Carolina A. Garcia-Baccino[1,2], Andres Legarra[3]* ⓘ, Ole F. Christensen[4], Ignacy Misztal[5] ⓘ, Ivan Pocrnic[5] ⓘ, Zulma G. Vitezica[3] ⓘ and Rodolfo J. C. Cantet[1,2] ⓘ

Abstract

Background: Metafounders are pseudo-individuals that encapsulate genetic heterozygosity and relationships within and across base pedigree populations, i.e. ancestral populations. This work addresses the estimation and usefulness of metafounder relationships in single-step genomic best linear unbiased prediction (ssGBLUP).

Results: We show that ancestral relationship parameters are proportional to standardized covariances of base allelic frequencies across populations, such as F_{st} fixation indexes. These covariances of base allelic frequencies can be estimated from marker genotypes of related recent individuals and pedigree. Simple methods for their estimation include naïve computation of allele frequencies from marker genotypes or a method of moments that equates average pedigree-based and marker-based relationships. Complex methods include generalized least squares (best linear unbiased estimator (BLUE)) or maximum likelihood based on pedigree relationships. To our knowledge, methods to infer F_{st} coefficients from marker data have not been developed for related individuals. We derived a genomic relationship matrix, compatible with pedigree relationships, that is constructed as a cross-product of $\{-1,0,1\}$ codes and that is equivalent (apart from scale factors) to an identity-by-state relationship matrix at genome-wide markers. Using a simulation with a single population under selection in which only males and youngest animals are genotyped, we observed that generalized least squares or maximum likelihood gave accurate and unbiased estimates of the ancestral relationship parameter (true value: 0.40) whereas the naïve method and the method of moments were biased (average estimates of 0.43 and 0.35). We also observed that genomic evaluation by ssGBLUP using metafounders was less biased in terms of estimates of genetic trend (bias of 0.01 instead of 0.12), resulted in less overdispersed (0.94 instead of 0.99) and as accurate (0.74) estimates of breeding values than ssGBLUP without metafounders and provided consistent estimates of heritability.

Conclusions: Estimation of metafounder relationships can be achieved using BLUP-like methods with pedigree and markers. Inclusion of metafounder relationships reduces bias of genomic predictions with no loss in accuracy.

Background

Metafounders are pseudo-individuals that describe relationships within and across pedigree base populations. The concept of metafounders provides a coherent framework for the theory of genomic evaluation [1]. Genomic evaluation in agricultural species often implies partially genotyped populations, i.e. some individuals are genotyped, using high-density genetic markers across the genome, others are not, and phenotypes may be recorded in either of the two subsets. An integrated solution called single-step genomic best linear unbiased prediction (ssGBLUP) has been proposed [2–4]. This solution uses the following integrated relationship matrix:

$$\mathbf{H} = \begin{pmatrix} \mathbf{A}_{11} - \mathbf{A}_{12}\mathbf{A}_{22}^{-1}\mathbf{A}_{21} + \mathbf{A}_{12}\mathbf{A}_{22}^{-1}\mathbf{G}\mathbf{A}_{22}^{-1}\mathbf{A}_{21} & \mathbf{A}_{12}\mathbf{A}_{22}^{-1}\mathbf{G} \\ \mathbf{G}\mathbf{A}_{22}^{-1}\mathbf{A}_{21} & \mathbf{G} \end{pmatrix},$$

*Correspondence: andres.legarra@inra.fr
[3] GenPhySE, INRA, INPT, ENVT, Université de Toulouse, 31326 Castanet-Tolosan, France
Full list of author information is available at the end of the article

with inverse:

$$\mathbf{H}^{-1} = \mathbf{A}^{-1} + \begin{pmatrix} \mathbf{0} & \mathbf{0} \\ \mathbf{0} & \mathbf{G}^{-1} - \mathbf{A}_{22}^{-1} \end{pmatrix},$$

where $\mathbf{G}$ is the genomic relationship matrix, $\mathbf{A}$ is the pedigree-based relationship matrix, and matrices $\mathbf{A}_{11}, \mathbf{A}_{12}, \mathbf{A}_{21}, \mathbf{A}_{22}$ are submatrices of $\mathbf{A}$ with labels 1 and 2 denoting non-genotyped and genotyped individuals, respectively.

Because genotyped animals are often not a random sample from the analyzed populations (they tend to be younger or selected), it was quickly acknowledged that a proper analysis requires specifying different means for genotyped and non-genotyped individuals for the trait under consideration. These different means can be considered as parameters of the model, which are either fixed [4] or random [5, 6] effects. In the latter case, the random variables induce covariances between individuals, a situation that is informally referred to as "compatibility" of genomic and pedigree relationships. In fact, compatibility implies equality of the average breeding value of the base population and of the genetic variance [7] across the different measures of relationships. Numerically, the problem appears as follows. The formulae for matrix $\mathbf{H}$ and its inverse contain $(\mathbf{G} - \mathbf{A}_{22})$ and $(\mathbf{G}^{-1} - \mathbf{A}_{22}^{-1})$ (assuming $\mathbf{G}$ is full rank), respectively. This suggests that if $\mathbf{G}$ and $\mathbf{A}_{22}$ differ too much, biases may appear.

Genomic relationships are usually computed in one of two manners: using "cross-products" [8] or "corrected identity-by-state (IBS)" [9]. Both depend critically on assumed allele frequencies at markers in the pedigree base population [10]. Base allele frequencies are often unavailable. However, for most purposes, allele frequencies are not of interest *per se* and can be treated as nuisance parameters that can be marginalized. Christensen [11] achieved an algebraic integration of allele frequencies, leading to a very simple covariance structure with allele frequencies in genomic relationships fixed at 0.5 (e.g., using genotypes coded as $\{-1,0,1\}$ in the cross-product method) and a parameter called γ that describes relationships between pedigree founders i.e. $\mathbf{A}_{base}^{(\gamma)} = \mathbf{I}\left(1 - \frac{\gamma}{2}\right) + \mathbf{1}\mathbf{1}'\gamma$ in the base population. A second parameter in Christensen's marginalisation is s, which is a measure of marker heterozygosity in the base population. Therefore, instead of inferring (thousands of) base allele frequencies, inference can be based on two simple parameters γ and s. Both can be estimated by maximizing the likelihood of observed genotypes. In addition, this approach considers the fact that pedigree depth is arbitrary and mostly based on historical availability of records.

Legarra et al. [1] showed the equivalence of the Christensen approach to the metafounder concept:

pseudo-individuals that encapsulate three ideas: (a) separate means for each base population [4, 12, 13], (b) randomness of these means [5] and (c) propagation of the randomness of these means to the progeny [11], while accommodating several populations with complex crosses, e.g. [14]. Legarra et al. [1] also generalized one relationship between founders (scalar γ) to several relationships between founders in the pedigree, i.e. ancestral relationships (matrix $\mathbf{\Gamma}$), and suggested simple methods to estimate them. Legarra et al. [1] showed that construction of $\mathbf{A}^{\mathbf{\Gamma}}$ from $\mathbf{\Gamma}$ and a pedigree reduces to the use of the tabular rules [15] for construction of relationships, and its inversion is achieved by inversion of $\mathbf{\Gamma}$ followed by Henderson's rules [16]. We provide an example of matrices $\mathbf{A}^{\mathbf{\Gamma}}$ and $\mathbf{\Gamma}$ in "Appendix". However, the performance of their model has not been tested so far, either for estimation of ancestral relationships or for genomic evaluation.

This work has two objectives. The first is to show that the structure of the metafounder approach yields an alternative parameterization and method for estimation of ancestral relationships. By doing so, we found that ancestral relationships are generalizations of Wright's F_{st} fixation index [17]. The second goal is to test, by simulation, (1) methods to estimate ancestral relationship parameters, (2) the quality of genomic predictions using metafounders, and (3) the quality of variance component estimation. For the second goal, the simulated population is undergoing selection and with a complete partially genotyped pedigree.

Methods
Relationship between metafounders and allele frequencies in the pedigree base population
Single population
Let $\mathbf{M}$ be a matrix of genotypes coded as gene content, i.e. $\{0,1,2\}$ and the genomic relationship matrix $\mathbf{G} = (\mathbf{M} - \mathbf{J})(\mathbf{M} - \mathbf{J})'/s$, with $\mathbf{J}$ a matrix of 1s, with reference alleles taken at random, so that the expected allele frequency p is 0.5 for a random locus [11]. In other words, the matrix $\mathbf{Z} = (\mathbf{M} - \mathbf{J})$ contains values of $\{-1,0,1\}$ for each genotype. In a single population, let γ be the relationship coefficient between pedigree founders or, equivalently, the self-relationship of the metafounder [1, 11]. Parameter s (defined above) is a measure of marker heterozygosity in the population. Ancestral relationships in γ explain, for instance, genomic relationships in $\mathbf{G} = (\mathbf{M} - \mathbf{J})(\mathbf{M} - \mathbf{J})'/s$ that are not captured by available pedigree; e.g. across nominally unrelated individuals. It will be shown later that this relationship γ is relative to a population with maximum heterozygosity and is analogous to an F_{st} fixation index [18].

Christensen [11] estimated the two parameters, γ and s, using maximum likelihood, whereas [1] suggested methods of moments. Closer inspection of Appendix A in [11] leads to the following developments that were not described in Christensen [11] (see "Appendix" of the present paper for more details).

Parameter γ is such that $\gamma = \frac{4Var(p_i)}{2Var(p_i)+E(2p_iq_i)}$, with $p_i = 1 - q_i$ the allele frequency at a random locus i. Parameter $s = n(2Var(p_i) + E(2p_iq_i))$, with n being the number of markers. However, $E(2p_iq_i) = 2E(p_i)E(q_i) - 2Var(p_i) = 0.5 - 2Var(p_i)$, such that if reference alleles are chosen at random across loci, then $E(p_i) = E(q_i) = 0.5$. From this it follows that:

$$s = \frac{n}{2} = \frac{number\ of\ markers}{2},$$

and the genomic relationship matrix is $\mathbf{G} = 2(\mathbf{M} - \mathbf{J})(\mathbf{M} - \mathbf{J})'/n$. Interestingly, this matrix is similar to a matrix of IBS relationships, that can be written as:

$$\mathbf{G}_{IBS} = (\mathbf{M} - \mathbf{J})(\mathbf{M} - \mathbf{J})'/n + \mathbf{1}\mathbf{1}',$$

so that $\mathbf{G}_{IBS} = \frac{1}{2}\mathbf{G} + \mathbf{1}\mathbf{1}'$ (see proof in "Appendix").

Substituting $E(2p_iq_i) = 0.5 - 2Var(p_i)$ into the expression $\gamma = \frac{4Var(p_i)}{2Var(p_i)+E(2p_iq_i)}$ gives: $\gamma = 8Var(p_i) = 8\sigma_p^2$, such that γ for a single population is eight times the variance of allele frequencies in the base population (this variance was described by Cockerham [19]). We stress that $Var(p_i) = \sigma_p^2$ to imply that σ_p^2 (and γ) is a parameter, the variance of allele frequencies across markers [10, 11, 20, 21]. However, s can be considered as equivalent to heterozygosity when all markers have an allele frequency of 0.5, that is, the maximum possible heterozygosity.

Multiple populations

In an analogous manner, the relationship between two metafounders b and b' is: $\gamma_{b,b'} = 8Cov(p_{b,i}, p_{b',i}) = 8\sigma_{p_b,p_{b'}}$, i.e., the covariance across loci between allele frequencies of two populations b and b'. This is almost tautological: the relationship (between two populations in this case) is the covariance between the gene content at a locus. Christensen et al. [6] implicitly show this in Appendix A of their paper. Cockerham [19] and Robertson [22] interpreted $4\sigma_{p_b,p_{b'}}$ as the coancestry between two populations and Fariello et al. [23] used $\sigma_{p_b,p_{b'}}$ to describe the divergence of populations. Several measures of genetic distance between populations have been developed (e.g. [24]), and most of them contain a term that is related, implicitly or explicitly, to $\sigma_{p_b,p_{b'}}$. In particular, the average square of the Euclidean distance can be written as $D^2 = E((p_b - p_{b'})^2) = -2\sigma_{p_b,p_{b'}}$. Thus, $\gamma_{b,b'} = -4D^2$.

Estimation
Estimation in a single population
Estimation of s is trivial, it is simply half the number of markers. Parameter γ is proportional to the variance of allele frequencies in the base population. If base population individuals were genotyped, computing allele frequencies and estimating γ would be trivial. In the next section, we propose methods when this is not the case, i.e. genotyped individuals are related and perhaps several generations away from the base population.

Assuming no pedigree structure i.e. naïve The simplest model assumes that genotyped individuals are unrelated and constitute the base population. For locus i, let $\mathbf{m}_i$ be a vector of gene contents in the form $\{0,1,2\}$, defined as before. The mean of this vector is $\mu_i = 2p_i$. For each locus, μ_i is estimated as the observed mean of $\mathbf{m}_i$, then $Var(\hat{\boldsymbol{\mu}})$ is computed as the empirical variance across loci of $\hat{\boldsymbol{\mu}} = (\hat{\mu}_1, \dots, \hat{\mu}_n)$, and because $p_i = \mu_i/2$, then $\hat{\sigma}_p^2 = Var(\hat{\boldsymbol{\mu}})/4$ and $\gamma = 8\hat{\sigma}_p^2 = 2Var(\hat{\boldsymbol{\mu}})$.

Considering pedigree structure At locus i, gene content can be seen as a quantitative trait mean of $\mathbf{m}_i$ in the base population equal to $2p_i$, where p_i is the allele frequency in the base population and the genetic variance is $2p_iq_i$ [25–27]. Cockerham [19] showed that the covariance of gene content of marker i between individuals j and k is a function of their relationship (A_{jk}): $Cov(m_{i,j}, m_{i,k}) = A_{jk}2p_iq_i$. A linear model can therefore be written as:

$$\mathbf{m}_i = \mathbf{1}\mu_i + \mathbf{W}\mathbf{u}_i + \mathbf{e},$$

where $\mathbf{W}$ is an incidence matrix relating individuals in the pedigree to observed genotypes, and $\mathbf{u}_i$ is the deviation of each individual from the mean μ_i for all individuals [25–27]. Assuming multivariate normality: $\boldsymbol{\mu} \sim N(\mathbf{0}, \mathbf{I}\sigma_\mu^2)$ and $\mathbf{u}_i \sim N(\mathbf{0}, \mathbf{A}(2p_iq_i)) = N(\mathbf{0}, \mathbf{A}\sigma_{m_i}^2)$.

Equivalently, for the set of genotyped individuals (labelled as "2"), $\mathbf{u}_{2,i} \sim N(\mathbf{0}, \mathbf{A}_{22}(2p_iq_i))$, where $\mathbf{A}_{22} = \mathbf{W}\mathbf{A}\mathbf{W}'$ is an additive relationship matrix that includes only the genotyped individuals. From this formulation, there are two possible strategies to estimate σ_μ^2.

Generalized least squares (GLS) This ignores the prior distribution of $\boldsymbol{\mu}$ and estimates each μ_i as a "fixed effect", using best linear unbiased estimator (BLUE) (or, equivalently, GLS) estimators of μ_i separately for each locus. One option is to use the $\mathbf{A}^{-1}$ spanning all the pedigree and mixed model equations [25–27]. Equivalently, the corresponding GLS expression is:

$$\hat{\mu}_i = \left(\mathbf{1}'\mathbf{A}_{22}^{-1}\sigma_{m_i}^{-2}\mathbf{1}\right)^{-1}\mathbf{1}'\mathbf{A}_{22}^{-1}\mathbf{m}_i\sigma_{m_i}^{-2} = \left(\mathbf{1}'\mathbf{A}_{22}^{-1}\mathbf{1}\right)^{-1}\mathbf{1}'\mathbf{A}_{22}^{-1}\mathbf{m}_i,$$

where $\left(\mathbf{1}'\mathbf{A}_{22}^{-1}\mathbf{1}\right)$ is the sum of elements of $\mathbf{A}_{22}^{-1}$, $\sigma_{m_i}^2 = 2p_iq_i$ and $\mathbf{1}'\mathbf{A}_{22}^{-1}\mathbf{m}_i$ is a weighted sum of genotypes.

Then, σ_μ^2 is estimated as $Var(\hat{\boldsymbol{\mu}})$, because $p_i = \mu_i/2$, $\hat{\sigma}_p^2 = \sigma_\mu^2/4$, and it follows that $\hat{\gamma} = 2\hat{\sigma}_\mu^2$.

Maximum likelihood If allele frequencies in the base population have a distribution, μ_i can be considered as drawn from a normal distribution, $\boldsymbol{\mu} \sim N(\mathbf{0}, \mathbf{I}\sigma_\mu^2)$. Thus σ_μ^2 is a variance component that can be estimated by maximum likelihood (ML). The equations for given values of σ_μ^2 and $\sigma_{m_i}^2 = 2p_iq_i$ are $\left(\mathbf{1}'\mathbf{A}_{22}^{-1}\sigma_{m_i}^{-2}\mathbf{1} + \sigma_\mu^{-2}\right)\hat{\mu}_i = \mathbf{1}'\mathbf{A}_{22}^{-1}\sigma_{m_i}^{-2}\mathbf{m}_i$. An expectation–maximization scheme [28] to obtain ML is as follows. Pick starting values for σ_μ^2 and $\sigma_{m_i}^2$. Iterate until convergence on:

1. For each marker i,

   (a) estimate $\hat{\mu}_i = \left(\mathbf{1}'\mathbf{A}_{22}^{-1}\sigma_{m_i}^{-2}\mathbf{1} + \sigma_\mu^{-2}\right)^{-1}\mathbf{1}'\mathbf{A}_{22}^{-1}\sigma_{m_i}^{-2}\mathbf{m}_i$,

   (b) store $PEV_i(\hat{\mu}_i) = \left(\sigma_\mu^{-2} + \mathbf{1}'\mathbf{A}_{22}^{-1}\sigma_{m_i}^{-2}\mathbf{1}\right)^{-1}$,

   (c) update $\sigma_{m_i}^2$ as $\hat{\sigma}_{m_i}^2 = 2\hat{p}_i\hat{q}_i$ with $\hat{p}_i = \hat{\mu}_i/2$;

2. Update σ_μ^2 as $\hat{\sigma}_\mu^2 = \frac{1}{n}\left(\hat{\boldsymbol{\mu}}'\hat{\boldsymbol{\mu}} + \sum PEV_i(\hat{\mu}_i)\right)$, where the second part of the expression corresponds to the trace $tr(\mathbf{IC})$, $\mathbf{I}$, the identity matrix, is the relationship structure across levels of $\boldsymbol{\mu}$ and $\mathbf{C}$ is the prediction error covariance matrix of $\hat{\boldsymbol{\mu}}$. As only the diagonal elements of $\mathbf{C}$ are needed in $tr(\mathbf{IC})$, its elements $PEV_i(\hat{\mu}_i)$ can be obtained separately from each single locus analysis.

At convergence, the estimate is $\hat{\gamma} = 2\hat{\sigma}_\mu^2$. This gives the same estimate as the method based on a Wishart likelihood function [11] with $s = n/2$ (results not shown).

Estimation in multiple populations

If t base populations are considered, the variance component σ_μ^2 generalizes to $\boldsymbol{\Sigma}_0$, a $t \times t$ matrix of variances and covariances between means $\mu_i^{[b]}$ for marker i in population b. Across populations,

$$\boldsymbol{\Sigma}_0 = \begin{pmatrix} \sigma_{\mu^{[1]}\mu^{[1]}}^2 & \sigma_{\mu^{[1]}\mu^{[2]}} & \cdots \\ \cdots & \sigma_{\mu^{[2]}\mu^{[2]}}^2 & \cdots \\ \cdots & \cdots & \cdots \end{pmatrix} \text{ and } \hat{\boldsymbol{\Gamma}} = 2\hat{\boldsymbol{\Sigma}}_0.$$

Assuming no pedigree structure

Naïve If relationships across individuals are ignored:

$$\mathbf{m}_i = \mathbf{Q}\boldsymbol{\mu}_i + \mathbf{e}_i,$$

where $\mathbf{Q}$ is a matrix, the rows of which sum to 1, and that assigns individuals to fractions of populations, and $\boldsymbol{\mu}_i$ is a vector with t elements for the average of each population. For each locus, $\boldsymbol{\mu}_i$ can be estimated using least squares

and the covariance matrix of $\boldsymbol{\mu}_i$ across loci gives an estimate of $\boldsymbol{\Sigma}_0$, e.g. for two populations $\hat{\boldsymbol{\Sigma}}_0 = Cov(\boldsymbol{\mu}^{[1]}, \boldsymbol{\mu}^{[2]})$, a two-by-two matrix.

Considering pedigree structure

If there are no crosses between individuals from different populations in the pedigree, the estimation of allele frequencies in each base population can be split in separate analyses by population b: $\mathbf{m}_i^b = \mathbf{1}\mu_i^{[b]} + \mathbf{W}^b\mathbf{u}_i^b + \mathbf{e}$, with $\mathbf{u}_i^b \sim N(\mathbf{0}, \mathbf{A}^b(2p_i(1-p_i)))$ and $\mathbf{A}^b$ the matrix of pedigree-based relationships among individuals in population b, and the analysis proceeds as in a single population. Then, $\hat{\boldsymbol{\Sigma}}_0$ is estimated as the observed matrix of covariances for $\hat{\mu}_i^b$ across loci.

When there are crosses, there are two alternatives.

Generalized least squares (GLS)

The first alternative [27] is to use a genetic groups model [12, 13], as $\mathbf{m}_i = \mathbf{Q}\boldsymbol{\mu}_i + \mathbf{W}\mathbf{u}_i + \mathbf{e}$, where $\mathbf{Q}_{k,b}$ contains the fraction of ancestry b in individual k. This ignores the fact that the variance of gene content, $(2p_iq_i)$, differs between breeds and crosses. The second, and more exact alternative, is to use the representation where the breeding values are split into within- and across-breed components [29]:

$$\mathbf{m}_i = \mathbf{Q}\boldsymbol{\mu}_i + \sum_b \mathbf{W}^b\mathbf{u}_i^b + \sum_{b,b',b>b'} \mathbf{W}^{b,b'}\mathbf{u}_i^{b,b'} + \mathbf{e},$$

with partial relationship matrices for vectors $\mathbf{u}_i^b$ and $\mathbf{u}_i^{b,b'}$. The BLUE's of $\boldsymbol{\mu}_i$ can be obtained and then $\hat{\boldsymbol{\Sigma}}_0$ estimated as above.

Maximum likelihood (ML)

Analogously to the single population case, an expectation–maximization updated estimate can be obtained using multiple-trait formulations [28], where *PEC* is the prediction error variance–covariance, e.g. with two populations:

$$\boldsymbol{\Sigma}_0 = \begin{pmatrix} \boldsymbol{\mu}^{[1]'}\boldsymbol{\mu}^{[1]} & \boldsymbol{\mu}^{[1]'}\boldsymbol{\mu}^{[2]} \\ \boldsymbol{\mu}^{[2]'}\boldsymbol{\mu}^{[1]} & \boldsymbol{\mu}^{[2]'}\boldsymbol{\mu}^{[2]} \end{pmatrix}.$$

Our implementation of this approach is as follows:

1. For each marker i:

   (a) estimate $\hat{\boldsymbol{\mu}}_i = \left(\boldsymbol{\Sigma}_0^{-1} + \mathbf{Q}'\mathbf{A}_{22}^{-1}\sigma_{m_i}^{-2}\mathbf{Q}\right)^{-1}\mathbf{Q}'\mathbf{A}_{22}^{-1}\sigma_{m_i}^{-2}\mathbf{m}_i$,

   (b) store $PEC_i(\hat{\boldsymbol{\mu}}_i) = \left(\boldsymbol{\Sigma}_0^{-1} + \mathbf{Q}'\mathbf{A}_{22}^{-1}\sigma_{m_i}^{-2}\mathbf{Q}\right)^{-1}$,

   (c) update $\sigma_{m_i}^2$ as $\hat{\sigma}_{m_i}^2 = 2\hat{p}_i^*(1-\hat{p}_i^*)$ with $\hat{p}_i^* = \frac{1}{Nb}\sum_{b=1,Nb}\frac{\hat{\mu}_i^b}{2}$;

2. Update $\mathbf{\Sigma}_0$ using cross-products within and across populations as, e.g., with two populations:

$$\hat{\mathbf{\Sigma}}_0 = \frac{1}{n}\left(\begin{pmatrix}\hat{\mathbf{\mu}}^{[1]'}\hat{\mathbf{\mu}}^{[1]} & \hat{\mathbf{\mu}}^{[1]'}\hat{\mathbf{\mu}}^{[2]} \\ \hat{\mathbf{\mu}}^{[2]'}\hat{\mathbf{\mu}}^{[1]} & \hat{\mathbf{\mu}}^{[2]'}\hat{\mathbf{\mu}}^{[2]}\end{pmatrix} + \sum_{i=1,n}PEC_i\right).$$

Step 1 includes an approximation in (1c) because we assume that $\sigma^2_{m_i} = 2p_iq_i$ is the same for all base populations, as in the GLS above, which could be further improved by using partial relationship matrices. This point will be addressed in future research.

Simulation

To assess the quality of genomic predictions using one metafounder, we simulated data using QMSim [30]. The simulation closely followed that in [5] to mimic a dairy cattle selection scheme scenario. A historical population undergoing mutation and drift was generated, followed by a recent population undergoing selection.

First, 100 generations of the historical population were generated with an effective population size of 100 during the first 95 generations, followed by a gradual expansion during the last five generations to an effective population size of 3000. Thirty chromosomes of 100 cM and 40,000 segregating biallelic markers distributed at random along the chromosomes in the first generation of the historical population were simulated. The 40,000 markers were resampled from a larger set of 90,000 markers in order to obtain allelic frequencies from a beta(2,2) distribution, similar to dairy cattle marker data, so that parameter γ had a true value around 0.40. There were 1500 QTL affecting the phenotype; QTL allele effects were sampled from a Gamma distribution with a shape parameter of 0.4. Mutation rate at the markers (recurrent mutation process) and QTL was assumed to be 2.5×10^{-5} per locus per generation [31]. We used a higher mutation rate than typical (10^{-8}, [32, 33]) to overcome the fact that QMSim is not a coalescent simulator. Phenotypes for a trait recorded only on females with a heritability of 0.30 were simulated.

Then, 10 overlapping generations of selection followed. In each generation, 200 males were mated with 2600 females to produce 2600 offspring by a positive assortative mating design based on EBV. Within the simulation, individuals were selected according to estimated breeding value (EBV) based on pedigree BLUP. In each generation, 40% of males and 20% of females were replaced by selected younger individuals. No restrictions were set to avoid or minimize inbreeding, so highly inbred individuals were found, as a result of strong selection and matings among highly-related individuals. A total of 100 individuals had an inbreeding coefficient higher than 0.20 (mainly found in the last generation), with some individuals having inbreeding coefficients higher than 0.40. True breeding values (TBV) and pedigree information were available for all 10 generations (28,800 individuals in the pedigree), phenotypes were available for all females except in the last generation (14,300 records). The 840 sires of females with phenotypic records were genotyped, as well as 2600 individuals in generation 9 (with records) and 2600 in generation 10 (without records). A total of 20 independent replicates were made. A two-step analysis was carried out using the simulated data. First, we compared several methods to estimate γ. Then, we tested the quality of genomic predictions using four methods (see section on genomic prediction methods), one of which included one metafounder.

Methods to estimate γ

Parameter γ was estimated using four estimation methods. First, the naïve method that does not consider the pedigree structure. Pedigree information was included in three methods: GLS, ML, and the method of moments (MM) in [1]. For a single population, the last method involves estimation of γ based on summary statistics of $\mathbf{A}_{22}$ (regular pedigree-relationship matrix for genotyped individuals) and $\mathbf{G}$ (the genomic relationship matrix).

Genomic prediction methods

The EBV of the selection candidates in generation 10 (genotyped and without phenotype records) were estimated using four methods. The first was the pedigree-based BLUP (PBLUP) based on phenotype and pedigree information. The second method was ssGBLUP, in which genomic information is also taken into account. We used the correction of [34] to equate genomic and pedigree average inbreeding and relationships, the default method used in most practical applications [34, 35]. However, the implementation that we used does not include inbreeding in the setup of $\mathbf{A}^{-1}$ [36], although it does consider inbreeding in $\mathbf{A}_{22}^{-1}$ (see below for use of these matrices). The third method was ssGBLUP that includes inbreeding in the setup of $\mathbf{A}^{-1}$ and of $\mathbf{A}_{22}^{-1}$ (ssGBLUP_F). The fourth method was ssGBLUP with the metafounder (ssGBLUP_M), using γ estimated by GLS since it turned out to be an accurate method to estimate $\mathbf{\Gamma}$ (see the Results section). The four methods used the following inverse relationship matrices: PBLUP: $\mathbf{A}^{-1}$; ssGBLUP: $\mathbf{H}^{-1} = \mathbf{A}^{-1} + \begin{pmatrix} 0 & 0 \\ 0 & \mathbf{G}_a^{-1} - \mathbf{A}_{22}^{-1} \end{pmatrix}$ where $\mathbf{G}_a$ is as in [34] and $\mathbf{A}^{-1}$ is constructed ignoring inbreeding [36]; ssGBLUP_F: same as ssGBLUP, with $\mathbf{A}^{-1}$ correctly constructed; ssGBLUP_M: $\mathbf{H}^{(\gamma)-1} = \mathbf{A}^{(\gamma)-1} + \begin{pmatrix} 0 & 0 \\ 0 & \mathbf{G}^{-1} - \mathbf{A}_{22}^{(\gamma)-1} \end{pmatrix}$ where

$\mathbf{G} = (\mathbf{M} - \mathbf{J})(\mathbf{M} - \mathbf{J})'/s$ with $s = n/2$ (see the "Methods" section) and $\mathbf{A}^{(\gamma)}$ is as in [1]. More details are given in "Appendix". For computation, we used blupf90 [37]. In the case of ssGBLUP_M, we constructed $\mathbf{H}^{(\gamma)-1}$ with own software and then used the option user_file in blupf90 (http://nce.ads.uga.edu/wiki/doku.php).

Quality of genomic prediction

Prediction quality was evaluated for all 2600 selection candidates in generation 10. The accuracy of the methods was measured as the Pearson correlation between TBV and EBV. Bias was calculated as the difference between the average TBV and average EBV with respect to the base population (i.e. to the solution of the metafounder for ssGBLUP_M or to 0 for the other methods). Thus, bias is related to estimated genetic progress in the selection candidates. The inflation (often also called bias) of the prediction method was quantified by the coefficient of regression of TBV on EBV. These two statistics correspond to the coefficients b_0 and b_1 in the Interbull validation method [38], which uses the regression $TBV = b_0 + b_1 EBV + e$. The mean square error (MSE) of prediction of EBV was calculated as the mean of the squared difference between TBV and EBV. An ideal method should have maximum accuracy, minimum MSE, zero bias, and a regression coefficient of 1. These are not only elegant statistical properties but also have relevance in livestock selection [39–41]. Changes in ranking of the selection candidates were also assessed by calculating the Spearman's rank correlation coefficients between EBV across methods.

In addition, the quality of variance component estimation was assessed by comparing estimated and simulated heritabilities. For this purpose, variance components were estimated by REML with remlf90 [37] based on the four methods (PBLUP, ssGBLUP, ssGBLUP_F, ssGBLUP_M).

Results

Estimation of γ

Figure 1 shows boxplots of the differences between the estimates of γ based on the four methods (MM, Naïve, ML and GLS) and the true values obtained by simulation, for each of the 20 replicates. The simulations were tailored to produce $\gamma = 0.40$. Methods ML and GLS estimated γ very accurately. Method MM clearly underestimated γ, whereas the Naïve method overestimated it. Based on these results, we used γ estimated by GLS for ssGBLUP_M for prediction. The effect of employing different values of γ in genomic prediction was assessed to quantify its impact on predictions. Using estimates of γ based on MM only slightly changed results. For example,

the accuracies and slopes of ssGBLUP_M were not affected up to the 4th digit (not shown).

Quality of genomic prediction

Correlations between TBV and EBV of candidates in generation 10 for each prediction methods are in Table 1 and Fig. 2a. Compared with PBLUP, ssGBLUP_F and ssGBLUP_M increased accuracy by approximately 23 absolute points. This shows an important improvement by including marker information in the prediction and the possibility of generating a small extra gain when also including the metafounder. Method ssGBLUP resulted in a small loss of accuracy compared to ssGBLUP_F and ssGBLUP_M.

Table 1 and Fig. 2b display the regression coefficient of TBV on EBV, which measures the degree of inflation for each prediction method and should be close to 1. PBLUP and ssGBLUP_F produced values closest to 1. Including genomic data in the prediction based on ssGBLUP resulted in regression coefficients lower than 1, but including the metafounder in ssGBLUP_M gave values closer to 1. Methods ssGBLUP_M and ssGBLUP_F displayed a lower standard deviation compared to the other two methods. Again, method ssGBLUP showed the highest variability.

Biases of EBV obtained with each prediction method are in Table 1 and Fig. 2c. Both PBLUP and ssGBLUP_M were unbiased, whereas ssGBLUP and ssGBLUP_F were biased. The bias was higher for ssGBLUP than for ssGBLUP_F, which was largely due to a single outlier; the median bias was roughly the same for ssGBLUP and ssGBLUP_F. The bias with ssGBLUP_F was equivalent to roughly 0.5 generations of genetic improvement or 0.4 standard genetic deviations. Finally, ssGBLUP_M had the lowest MSE (closer to zero), followed by ssGBLUP_F (Table 1).

Ranking of EBV

The methods were also compared based on rank correlations of EBV with TBV and between methods. A rank correlation of 1 implies that the same candidates would be selected. Results are in Table 2. Rank correlations with TBV were similar to the Pearson correlations in Table 1. Selection decisions differed only slightly when using ssGBLUP, ssGBLUP_F or ssGBLUP_M. Note, however, that this table reports rank correlations among young selection candidates in the last generation and does not address comparisons across generations (e.g. old vs. young animals), which is sensitive to the biases that are reflected in Table 1 [41]. For instance, all young animals would be overestimated by 0.11 with ssGBLUP_F, which results in these young animals looking better than proven

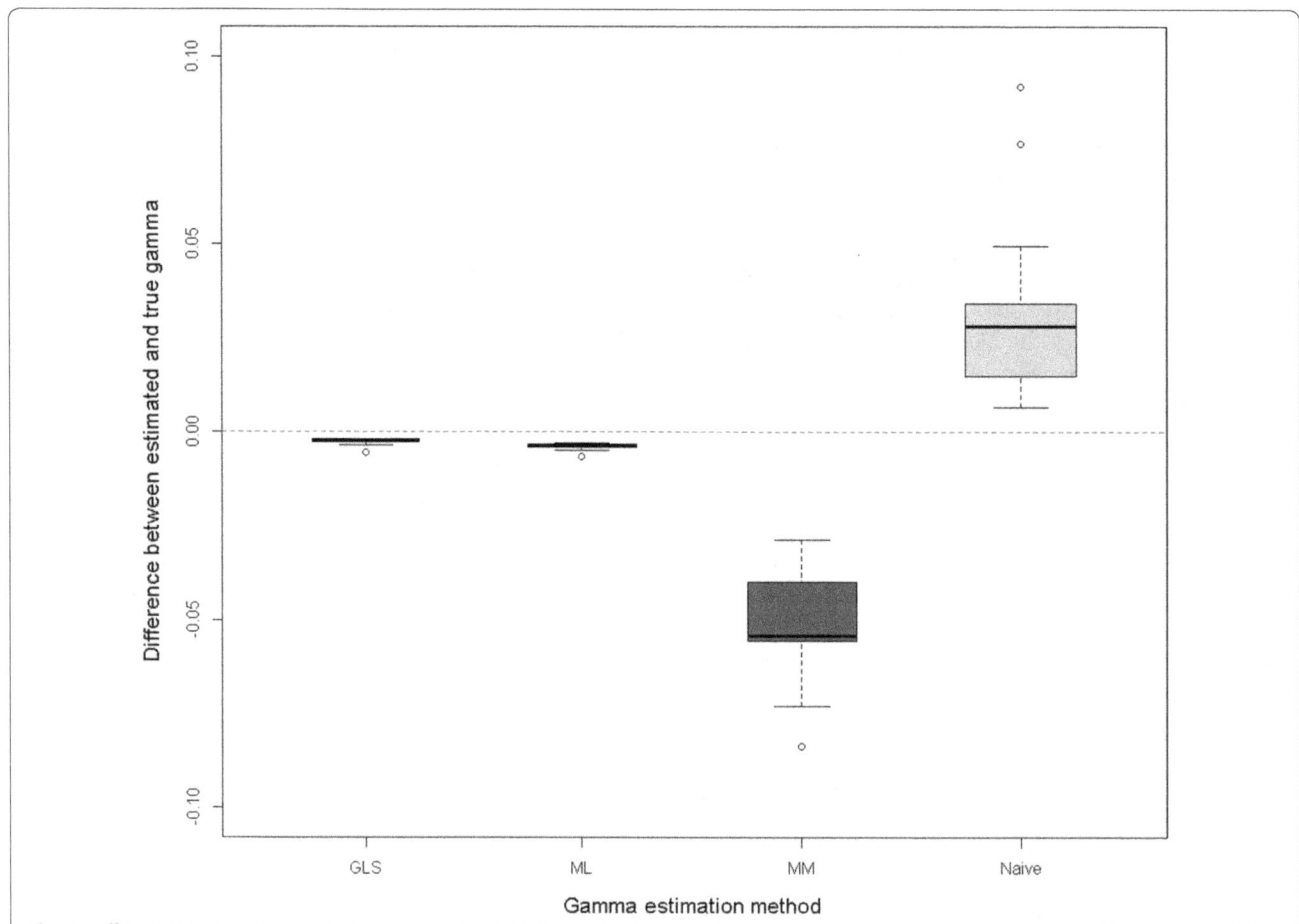

Fig. 1 Differences between estimated and true Gamma, across 20 simulation replicates. Gamma was estimated by generalized least squares (GLS), maximum likelihood (ML), method of moments (MM) and the Naive method

sires, which had an accuracy of essentially 1 and no bias. Depending on the selection scheme, this may lead to less than optimal selection decisions.

Estimation of variance components

Figure 3 shows estimates of heritability obtained with three of the four methods (PBLUP, ssGBLUP_F and ssGBLUP_M). The estimates obtained using ssGBLUP

did not converge for six of the 20 simulation replicates. Convergence was achieved in those cases by weighting the submatrix $\mathbf{A}_{22}^{-1}$ in $\mathbf{H}^{-1}$ by $\omega = 0.7$ instead of 1 [42] but poor quality estimates were obtained and are, therefore, not reported.

Estimates were generally lower than the simulated true heritability (0.30). The lowest estimates were obtained with ssGBLUP_F. Including the metafounder improved estimates compared to ssGBLUP_F and reduced variability of estimates compared to PBLUP.

Discussion

In this work, we have addressed the complex issue of conciliation of marker and pedigree information in genetic evaluation. Powell et al. [43] argued that both IBS (at the markers) and identity-by-descent (IBD) are compatible notions because they are both measures of identity at causal genes. However, incompatibility appears when mixing both types of relationships [5, 34, 44, 45]. Legarra [7] suggested that, in order to compare genetic variance across IBD, IBS or other measures of relationships,

Table 1 Accuracy (correlation between TBV and EBV), inflation (regression coefficient of TBV on EBV), bias [average (EBV–TBV)] and mean square error (MSE) for each prediction methods

Prediction method	Accuracy	Inflation	Bias	MSE
PBLUP	0.51 (0.05)	0.98 (0.06)	−0.0003 (0.03)	0.206 (0.01)
ssGBLUP	0.72 (0.03)	0.89 (0.19)	0.2169 (0.04)	0.159 (0.03)
ssGBLUP_F	0.74 (0.02)	0.99 (0.04)	0.1167 (0.04)	0.141 (0.01)
ssGBLUP_M	0.74 (0.02)	0.94 (0.04)	0.0094 (0.03)	0.125 (0.01)

Averages across 20 replicates with standard deviations in parenthesis

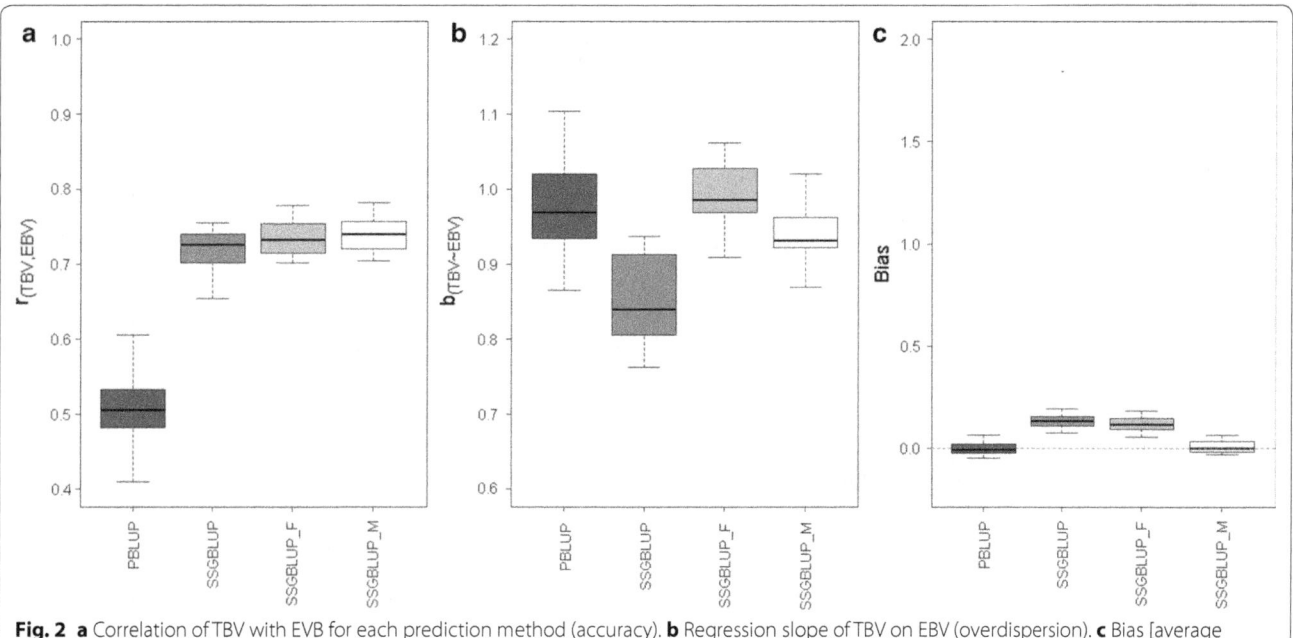

Fig. 2 **a** Correlation of TBV with EVB for each prediction method (accuracy). **b** Regression slope of TBV on EBV (overdispersion). **c** Bias [average (EBV–TBV)]

Table 2 Spearman correlations among TBV and the four EBV for each prediction methods

	EBV PBLUP	EBV ssGB-LUP	EBV ssGBLUP_F	EBV ssGBLUP_M
TBV	0.49 (0.06)	0.71 (0.02)	0.72 (0.03)	0.73 (0.02)
EBV PBLUP		0.56 (0.05)	0.62 (0.04)	0.64 (0.04)
EBV ssGBLUP			0.99 (0.01)	0.98 (0.01)
EBV ssGBLUP_F				0.99 (0.002)

Averages across 20 replicates with standard deviations in parenthesis

a common reference must be chosen. Similar (but not identical) to [43], in this work we used a fixed reference (**G** constructed as a cross-product of $\{-1,0,1\}$ genotypic codes) and tailored **A** (IBD, pedigree) to fit **G** (IBS, markers). Compared to previous approaches, using a fixed reference has the advantage that genomic relationships are immutable (i.e. adding more genotyped individuals to the database does not change the existing relationships) and they do not depend on pedigree depth, which by construction is always limited and, in animal breeding, often heterogeneous. Our approach is in fact very similar to using IBS as measure of identity. We used a genomic relationship matrix $\mathbf{G} = 2(\mathbf{M} - \mathbf{J})(\mathbf{M} - \mathbf{J})'/n$, whereas the matrix of IBS is $\mathbf{G}_{IBS} = \mathbf{G}/2 + \mathbf{11}'$ (see proof in "Appendix"). In GBLUP with associated variance component estimation, when all animals are genotyped, using a model with $\mathbf{G}_{IBS}$ or the **G** matrix proposed here

yields identical EBV, as the term ½ in $\mathbf{G}/2$ gets absorbed into the variance component and the constant $\mathbf{11}'$ gets absorbed into the fixed part of the linear mixed model [7, 46]. However, matrix **G** rather than $\mathbf{G}_{IBS}$ must be used in ssGBLUP_M because $\mathbf{G}_{IBS}$ is not compatible with pedigree relationships. In [4], the (fixed effect) intercept term μ_g models, identical to [5], the difference between genetic values of individuals in the base and genotyped individuals. These intercept terms play therefore a similar role as metafounders.

Easy estimation of ancestral relationships

Derivations in the Theory section show that estimation of ancestral relationships based on γ (one base population) and $\boldsymbol{\Gamma}$ (several base populations) can be framed within the classic linear model approach of quantitative genetics [19], which has recently been used for gene content [14, 25–27]. This approach is easy to understand and compute. Also, $\boldsymbol{\Gamma}$ can be understood, just like heritability, as an unobserved base population parameter that does not change with additional data (although its estimate may change). Therefore, an accurate estimate of $\boldsymbol{\Gamma}$ can be used repeatedly without the need for re-estimation, as is customary in livestock genetic evaluation. This contrasts with "centering" of marker covariates, which changes with every new genotype. If all base allele frequencies were known exactly, then there should be no need to use metafounders, as relationship matrices can be appropriately constructed [14].

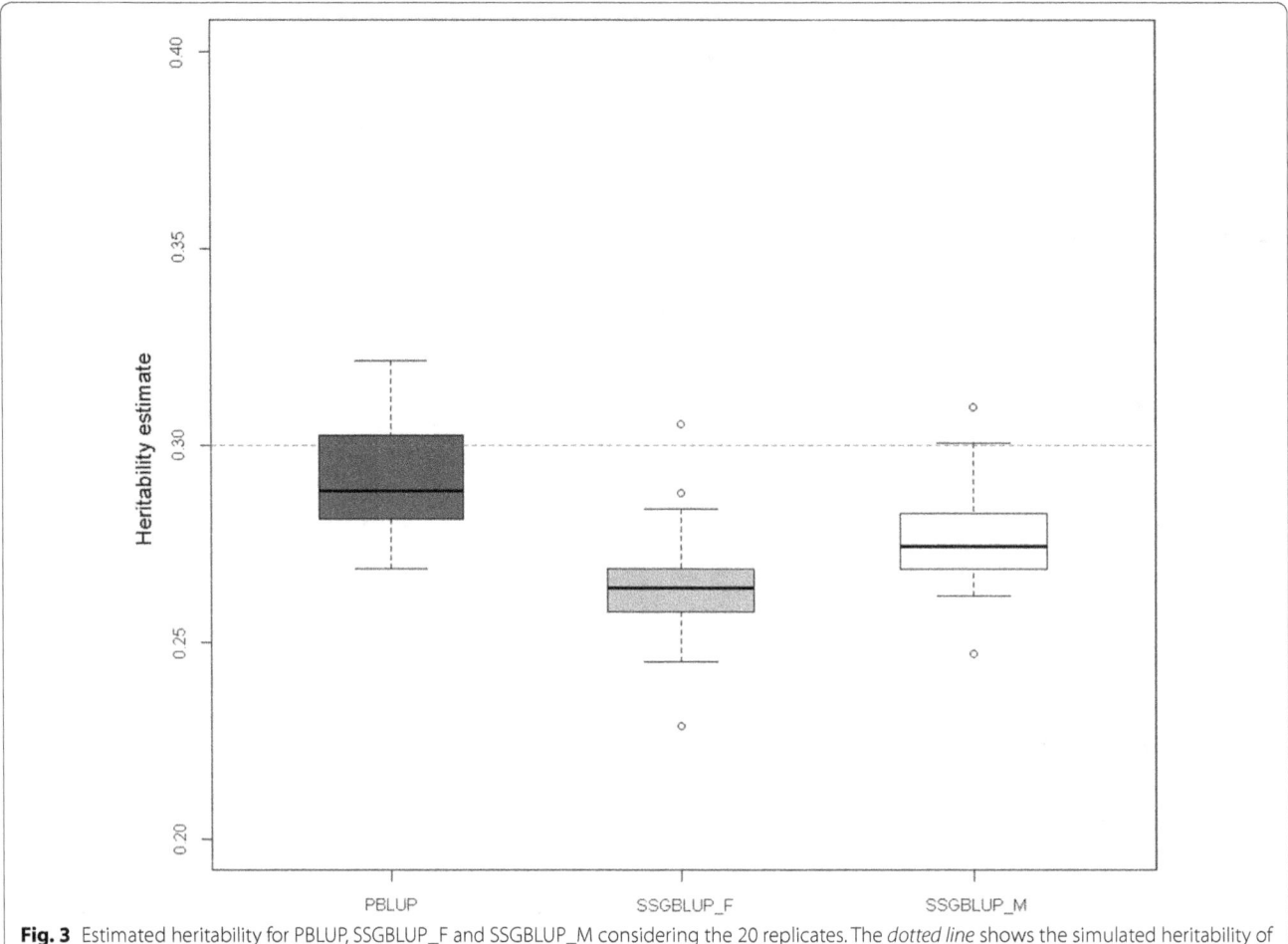

Fig. 3 Estimated heritability for PBLUP, SSGBLUP_F and SSGBLUP_M considering the 20 replicates. The *dotted line* shows the simulated heritability of 0.30

In the work presented here, the simplest methods (Naïve and method of moments) yielded biased (upwards and downwards, respectively) estimates of γ; the naïve method because it ignores that allele frequencies tend to drift to their extreme values as generations progress, and the method of moments because it implicitly assumes that genotyped individuals are a random sample from a particular generation.

Equivalence of ancestral relationships with second moments of allele frequencies also shows a strong relation with population genetics theory, which will be detailed in the next paragraph.

Relationship between metafounders parameter γ and F_{st} fixation index

The fixation index F_{st} [17] is a measure of diversity of a set of populations with respect to a reference population, usually the pool of all populations. In this approach, each population is assumed to be a random sample from all possible populations that could be sampled according to

the evolutionary process described by F_{st}. Conceptually, F_{st} is a parameter to be estimated [18, 19], and it is not a statistic computed from the data. The usual definition of F_{st} for a particular biallelic locus is:

$$F_{st} = \frac{\sigma_p^2}{\bar{p}(1 - \bar{p})},$$

where σ_p^2 is the variance of allelic frequencies across populations and $\bar{p}$ is the allele frequency of the conceptual combined population. If we consider that the variance of allele frequencies applies *across* loci and not *across* populations, it follows that $\bar{p} = 0.5$ because reference alleles are taken at random. In this case:

$$F_{st} = \frac{\sigma_p^2}{\bar{p}(1 - \bar{p})} = \frac{\sigma_p^2}{0.5^2} = 4\sigma_p^2 = \frac{\gamma}{2}.$$

Our interpretation of this link between F_{st} and γ is as follows. Jacquard [47] called $\frac{\gamma}{2}$ the "inbreeding coefficient of a population". Cockerham [16] modelled $\frac{\gamma}{2} = \theta_l = F_{st}$ as an intraclass correlation, "the coancestry of the line with itself", in other words, the probability that two gametes taken at random from the population are identical. Thus, it makes perfect sense to consider that the additive relationship (which is twice the coancestry value) of a group with itself is $\gamma = 2\theta_l = 8\sigma_p^2$. This is the interpretation of the $\frac{\gamma}{2}$ coefficient in Legarra et al. [1]. Note that the assumption that $\bar{p} = 0.5$ is automatically fulfilled if reference alleles are chosen at random across loci (i.e., they are neither the most frequent nor the least observed allele).

Alternatively, [1] showed that for a population with self-relationships equal to γ, the average heterozygosity is $1 - \frac{\gamma}{2}$, i.e. the variance is reduced by an amount equal to $\frac{\gamma}{2}$ from the conceptual population with heterozygosity 1. Thus $\frac{\gamma}{2}$ can be interpreted as F_{st} if the F_{st} is taken as a measure of homozygosity.

Consequences of using metafounders in genomic evaluation

Genomic estimates of breeding values are invariant to allele coding [46] when all individuals are genotyped. However, this is not the case when pedigree and marker informations are combined, as in ssGBLUP. In this work, we have shown that, even in the presence of complete pedigree and a single base population, use of metafounders in ssGBLUP_M leads to slightly more inflated and less biased EBV, lower MSE, and nearly unbiased estimates of heritability compared to ssGBLUP_F. Bias, defined as E(EBV–TBV), is typically overlooked in genomic prediction, but in an example of biased evaluation, Henderson [48] recognized that "sires of later generations appeared to be under-evaluated relative to older sires". Overdispersion, also called bias in recent literature (e.g. [38]), may also have a dramatic impact in practice [39–41] and the trade-off between bias and variance needs further study. For instance, Vitezica et al. [5] found that ssGBLUP_F was unbiased but had some overdispersion, which likely depends on the data structure, including which individuals are genotyped.

In addition, use of metafounders allows a clear definition of genomic relationships because relationships do not depend on pedigree depth or completeness or on changes in allele frequencies as new data is added. In addition, a high-dimensional parameter (i.e. base allele frequencies) is substituted by a low-dimensional one (matrix $\mathbf{\Gamma}$).

The poor performance of ssGBLUP compared to ssGBLUP_F is likely due to the presence of highly inbred individuals because ssGBLUP ignored inbreeding in the setup of $\mathbf{A}^{-1}$. This relates to the interpretation of

parameter ω, as used in early studies of ssGBLUP [42]. An application of ssGBLUP for type traits in Holstein [42] experienced convergence problems, which were eliminated when $\mathbf{A}_{22}^{-1}$ was multiplied by $\omega = 0.7$ and which increased accuracy of predictions. However, the nature of parameter ω was not known [49]. In those studies, the inverse of the numerator relationship matrix $\mathbf{A}^{-1}$ was constructed using Henderson's rules while ignoring inbreeding [36], while the submatrix $\mathbf{A}_{22}^{-1}$ included inbreeding. As a result, the elements in the latter matrix were too large. In addition, genotyped animals were on average unrelated in $\mathbf{G}$ but not in $\mathbf{A}_{22}$, which can be corrected by scaling $\mathbf{G}$, as in [5]. However, this resulted in the elements in $\mathbf{A}_{22}^{-1}$ to be too large for younger animals relative to $\mathbf{G}$. Both these problems are partially circumvented by putting a weight $\omega < 1$ on $\mathbf{A}_{22}^{-1}$. When $\mathbf{A}^{-1}$ was constructed while considering inbreeding, the optimal value of ω in an analysis of Holstein dairy cattle increased from 0.7 to 0.9 (Masuda, personal communication, 2016). However, the metafounder approach provides a more principled solution to this problem. Also, following these experiences, $\mathbf{A}^{-1}$ should always be constructed while considering inbreeding to avoid infrequent but pathological problems.

Conclusions

Metafounders have relationships that are closely related to F_{st} fixation indices and proportional to covariances of allele frequencies in base populations. Use of metafounders can be simplified by new methods to estimate the covariance of base allele frequencies. We verified by simulation of a selected population that, in a single population, both GLS and ML are unbiased and computationally efficient. In the same simulation, use of metafounders in ssGBLUP led to more accurate and less biased evaluations, and also to more accurate estimates of genetic parameters. We propose a genomic relationship matrix that refers to a population with ideal base allele frequencies equal to 0.5. This matrix is similar to an IBS relationship matrix (up to scale factors), does not change with new data, and is compatible with pedigree data if metafounders are used. In the simulated data, pedigrees were perfectly known. Future work with real datasets in more complex settings—purebreds and their crosses [50, 51], and selected populations with unknown parent groups [13] will investigate the feasibility and accuracy, in practice, of using metafounders in ssGBLUP.

Authors' contributions
AL and OFC derived the theory with help from ZGV and CAGB. All authors agreed on scenarios to be tested. CAGB programmed and run all the simulations, with substantial input from IP and IM. The initial version of the manuscript was written by CAGB and AL and then completed by all authors. All authors read and approved the final manuscript.

Author details
[1] Departamento de Producción Animal, Facultad de Agronomía, Universidad de Buenos Aires, C1417DSE Buenos Aires, Argentina. [2] Instituto de Investigaciones en Producción Animal - Consejo Nacional de Investigaciones Científicas y Técnicas, Buenos Aires, Argentina. [3] GenPhySE, INRA, INPT, ENVT, Université de Toulouse, 31326 Castanet-Tolosan, France. [4] Center for Quantitative Genetics and Genomics, Department of Molecular Biology and Genetics, Aarhus University, 8830 Tjele, Denmark. [5] Animal and Dairy Science, University of Georgia, Athens, GA 30602, USA.

Acknowledgements
We thank S. Boitard and B. Servin for discussions concerning F_{st} and all members of AdMixSel project. We acknowledge suggestions and corrections from two anonymous referees.

Competing interests
The authors declare that they have no competing interests.

Funding
CAGB, SML and RJCC were partially funded by grants FONCyT PICT 2013-1661, UBACyT 861/2011 and PIP CONICET 833/2013. This work was partially financed by the AdMixSel project of the INRA SELGEN metaprogram (CAGB, AL and ZGV) as well as INP Toulouse (CAGB, AL). The project was partly supported by the Toulouse Midi-Pyrenees Bioinformatics platform. Reviewers and editors are acknowledged for useful comments and corrections.

Appendix

The appendix contains examples, details and algebraic developments that were not detailed in the main text.

Example of relationship matrix with one metafounder

Consider the pedigree:

1	0	0
2	1	1
3	1	1
4	2	3
5	2	4

where 1 is a metafounder with $\gamma = a_{1,1} = 0.2$. Using the tabular method [15], $a_{2,2} = 1 + a_{1,1}/2 = 1.1$ and $a_{1,2} = 0.5(a_{1,sire(2)} + a_{1,dam(2)}) = 0.5(a_{1,1} + a_{1,1}) = 0.2$. Proceeding with the tabular method, $\mathbf{A}^{(\gamma)}$ is:

0.2000	0.2000	0.2000	0.2000	0.2000
0.2000	1.1000	0.2000	0.6500	0.8750
0.2000	0.2000	1.1000	0.6500	0.4250
0.2000	0.6500	0.6500	1.1000	0.8750
0.2000	0.8750	0.4250	0.8750	1.3250

with inverse $\mathbf{A}^{(\gamma)-1}$, that can be obtained by inverting γ and using Henderson's rules [1, 16]:

7.2222	−1.1111	−1.1111	0.0000	0.0000
−1.1111	2.2222	0.5556	−0.5556	−1.1111
−1.1111	0.5556	1.6667	−1.1111	0.0000
0.0000	−0.5556	−1.1111	2.7778	−1.1111
0.0000	−1.1111	0.0000	−1.1111	2.2222

These compare with regular $\mathbf{A}$ that can be obtained by setting $\gamma = 0$. In this case, individual 1 is an unknown parent group and its "relationships" have been set to 0 for presentation:

0.0000	0.0000	0.0000	0.0000	0.0000
0.0000	1.0000	0.0000	0.5000	0.7500
0.0000	0.0000	1.0000	0.5000	0.2500
0.0000	0.5000	0.5000	1.0000	0.7500
0.0000	0.7500	0.2500	0.7500	1.2500

and the inverse relationship matrix including the unknown parent group [13] is $\mathbf{A}^{-1}$:

2.0000	−1.0000	−1.0000	0.0000	0.0000
−1.0000	2.0000	0.5000	−0.5000	−1.0000
−1.0000	0.5000	1.5000	−1.0000	0.0000
0.0000	−0.5000	−1.0000	2.5000	−1.0000
0.0000	−1.0000	0.0000	−1.0000	2.0000

Analytical derivation of γ and s

For a particular population, the genetic variance–covariance structure is a function of two parameters η_1 and η_2 : $\gamma = \frac{4\eta_1}{2\eta_1 + \eta_2}$ and $s = n(2\eta_1 + \eta_2)$ (n being the number of markers) which depend on the allelic frequencies Appendix A in [11]. With p_j being the allelic frequencies across the $j = 1 \ldots n$ loci, these parameters do not depend on j and are equal to:

$$\eta_1 = Var(p_j),$$

$$\eta_2 = E(2p_jq_j),$$

with $q = 1 - p$.

Now, we use the following developments.

$$E(pq) = E(p(1-p)) = E(p) - E(p^2). \tag{1}$$

Since we have $Var(p) = E(p^2) - E(p)^2$, we obtain $E(p^2) = Var(p) + E(p)^2$. We also have $E(q) = 1 - E(p)$. Substituting $E(p^2)$ in Eq. (1) gives:

$$E(pq) = E(p) - Var(p) - E(p)^2$$
$$= E(p)(1 - E(p)) - Var(p) = E(p)E(q) - Var(p).$$

If markers are biallelic and labeled at random $E(p) = E(q) = 0.5$. So the equation above gives $E(pq) = 0.25 - Var(p)$. From this we obtain:

$$2\eta_1 + \eta_2 = 2Var(p_j) + 0.5 - 2Var(p_j) = 0.5,$$

and therefore

$$s = n(2\eta_1 + \eta_2) = \frac{n}{2}, \tag{2}$$

or, in other words, s is half the number of markers. Furthermore,

$$\gamma = \frac{4\eta_1}{2\eta_1 + \eta_2} = \frac{4\eta_1}{0.5} = 8Var(p_j) = 8\sigma_p^2, \qquad (3)$$

so that γ for a single population is eight times the variance of allelic frequencies at the base population.

Equivalences of genomic relationship matrices

The matrix $\mathbf{G}$ described in [11] and in this paper can be written as:

$$\mathbf{G} = \frac{2}{n}(\mathbf{M} - \mathbf{J})(\mathbf{M} - \mathbf{J})',$$

where $\mathbf{M}$ contains genotypes coded as $\{0,1,2\}$ and $\mathbf{J}$ is a matrix of 1s. The purpose of this paragraph is to show the linear relationship of this matrix with a matrix describing IBS coefficients, in fact $\mathbf{G}_{IBS} = \frac{1}{2}\mathbf{G} + \mathbf{11}'$. The terms in $\mathbf{G}_{IBS}$ are usually described in terms of identities or countings (i.e. [9, 10, 52]):

$$G_{IBS_{ij}} = \frac{1}{n}\sum_{m=1}^{n} 2\frac{\sum_{k=1}^{2}\sum_{l=1}^{2} I_{kl}}{4},$$

where I_{kl} measures the identity (with value 1 or 0) of allele k in individual i with allele l in individual j, and single-locus identity measures are averaged across k loci. There is an algebraic expression for this "counting". Toro et al. [10] in their Eq. (1) show that, for biallelic markers, for a locus k (omitted in the notation for clarity):

$$f_{M_{ij}} = \frac{m_i}{2}\frac{m_j}{2} + \left(1 - \frac{m_i}{2}\right)\left(1 - \frac{m_j}{2}\right), \qquad (4)$$

for coancestry (half relationship) $f_{M_{ij}}$ of individuals i and j, where $m/2$ is the "gene frequency" of the individual (half the gene content (m), i.e. $\{0,1/2,1\}$ for the three genotypes).

In order to prove $\mathbf{G}_{IBS} = \frac{1}{2}\mathbf{G} + \mathbf{11}'$, first we translate the equation in [10] to the more familiar scale of relationships $g_{IBS_{ij}} = 2f_{M_{ij}}$ and gene contents m. Thus:

$$g_{IBS_{ij}} = 2f_{M_{ij}} = 2\left(\frac{m_i}{2}\frac{m_j}{2} + \left(\frac{2}{2} - \frac{m_i}{2}\right)\left(\frac{2}{2} - \frac{m_j}{2}\right)\right)$$

$$g_{IBS_{ij}} = m_i m_j - m_i - m_j + 2.$$

This expression can be easily verified in a table with the nine possible genotypes:

	AA	Aa	aa
AA	2	1	0
Aa	1	1	1
aa	0	1	2

Also,

$$g_{IBS_{ij}} = m_i m_j - m_i - m_j + 2 = (m_i - 1)(m_j - 1) + 1,$$

which extends to all individuals and averaged across loci can be written as:

$$\mathbf{G}_{IBS} = \frac{1}{n}(\mathbf{M} - \mathbf{J})(\mathbf{M} - \mathbf{J})' + \mathbf{11}'.$$

Thus, matrix $\mathbf{G}_{IBS} = \frac{1}{n}(\mathbf{M} - \mathbf{J})(\mathbf{M} - \mathbf{J})' + \mathbf{11}'$ and because $\mathbf{G} = \frac{2}{n}(\mathbf{M} - \mathbf{J})(\mathbf{M} - \mathbf{J})'$ it follows that $\mathbf{G}_{IBS} = \frac{1}{2}\mathbf{G} + \mathbf{11}'$. The equivalence can also be verified by noting that, for all nine genotypes, the cross-product $(m_i - 1)(m_j - 1)$ in the following table is identical to $g_{IBS_{ij}} - 1$ in the previous table.

	AA	Aa	aa
AA	1	0	−1
Aa	0	0	0
Aa	−1	0	1

Computation of the different H matrices

For ssGBLUP and ssGBLUP_F, matrix $\mathbf{H}^{-1}$ is constructed as follows [2, 3]:

$$\mathbf{H}^{-1} = \mathbf{A}^{-1} + \begin{pmatrix} \mathbf{0} & \mathbf{0} \\ \mathbf{0} & \mathbf{G}_a^{*-1} - \mathbf{A}_{22}^{-1} \end{pmatrix},$$

with $\mathbf{G}_a^* = 0.95\mathbf{G}_a + 0.05\mathbf{A}_{22} = 0.95(a + b\mathbf{G}) + 0.05\mathbf{A}_{22}$ and $\mathbf{G} = \frac{(\mathbf{M}-\mathbf{P})(\mathbf{M}-\mathbf{P})}{2\sum p_i q_i}$ as in [8], $\mathbf{M}$ contains genotypes coded as $\{0,1,2\}$ and $\mathbf{P}$ contains twice allelic frequencies p_i. These are computed from the observed genotypes so that $2p_i$ is equal to the mean of the i-th column of $\mathbf{M}$. Constants a and b are such that the full-matrix and diagonal averages of $\mathbf{G}_a$ and $\mathbf{A}_{22}$ are the same [34] in order to make the two matrices compatible. The use of the weights 0.95 and 0.05 is in order to make $\mathbf{G}_a$ invertible. Matrix $\mathbf{A}^{-1}$ should be constructed using contributions with values described in the table below (i.e. [53]):

No parent known	1
One parent known	$\left(0.75 - \frac{F_{known}}{4}\right)^{-1}$
Two parents known	$\left(0.5 - \frac{F_{sire}}{4} - \frac{F_{dam}}{4}\right)^{-1}$

Or, in a more compact way $\left(0.5 - \frac{F_{sire}}{4} - \frac{F_{dam}}{4}\right)^{-1}$ with $F_{unknown} = -1$.

ssGBLUP uses the defaults in blupf90 suite of programs (random_type *add_animal*). ssGBLUP uses the simple method to create $\mathbf{A}^{-1}$, a method which pretends that, in all cases, inbreeding in expressions above is $F = 0$.

ssGBLUP_F uses $\mathbf{H}^{-1}$ as above but constructs $\mathbf{A}^{-1}$ correctly (blupf90 random_type *add_an_upginb*), using the rules above.

ssGBLUP_M uses the blupf90 random_type *user_file* to consider the following relationship matrix, which was constructed externally:

$$\mathbf{H}^{(\Gamma)-1} = k\left(\mathbf{A}^{(\Gamma)-1} + \begin{pmatrix} \mathbf{0} & \mathbf{0} \\ \mathbf{0} & \mathbf{G}^{*-1} - \mathbf{A}_{22}^{(\Gamma)-1} \end{pmatrix}\right),$$

with $\mathbf{G}^* = 0.95\mathbf{G} + 0.05\mathbf{A}_{22}^{(\Gamma)}$ (basically to make $\mathbf{G}$ invertible), $\mathbf{G} = \frac{1}{s}(\mathbf{M} - \mathbf{J})(\mathbf{M} - \mathbf{J})'$ and $s = n/2$, $\mathbf{M}$ contains genotypes coded as $\{0,1,2\}$, n is the number of markers, $\mathbf{A}^{(\Gamma)-1}$ and $\mathbf{A}_{22}^{(\Gamma)-1}$ are constructed with own programs as in [1] using the estimated value of $\mathbf{\Gamma}$. Inbreeding is fully considered in both matrices $\mathbf{A}^{(\Gamma)-1}$ and $\mathbf{A}_{22}^{(\Gamma)-1}$. The constant $k = 1 - \frac{\gamma}{2}$ puts the genetic variance associated to metafounders (i.e. to "related" founders) on the same scale as regular "unrelated" founders in $\mathbf{A}$ or $\mathbf{H}$ [1].

References

1. Legarra A, Christensen OF, Vitezica ZG, Aguilar I, Misztal I. Ancestral relationships using metafounders: finite ancestral populations and across population relationships. Genetics. 2015;200:455–68.
2. Legarra A, Aguilar I, Misztal I. A relationship matrix including full pedigree and genomic information. J Dairy Sci. 2009;92:4656–63.
3. Christensen OF, Lund MS. Genomic prediction when some animals are not genotyped. Genet Sel Evol. 2010;42:2.
4. Fernando RL, Dekkers JC, Garrick DJ. A class of Bayesian methods to combine large numbers of genotyped and non-genotyped animals for whole-genome analyses. Genet Sel Evol. 2014;46:50.
5. Vitezica Z, Aguilar I, Misztal I, Legarra A. Bias in genomic predictions for populations under selection. Genet Res (Camb). 2011;93:357–66.
6. Christensen OF, Legarra A, Lund MS, Su G. Genetic evaluation for three-way crossbreeding. Genet Sel Evol. 2015;47:98.
7. Legarra A. Comparing estimates of genetic variance across different relationship models. Theor Popul Biol. 2016;107:26–30.
8. VanRaden PM. Efficient methods to compute genomic predictions. J Dairy Sci. 2008;91:4414–23.
9. Ritland K. Estimators for pairwise relatedness and individual inbreeding coefficients. Genet Res (Camb). 1996;67:175–85.
10. Toro MÁ, García-Cortés LA, Legarra A. A note on the rationale for estimating genealogical coancestry from molecular markers. Genet Sel Evol. 2011;43:27.
11. Christensen OF. Compatibility of pedigree-based and marker-based relationship matrices for single-step genetic evaluation. Genet Sel Evol. 2012;44:37.
12. Thompson R. Sire evaluation. Biometrics. 1979;35:339–53.
13. Quaas RL. Additive genetic model with groups and relationships. J Dairy Sci. 1988;71:1338–45.
14. Makgahlela ML, Strandén I, Nielsen US, Sillanpää MJ, Mäntysaari EA. Using the unified relationship matrix adjusted by breed-wise allele frequencies in genomic evaluation of a multibreed population. J Dairy Sci. 2014;97:1117–27.
15. Emik LO, Terrill CE. Systematic procedures for calculating inbreeding coefficients. J Hered. 1949;40:51–5.
16. Henderson CR. A simple method for computing the inverse of a numerator relationship matrix used in prediction of breeding values. Biometrics. 1976;32:69–83.
17. Wright S. Isolation by distance. Genetics. 1943;28:114–38.
18. Holsinger KE, Weir BS. Genetics in geographically structured populations: defining, estimating and interpreting F(ST). Nat Rev Genet. 2009;10:639–50.
19. Cockerham CC. Variance of gene frequencies. Evolution. 1969;23:72–84.
20. Wright S. Evolution in Mendelian populations. Genetics. 1931;16:97–159.
21. Crow J, Kimura M. An introduction to population genetics theory. New York: Harper and Row; 1970.
22. Robertson A. Gene frequency distributions as a test of selective neutrality. Genetics. 1975;81:775–85.
23. Fariello MI, Boitard S, Naya H, SanCristobal M, Servin B. Detecting signatures of selection through haplotype differentiation among hierarchically structured populations. Genetics. 2013;193:929–41.
24. Laval G, SanCristobal M, Chevalet C. Measuring genetic distances between breeds: use of some distances in various short term evolution models. Genet Sel Evol. 2002;34:481–508.
25. McPeek MS, Wu X, Ober C. Best linear unbiased allele-frequency estimation in complex pedigrees. Biometrics. 2004;60:359–67.
26. Gengler N, Mayeres P, Szydlowski M. A simple method to approximate gene content in large pedigree populations: application to the myostatin gene in dual-purpose Belgian Blue cattle. Animal. 2007;1:21–8.
27. Forneris NS, Legarra A, Vitezica ZG, Tsuruta S, Aguilar I, Misztal I, et al. Quality control of genotypes using heritability estimates of gene content at the marker. Genetics. 2015;199:675–81.
28. Mäntysaari E, Van Vleck LD. Restricted maximum likelihood estimates of variance components from multitrait sire models with large number of fixed effects. J Anim Breed Genet. 1989;106:409–22.
29. Garcia-Cortes LA, Toro M. Multibreed analysis by splitting the breeding values. Genet Sel Evol. 2006;38:601–15.
30. Sargolzaei M, Schenkel FS. QMSim: a large-scale genome simulator for livestock. Bioinformatics. 2009;25:680–1.
31. Solberg TR, Sonesson AK, Woolliams JA, Meuwissen THE. Genomic selection using different marker types and densities. J Anim Sci. 2008;86:2447–54.
32. Hickey JM, Gorjanc G. Simulated data for genomic selection and genome-wide association studies using a combination of coalescent and gene drop methods. G3 (Bethesda). 2012;2:425–7.
33. MacLeod IM, Hayes BJ, Goddard ME. The effects of demography and long-term selection on the accuracy of genomic prediction with sequence data. Genetics. 2014;198:1671–84.
34. Christensen O, Madsen P, Nielsen B, Ostersen T, Su G. Single-step methods for genomic evaluation in pigs. Animal. 2012;6:1565–71.
35. Masuda Y, Misztal I, Tsuruta S, Legarra A, Aguilar I, Lourenco DAL, et al. Implementation of genomic recursions in single-step genomic best linear unbiased predictor for US Holsteins with a large number of genotyped animals. J Dairy Sci. 2016;99:1968–74.
36. Mehrabani-Yeganeh H, Gibson JP, Schaeffer LR. Including coefficients of inbreeding in BLUP evaluation and its effect on response to selection. J Anim Breed Genet. 2000;117:145–51.
37. Misztal I, Tsuruta S, Strabel T, Auvray B, Druet T, Lee DH. BLUPF90 and related programs (BGF90). In: Proceedings of the 7th World Congress on Genetics Applied to Livestock Production, 19–23 Aug 2002, Montpellier. 2002. CD-ROM communication no. 28-07.
38. Mantysaari E, Liu Z, VanRaden P. Interbull validation test for genomic evaluations. Interbull Bull. 2010;41:17–22.
39. Sargolzaei M, Chesnais J, Schenkel FS. Assessing the bias in top GPA bulls. 2012. cgil.uoguelph.ca/dcbgc/Agenda1209/DCBGC1209_Bias_Mehdi.pdf. Accessed 21 July 2016.
40. Spelman RJ, Arias J, Keehan MD, Obolonkin V, Winkelman AM, Johnson DL, et al. Application of genomic selection in the New Zealand dairy cattle industry. In: Proceedings of the 9th World Congress on Genetics Applied to Livestock Production, 1–6 Aug 2010, Leipzig. 2010.
41. Winkelman AM, Johnson DL, Harris BL. Application of genomic evaluation to dairy cattle in New Zealand. J Dairy Sci. 2015;98:659–75.
42. Tsuruta S, Misztal I, Aguilar I, Lawlor T. Multiple-trait genomic evaluation of linear type traits using genomic and phenotypic data in US Holsteins. J Dairy Sci. 2011;94:4198–204.
43. Powell JE, Visscher PM, Goddard ME. Reconciling the analysis of IBD and IBS in complex trait studies. Nat Rev Genet. 2010;11:800–5.
44. Harris BL, Johnson DL. Genomic predictions for New Zealand dairy bulls and integration with national genetic evaluation. J Dairy Sci. 2010;93:1243–52.
45. Meuwissen THE, Luan T, Woolliams JA. The unified approach to the use of genomic and pedigree information in genomic evaluations revisited. J Anim Breed Genet. 2011;128:429–39.

46. Strandén I, Christensen OF. Allele coding in genomic evaluation. Genet Sel Evol. 2011;43:25.

47. Jacquard A. The genetic structure of populations. Berlin: Springer; 1974.

48. Henderson C. Sire evaluation and genetic trends. J Anim Sci. 1973: symposium 10-41. doi:10.2527/1973.1973Symposium10x.

49. Misztal I, Vitezica ZG, Legarra A, Aguilar I, Swan AA. Unknown-parent groups in single-step genomic evaluation. J Anim Breed Genet. 2013;130:252–8.

50. Christensen OF, Madsen P, Nielsen B, Su G. Genomic evaluation of both purebred and crossbred performances. Genet Sel Evol. 2014;46:23.

51. Lourenco DAL, Tsuruta S, Fragomeni BO, Chen CY, Herring WO, Misztal I. Crossbreed evaluations in single-step genomic best linear unbiased predictor using adjusted realized relationship matrices. J Anim Sci. 2016;94:909–19.

52. Nejati-Javaremi A, Smith C, Gibson JP. Effect of total allelic relationship on accuracy of evaluation and response to selection. J Anim Sci. 1997;75:1738–45.

53. Meuwissen THE, Luo Z. Computing inbreeding coefficients in large populations. Genet Sel Evol. 1992;24:305–13.

6

Divergent selection-induced obesity alters the composition and functional pathways of chicken gut microbiota

Jinmei Ding[1†], Lele Zhao[1,5†], Lifeng Wang[3†], Wenjing Zhao[1], Zhengxiao Zhai[1], Li Leng[2], Yuxiang Wang[2], Chuan He[1], Yan Zhang[4], Heping Zhang[3], Hui Li[2] and He Meng[1*]

Abstract

Background: The gastrointestinal tract is populated by a complex and vast microbial network, with a composition that reflects the relationships of the symbiosis, co-metabolism, and co-evolution of these microorganisms with their host. The mechanism that underlies such interactions between the genetics of the host and gut microbiota remains elusive.

Results: To understand how genetic variation of the host shapes the gut microbiota and interacts with it to affect the metabolic phenotype of the host, we compared the abundance of microbial taxa and their functional performance between two lines of chickens (fat and lean) that had undergone long-term divergent selection for abdominal fat pad weight, which resulted in a 4.5-fold increase in the fat line compared to the lean line. Our analysis revealed that the proportions of *Fusobacteria* and *Proteobacteria* differed significantly between the two lines (8 vs. 18% and 33 vs. 24%, respectively) at the phylum level. Eight bacterial genera and 11 species were also substantially influenced by the host genotype. Differences between the two lines in the frequency of host alleles at loci that influence accumulation of abdominal fat were associated with differences in the abundance and composition of the gut microbiota. Moreover, microbial genome functional analysis showed that the gut microbiota was involved in pathways that are associated with fat metabolism such as lipid and glycan biosynthesis, as well as amino acid and energy metabolism. Interestingly, citrate cycle and peroxisome proliferator activated receptor (PPAR) signaling pathways that play important roles in lipid storage and metabolism were more prevalent in the fat line than in the lean line.

Conclusions: Our study demonstrates that long-term divergent selection not only alters the composition of the gut microbiota, but also influences its functional performance by enriching its relative abundance in microbial taxa. These results support the hypothesis that the host and gut microbiota interact at the genetic level and that these interactions result in their co-evolution.

Background

The development of sequencing technologies for application in metagenomics has increased our capacity to investigate the composition and dynamics of the microbial communities that harbor diverse habitats [1]. The gastrointestinal tract is populated by a complicated and vast microbial network that influences the health and development of the host organism in numerous aspects [2, 3]. The gut microbial composition can be viewed as a polygenic trait, that not only produces essential products and forms a barrier against pathogens, but also has multiple functions in physiology, metabolism, immunity, development, and behavior of the host [4–6]. The gut microbiota causes the suppression of the circulating lipoprotein lipase inhibitor that results in increased lipoprotein lipase activity, which in turn results in a significant

*Correspondence: menghe@sjtu.edu.cn
†Jinmei Ding, Lele Zhao and Lifeng Wang contributed equally to this work
[1] Department of Animal Science, School of Agriculture and Biology, Shanghai Jiao Tong University, Shanghai Key Laboratory of Veterinary Biotechnology, Shanghai 200240, People's Republic of China
Full list of author information is available at the end of the article

increase in body fat deposition in the host [7]. Suppression of the expression of these genes by direct action of the gut microbiota on the villi epithelia also causes increased lipoprotein lipase activity, which leads to increased triglyceride uptake and peripheral fat storage [8]. These findings are in agreement with previous studies in other chicken populations selected for high or low body fat [9, 10] and show that the gut microbiota affects energy uptake from the diet and energy storage in the host [7]. In our previous studies, in order to quantify the influence of genetic variation of the host on the structure of the gut microbiota, the abundance of gut microbiota was considered as a quantitative trait of the host, and we calculated the heritability of abundance of specific microorganisms in the gut microbiota. A few bacterial families of the microbiota had a moderate heritability, which indicated that the host genetics has an effect on the composition of the gut microbiota. Concurrently, we calculated the genetic correlations between specific microorganisms in the gut microbiota to examine if the genetics of the host is involved in the interactions between microorganisms in the gut microbiota. Significant genetic correlations between microorganisms in the gut microbiota were observed. Further analysis showed that such genetic correlations can be altered by genetic variation of the host. These results imply the importance of the host genetic background on the interactions between the microorganisms in the gut microbiota [11, 12]. However, the interactional mechanism between gut microbiota and genetic variation of the host genome has remained obscure. Until now, most studies focused on microbial taxa instead of microbial functional performance to understand the interactions between host genetics and gut microbiota.

Many factors influence the mechanism of the interactions between the host and the gut microbiota [13, 14]. Thus, choosing a model organism that is maintained in a controlled environment should enhance our understanding of the relationships between gut microbiota and host genetic factors. The chicken, which bridges the evolutionary gap between mammals and reptiles, serves as an important experimental model organism for the extant avian species due to the characteristics of its less complex gut microbiota and minimal maternal effect. Here, we analyzed and compared the function and classification of gut microbiota from two divergently selected lines of chickens, i.e. a fat line and a lean line. These lines originated from a single commercial grandsire line and underwent long-term (15 generations) divergent selection for abdominal fat percentage (AFP) and plasma very-low-density lipoprotein (VLDL) concentration. At 7 weeks of age, the mean adipocyte diameter in the fat line was 1.3 times wider than in the lean line, and the number of fat cells was 2.4 times larger in the fat line than in the lean line [15]. The long-term divergent selection also resulted in a 4.5-fold increase in abdominal fat pad weight in the fat line [16]. A total of 230 genes were found to be differentially expressed in the lean and fat lines; these genes are mainly related to signal transduction, tumorigenesis, immunity, and lipid and energy metabolism [17]. The two lines carry two main haplotypes with completely opposite single nucleotide polymorphism (SNP) alleles and a recombinant haplotype with nearly equal frequency in the 0.73-Mb *PC1/PCSK1* region of the Z chromosome. Genome-wide association analysis revealed that nearly all regions with evidence of selection signatures had SNP effects on abdominal fat weight and percentage [18].

Methods
Animals and samples collection
Two chicken lines (fat and lean lines) that were divergently selected for abdominal fat content (AFP) and plasma very-low-density lipoprotein (VLDL) were used in this study. Throughout all generations, they were maintained at the same location and reared on the same diets. Fecal samples were collected at 35 weeks of age from 29 fat line males, 26 lean line males, 27 fat line females, and 27 lean line females, for a total of 109 individuals from the 15th generation. The fecal samples were stored at −80 °C after collection. Animals were cared for in accordance with the Institute for Laboratory Animal Research (ILAR) guide for Care and Use of Laboratory Animals at Shanghai Jiao Tong University, China.

Gut microbial 16S rDNA sequencing
Fecal microbial genomic DNA extraction and 16S rDNA amplification and sequencing were performed as previously reported in [11]. A QIAmp DNA Stool Mini Kit (Qiagen, cat#51504) was used for microbial genomic DNA extraction. Extracted DNA was measured using a nanodrop spectrophotometer (Thermo Fisher Scientific) to assess DNA quantity and quality. The V4 hypervariable region of the 16S rDNA gene was PCR-amplified from microbiota genomic DNA using sample-specific sequence barcode fusion primers (forward 5′AYTGGGYDTAAA GNG 3′, reverse 5′ TACNVGGGTATCTAATCC 3′). PCR reactions and PCR product purification were performed as previously reported in [11]. Purified PCR products from the 109 samples were combined at equal concentrations and used to construct a metagenomic library using Illumina TruSeq sample preparation kit (Illumina, USA) according to the manufacturer's protocol. Sequencing was carried out by the Shanghai Personal Biotechnology Limited Company (Shanghai, P. R. China) using an Illumina MiSeq (Illumina, USA) sequencing platform. Sequence reads were quality-checked and removed based on the

following criteria: reads that (1) contained ambiguous bases, (2) had an average phred score lower than 25, (3) contained a homopolymer run that exceeded 6, (4) contained mismatches in the primers, and (5) had sequence lengths that were outside the limits of 200 and 1000 bp. The filtered sequences with an overlap longer than 10 bp between Read 1 and Read 2 and without mismatches were assembled according to their overlapping sequences. Reads that could not be assembled were discarded. The barcode and sequencing primers were trimmed from each sequence.

Analysis of classification and abundance

Based on the V4 region of the 16S rDNA sequence that passed the quality criteria, 2,301,532 amplicons were used for this study, with an average of 21,115 amplicons for each sample (ranging from 12,137 to 30,067) [see Additional file 1: Table S1]. The average sequenced amplicon length was 225 bp. Following filtering, each sample's trimmed and filtered sequences were submitted to Metagenome Rapid Annotation using Subsystem Technology (MG-RAST) [19] and compared to the Ribosomal database project databases (RDP) [20] using the best hit classification option to classify the abundance count of each taxon. The metagenome sequences used in this paper are publicly available from MG-RAST under the project name "fatandleanchicken". Data were generated at the species level, using cutoffs for the parameter classification at 8 for maximum e-value, 98% for minimum percentage identity, and 120 bp for minimum alignment length. A total of 37,590 taxa on the phylum, class, order, family, genus and species levels were annotated [see Additional file 2: Table S2]. Taxa that were present in at least 28 samples were considered as commonly existing classifications; 51 genera and 109 species met that criterion and their abundance counts were used for further analysis.

The taxon abundance counts were log2 transformed and normalized by subtracting the mean of all transformed values and dividing by the standard deviation of all log-transformed values for the given sample. After this procedure, the abundance profiles for all samples exhibited a mean of 0 and a standard deviation of 1. In order to detect if host genetic factors influence gut microbiota, T test was performed between fat and lean lines for specific microbes using Microsoft Excel, with adjustment of p values by Benjamini Hochberg FDR (FDR < 0.05) [21]. Alpha-diversity analysis was performed in mothur 1.31.2 [22] with the alpha-diversity.py script to calculate the index of chao1 and Shannon.

Sequencing of the whole microbial genome

Microbial genomic DNA of three females from each fat and lean line was used to construct whole microbial genome sequencing libraries with insert sizes of 300 and 400 bp. Each library was sequenced by high-throughput sequencing at 2×100 bp using the Illumina HiSeq 2000 (Illumina, USA). Eighty percent of the whole microbial genome sequence data with paired-end Illumina sequences were accounted for across all samples. A data cleaning process was applied to all samples. Low-quality reads, and low-compositional-complexity reads were removed. An average of 37.9 million reads per sample were used in the analysis. The DNA sequences are publicly available in MG-RAST under the project name "Hiseqchicken-six".

Annotation of microbial function

Quality-filtered reads were submitted to MG-RAST and compared to the Kyoto Encyclopedia of Genes and Genomes (KEGG) database [23] using the 'all annotation' option for functional annotation with a maximum e-value cutoff of 1e-5, a minimum percent identity cutoff of 90%, and a minimum alignment length cutoff of 20 amino acids. Functional pathways, which had a relative abundance that was greater than 0.1% and for at least two samples, were chosen for further analysis. The relative abundance of each functional pathway was normalized within each sample. Clustering analysis was performed by Cluster 3.0 and Java Treeview [24] and differential analysis was evaluated by STAMP v2.0 [25] between fat and lean lines for abundance of each functional pathway by applying the two-side Welch's t-test [26] and Benjamini-Hochberg FDR correction (FDR < 0.05).

Results

Diversity of gut microbial composition between the fat and lean lines

16S rDNA amplicon sequencing was used to analyze the microbial diversity and abundance in the gut microbiota of the fat and lean chicken lines. Alpha diversity results suggested that the richness and diversity of gut microbiota were influenced by the long-term divergent selection [see Additional file 3: Figure S1]. Four major phyla dominated the chicken gut bacterial community; *Firmicutes* was the most predominant phylum, followed by *Proteobacteria*, *Fusobacteria*, and *Actinobacteria* (Fig. 1a). Consistent with previous studies related to avian microbial diversity, *Firmicutes* and *Proteobacteria* were the main ubiquitous members in the gut microbiota, but more *Fusobacteria* were classified compared with several other avian gut microbial studies [27–29]. The gut microbial composition differed between the fat and lean lines. The percentage of *Fusobacteria* was significantly lower in the fat line (8%) than in the lean line (18%). Conversely, the percentage of *Proteobacteria* was 33% in the fat line and approximately 24% in the lean line (Fig. 1a). At the genus

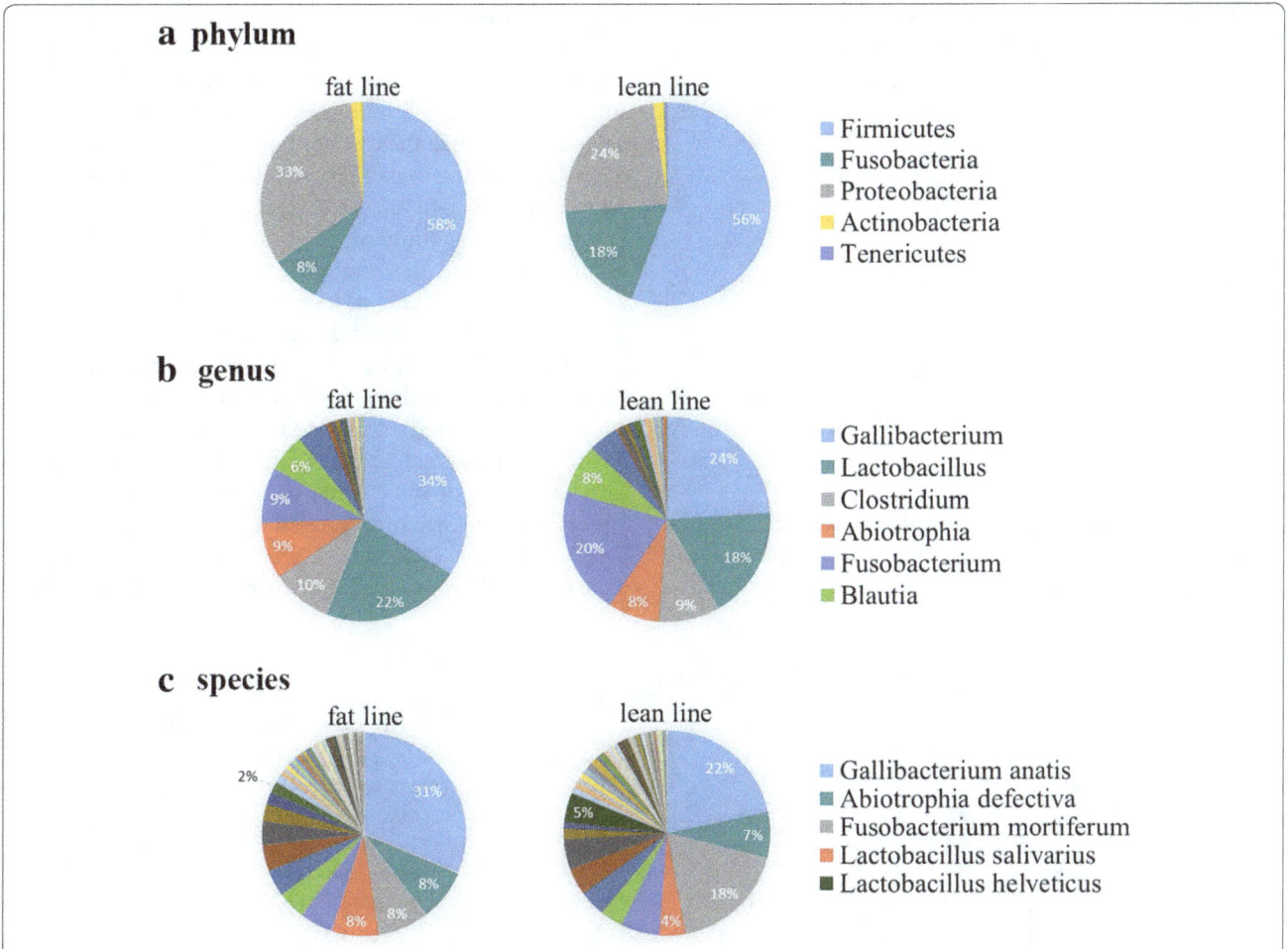

Fig. 1 Aggregate microbiota composition at different levels in the fat and lean lines. **a** Phylum level, **b** genus level, **c** species level. Only major taxonomic groups are shown

level, *Gallibacterium,* which belongs to the phylum of *Proteobacteria* and comprises the *Gallibacterium anatis* species, was the most abundant genus in chicken gut microbiota (Fig. 1c). The genus *Fusobacterium,* belonging to the phylum of *Fusobacteria,* was in lower proportion in the fat line (9%) than in the lean line (20%) (Fig. 1b). The analysis showed that one (*Proteobacteria*) of the eight phyla [see Additional file 4: Table S3], eight of the 52 genera (Table 1) and 11 species [see Additional file 5: Table S4] were significantly influenced by the genetics of the host.

The effect of host genetics on gene functional enrichment of gut microbiota

In order to investigate the influence of host genetic variation on the functional performance of the microbiota, we sequenced the whole gut microbial genome using three

biological replicates from each line. Based on the associated KEGG orthologous group markers, we compared predicted microbial functions between the fat and lean lines and detected that amino acid metabolism, energy metabolism, lipid metabolism, and cell motility were nearly twofold more enriched in the lean line than in the fat line (Fig. 2). Pathways that were more enriched in the fat line included translation, signal transduction mechanisms, metabolism of terpenoids and polyketides, protein folding and degradation, biosynthesis of secondary metabolites, and cancers (Fig. 2). These results are consistent with the previous findings of a study on obese rats [30].

Based on the analysis of whole microbial genome sequencing data, we observed that enriched markers were frequently involved in the functional pathways of inositol phosphate metabolism, antigen processing and

Table 1 Comparison of bacterial genus abundance in the gut microbiota between the fat and lean lines

Phylum	Genus	Relative fold change[a] Fat versus lean line	p value (*p < 0.05, **p < 0.01)
Actinobacteria	*Rothia*	1.28	0.004**
	Micrococcus	1.20	0.009**
Bacteroidetes	*Bacteroides*	−1.08	0.019*
Proteobacteria	*Gallibacterium*	1.25	0.011*
Tenericutes	*Acholeplasma*	−1.19	0.03*
Firmicutes	*Aerococcus*	1.14	0.037*
	Pectinatus	−1.27	0.003**
	Selenomonas	1.17	0.04*

[a] + fat/lean; − lean/fat

presentation, and phosphonate and phosphinate metabolism in the lean line. In contrast, the gut microbiota of the fat line showed enrichment in citrate cycle, other types of o-glycan biosynthesis, peroxisome proliferator activated receptor (PPAR) signaling pathway, carbon fixation in photosynthetic organisms, ribosomes, and cell adhesion molecules (Fig. 3). A hierarchy cluster heatmap was generated to visualize the distribution of microbial functions in the fat and lean lines (Fig. 4). The microbial functions were also matched to the microbial metabolic pathway results from the study on obese mice [31]. The heatmap results suggested that aminotransferase, arginine decarboxylase, cytochrome o ubiquinol oxidase subunit III, and 1-phosphatidylinositol-3-phosphate 5-kinase, which are involved in amino acid metabolism, energy metabolism, and carbohydrate metabolism respectively, were more abundant in the lean line than in the fat line (Fig. 4) and [see Additional file 6: Table S5]. Compared to the lean line, the gut microbiota in the fat line had a higher functional performance related to bacitracin transport system permease protein, citrate (pro-3s)-lyase ligase, and ribonucleoside-diphosphate reductase alpha chain,

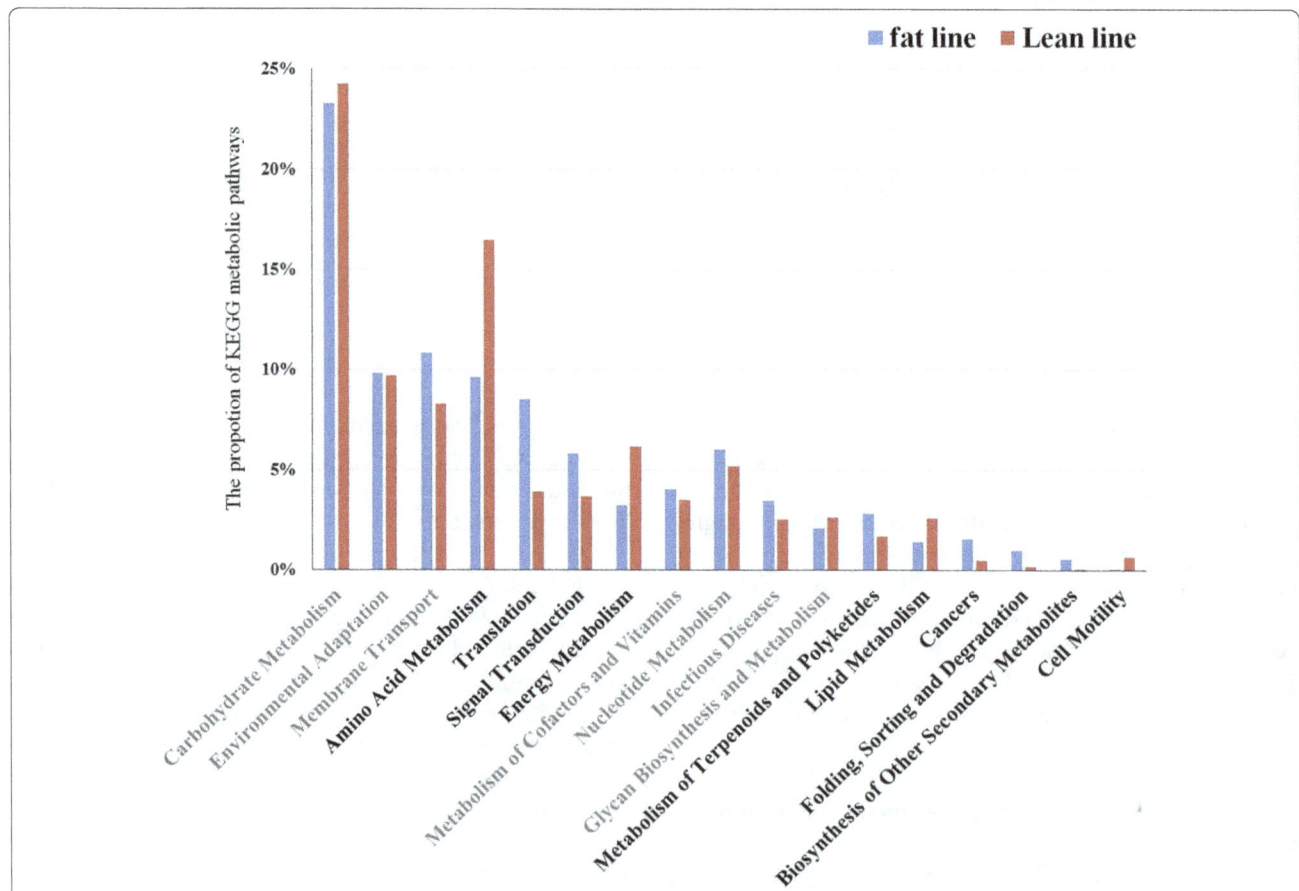

Fig. 2 Distribution of KEGG metabolic pathways in the fat and lean lines. Profile *bar plots* show the relative proportion of each metabolic pathway. The pathways labeled in *black* were differentially expressed (fold change >1.5)

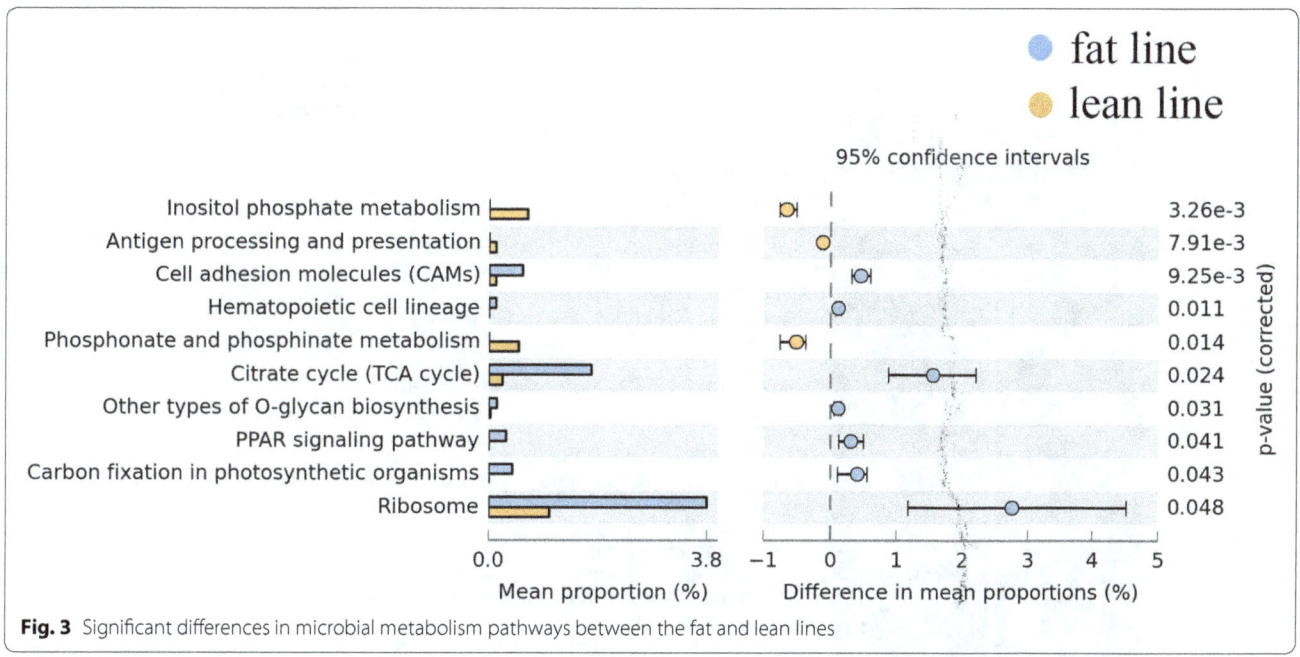

Fig. 3 Significant differences in microbial metabolism pathways between the fat and lean lines

which are respectively involved in immune system diseases, signal transduction and nucleotide metabolism (Fig. 4) and [see Additional file 6: Table S5].

Discussion

Previous studies reported that the genetics of the host can influence the abundance and composition of gut microbiota. In this study, significant differences in 11 microbial species were observed between the fat and lean lines [see Additional file 5: Table S4]. Among these species, *Pectinatus frisingensis*, *Lactobacillus salivarius*, and *Micrococcus sp. SMCC ZAT352* were found to be associated with adipogenesis. For example, *P. frisingensis* synthesizes lipopolysaccharide with polymeric O-specific chains that are related to host obesity [32], *L. salivarius* can modify the fecal microbiota, which in turn affects metabolic pathways in obese chickens and humans [33, 34], and *Micrococcus* is involved in lipolytic activity, which shows a positive correlation with fatty acid biosynthesis [35]. Although 16S rDNA amplicon sequencing was the primary method used to analyze microbial diversity, we also used the computation tool PICRUSTs [36] to predict microbial community functions [see Additional file 7]. Functional prediction results revealed that signal transduction mechanisms and fatty acid biosynthesis were more abundant in the fat line than in the lean line and this was consistent with the results of the microbial

composition of the gut microbiota [see Additional file 5: Table S4 and Additional file 8: Figure S2].

Several studies have shown that multiple transcription factors and signaling pathways are involved in the regulation of adipogenesis [37–39]. PPAR plays an important role in adipogenesis, adipocyte gene expression, and fat cell differentiation, which promote lipid storage and metabolism [40, 41]. Moreover, the PPAR signaling axis is also a potential target for the modulation of adipogenesis [42]. Interestingly, our whole microbial genome sequencing results suggested that, compared to the lean line, the PPAR signal pathway of gut microbiota in the fat line had a significantly higher functional performance (Fig. 4). This suggests the possibility that the PPAR signal pathway may also be involved in lipid storage. The citrate cycle is another key metabolic pathway that unifies carbohydrate, lipid, and protein metabolism. A significant correlation between citrate synthase level and obesity, together with a decreased activity of this enzyme in the mitochondria of human omental adipose tissue, were reported in obese humans [43]. Previous studies showed that citrate synthase activity was suppressed in obese mice, resulting in excessive carbon flow into the citrate cycle prompting energy storage [44]. Gut microbiota appears to play a key role in the development and progression of obesity, together with changes in citrate synthase activity [45, 46]. In this study, analysis of the results of whole microbial genome sequencing suggested that enrichment in the microbial function that

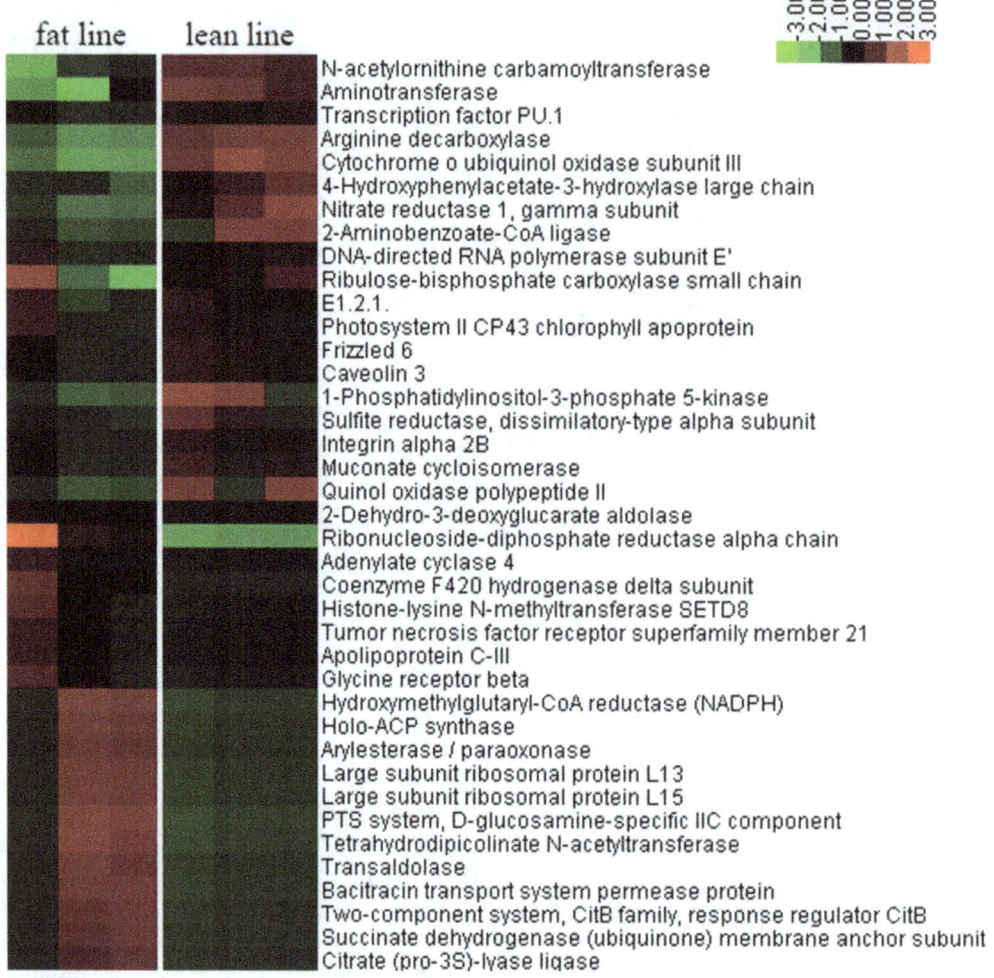

Fig. 4 Heatmap of microbial function pathways in the fat and lean lines. *Colors* reflect relative abundance from low (*green*) to high (*red*); detailed categories for each gene are in Table S5 [see Additional file 6: Table S5]

relates to citrate cycle was significantly different between the fat and lean lines (Fig. 4). We have reasons to believe that microbes undertake many metabolic tasks, and that functional interactions between host genetic factors and gut microbiota are inevitable.

Conclusions

We found that long-term divergent selection for abdominal fat has considerable influence on the abundance and composition of gut microbiota by altering the frequencies of obesity-related alleles. Furthermore, whole microbial genome sequencing results revealed that functional activities of the microbiota, such as those related to the citrate cycle and PPAR signaling pathway, differed significantly between the fat and lean lines and were affected by the gut microbiota and by differences in frequencies of host alleles. Our results provide further evidence for the hypothesis that host genetic factors interact and co-evolve with gut microbiota.

Additional files

Additional file 1: Table S1. Summary of sequencing data for all samples.

Additional file 2: Table S2. Numbers of taxa at each level.

Additional file 3: Figure S1. Alpha diversity of bacteria in the gut micro-biota of fat and lean lines. *Boxes* indicate the IQR (75th to 25th of the data). The median value is shown as a line within the *box* and the mean value as a *star*. Whiskers extend to the most extreme value within 1.5 * IQR. Outliers are shown as *crosses*. Higher chao1 suggests greater richness of microbes. Higher Shannon suggests greater diversity of microbes.

Additional file 4: Table S3. Comparison of microorganisms in the gut microbiota at the phylum level between the fat and lean lines. This table lists the relative fold change and *p* value of the differences in microorganisms at the phylum level between the fat and lean lines.

Additional file 5: Table S4. Comparison of microorganisms in the gut microbiota at the species level between the fat and lean lines. This table lists the relative fold change and *p* value of the differences in microorganisms in the gut microbiota at the species level between the fat and lean lines.

Additional file 6: Table S5. Corresponding metabolic pathways of the significant functions in the heatmap (related to Fig. 4). This table lists the corresponding metabolic pathways that are in Fig. 4.

Additional file 7. Prediction of microbial functions. This file describes the method for functional prediction based on 16S rDNA sequencing data.

Additional file 8: Figure S2. Predicted functional pathways in fat and lean lines based on 16S rDNA sequencing data.

Authors' contributions

JD, YZ and HM wrote the manuscript. JD and LZ performed statistical analysis and prepared the necessary scripts. JD, HZ, HL and HM conceived and designed the experimental procedure and supervised the study. LW, WZ, ZZ, LL, YW and CH participated in sample collection, DNA extraction, and data processing. All authors read and approved the final manuscript.

Author details

[1] Department of Animal Science, School of Agriculture and Biology, Shanghai Jiao Tong University, Shanghai Key Laboratory of Veterinary Biotechnology, Shanghai 200240, People's Republic of China. [2] College of Animal Science and Technology, Northeast Agricultural University, Harbin 150030, People's Republic of China. [3] College of Food Science and Engineering, Inner Mongolia Agricultural University, Key Laboratory of Dairy Biotechnology and Engineering, Hohhot 010018, People's Republic of China. [4] Shanghai Personal Biotechnology Limited Company, Shanghai 200231, People's Republic of China. [5] Shanghai Animal Disease Control Center, Shanghai 201103, People's Republic of China.

Acknowledgements
The authors would like to thank Christa F. Honaker for editing the manuscript.

Competing interests
The authors declare that they have no competing interests.

Funding
This study was supported by the National Science Foundation of China (Grant No. 31572384) and the National High Technology Research and Development Program of China (Grant No. 2011AA100901).

References

1. Waldor MK, Tyson G, Borenstein E, Ochman H, Moeller A, Finlay BB, et al. Where next for microbiome research? PLoS Biol. 2015;13:e1002050.
2. Turnbaugh PJ, Hamady M, Yatsunenko T, Cantarel BL, Duncan A, Ley RE, et al. A core gut microbiome in obese and lean twins. Nature. 2009;457:480–4.
3. Turnbaugh PJ, Gordon JI. The core gut microbiome, energy balance and obesity. J Physiol. 2009;587:4153–8.
4. Ley RE, Backhed F, Turnbaugh PJ, Lozupone CA, Knight RD, Gordon JI. Obesity alters gut microbial ecology. Proc Natl Acad Sci USA. 2005;102:11070–5.
5. Ley RE, Peterson DA, Gordon JI. Ecological and evolutionary forces shaping microbial diversity in the human intestine. Cell. 2006;124:837–48.
6. Benson AK, Kelly SA, Legge R, Ma F, Low SJ, Kim J, et al. Individuality in gut microbiota composition is a complex polygenic trait shaped by multiple environmental and host genetic factors. Proc Natl Acad Sci USA. 2010;107:18933–8.
7. Backhed F, Ding H, Wang T, Hooper LV, Koh GY, Nagy A, et al. The gut microbiota as an environmental factor that regulates fat storage. Proc Natl Acad Sci USA. 2004;101:15718–23.
8. Wolf G. Gut microbiota: a factor in energy regulation. Nutr Rev. 2006;64:47–50.
9. Simon J, Leclercq B. Longitudinal study of adiposity in chickens selected for high or low abdominal fat content: further evidence of a glucose-insulin imbalance in the fat line. J Nutr. 1982;112:1961–73.
10. Hermier D, Quignard-Boulangé A, Dugail I, Guy G, Salichon MR, Brigant L, et al. Evidence of enhanced storage capacity in adipose tissue of genetically fat chickens. J Nutr. 1989;119:1369–75.
11. Zhao LL, Wang G, Siegel P, He C, Wang H, Zhao WJ, et al. Quantitative genetic background of the host influences gut microbiomes in chickens. Sci Rep. 2013;3:1163.
12. Meng H, Zhang Y, Zhao LL, Zhao WJ, He C, Honaker CF, et al. Body weight selection affects quantitative genetic correlated responses in gut microbiota. PLoS One. 2014;9:e89862.
13. Turnbaugh PJ, Backhed F, Fulton L, Gordon JI. Diet-induced obesity is linked to marked but reversible alterations in the mouse distal gut microbiome. Cell Host Microbe. 2008;3:213–23.
14. Dominguez-Bello MG, Costello EK, Contreras M, Magris M, Hidalgo G, Fierer N, et al. Delivery mode shapes the acquisition and structure of the initial microbiota. Proc Natl Acad Sci USA. 2010;107:11971–5.
15. Guo L, Sun B, Shang Z, Leng L, Wang Y, Wang N, et al. Comparison of adipose tissue cellularity in chicken lines divergently selected for fatness. Poult Sci. 2011;90:2024–34.
16. Zhang H, Wang SZ, Wang ZP, Da Y, Wang N, Hu XX, et al. A genome-wide scan of selective sweeps in two broiler chicken lines divergently. BMC Genomics. 2012;13:704.
17. Wang HB, Li H, Wang QG, Zhang XY, Wang SZ, Wang YX, et al. Profiling of chicken adipose tissue gene expression by genome array. BMC Genomics. 2007;8:193.
18. Zhang H, Hu XX, Wang ZP, Zhang YD, Wang SZ, Wang N, et al. Selection signature analysis implicates the PC1/PCSK1 region for chicken abdominal fat content. PLoS One. 2012;7:e40736.
19. Meyer F, Paarmann D, D'Souza M, Olson R, Glass EM, Kubal M, et al. The metagenomics RAST server—a public resource for the automatic phylogenetic and functional analysis of metagenomes. BMC Bioinformatics. 2008;9:386.
20. Cole JR, Wang Q, Fish JA, Chai B, McGarrell DM, Sun Y, et al. Ribosomal database project: data and tools for high throughput rRNA analysis. Nucleic Acids Res. 2014;42:D633–42.
21. Benjamini Y, Hochberg Y. Controlling the false discovery rate: a practical and powerful approach to multiple testing. J R Stat Soc B. 1995;57:289–300.
22. Schloss PD, Westcott SL, Ryabin T, Hall JR, Hartmann M, Hollister EB, et al. Introducing mothur: open-source, platform-independent, community-supported. Appl Environ Microbiol. 2009;75:7537–41.
23. Kanehisa M, Goto S, Sato Y, Kawashima M, Furumichi M, Tanabe M. Data, information, knowledge and principle: back to metabolism in KEGG. Nucleic Acids Res. 2014;42:D199–205.
24. Saldanha AJ. Java Treeview—extensible visualization of microarray data. Bioinformatics. 2004;20:3246–8.

25. Parks DH, Beiko RG. Identifying biologically relevant differences between metagenomic communities. Bioinformatics. 2010;26:715–21.

26. Welch BL. The generalisation of student's problems when several different population variances are involved. Biometrika. 1947;34:28–35.

27. Lu J, Domingo JS. Turkey fecal microbial community structure and functional gene diversity revealed by 16S rRNA gene and metagenomic sequences. J Microbiol. 2008;46:469–77.

28. Danzeisen JL, Kim HB, Isaacson RE, Tu ZJ, Johnson TJ. Modulations of the chicken cecal microbiome and metagenome in response to anticoccidial and growth promoter treatment. PLoS One. 2011;6:e27949.

29. Waite DW, Taylor MW. Characterizing the avian gut microbiota: membership, driving influences, and potential function. Front Microbiol. 2014;5:223.

30. An Y, Xu W, Li H, Lei H, Zhang L, Hao F, et al. High-fat diet induces dynamic metabolic alterations in multiple biological matrices of rats. J Proteome Res. 2013;12:3755–68.

31. Turnbaugh PJ, Ley RE, Mahowald MA, Magrini V, Mardis ER, Gordon JI. An obesity-associated gut microbiome with increased capacity for energy harvest. Nature. 2006;444:1027–31.

32. Vinogradov E, Li J, Sadovskaya I, Jabbouri S, Helander I. The structure of the carbohydrate backbone of the lipopolysaccharide of pectinatus frisingensis strain VTT E-79104. Carbohydr Res. 2004;339:1637–42.

33. Guban J, Korver DR, Allison GE, Tannock GW. Relationship of dietary antimicrobial drug administration with broiler performance, decreased population levels of *Lactobacillus salivarius*, and reduced bile salt deconjugation in the ileum of broiler chickens. Poult Sci. 2006;85:2186–94.

34. Larsen N, Vogensen FK, Gobel RJ, Michaelsen KF, Forssten SD, Lahtinen SJ, et al. Effect of *Lactobacillus salivarius* Ls-33 on fecal microbiota in obese adolescents. Clin Nutr. 2013;32:935–40.

35. Coppola R, Iorizzo M, Saotta R, Sorrentino E, Grazia L. Characterization of micrococci and staphylococci isolated from soppressata molisana, a southern Italy fermented sausage. Food Microbiol. 1997;14:47–53.

36. Langille MGI, Zaneveld J, Caporaso JG, McDonald D, Knights D, Reyes JA, et al. Predictive functional profiling of microbial communities using 16S rRNA marker. Nat Biotechnol. 2013;31:814–21.

37. Shi H, Wang Q, Wang Y, Leng L, Zhang Q, Shang Z, et al. Adipocyte fatty acid-binding protein: an important gene related to lipid metabolism in chicken adipocytes. Comp Biochem Physiol B Biochem Mol Biol. 2010;157:357–63.

38. Wang L, Di LJ, Noguchi CT. AMPK is involved in mediation of erythropoietin influence on metabolic activity and reactive oxygen species production in white adipocytes. Int J Biochem Cell Biol. 2014;54:1–9.

39. Wang L, Di LJ. Wnt/β-catenin mediates AICAR effect to increase GATA3 expression and inhibit adipogenesis. J Biol Chem. 2015;290:29759.

40. Vidal-Puig AJ, Considine RV, Jimenez-Linan M, Werman A, Pories WJ, Caro JF, et al. Peroxisome proliferator-activated receptor gene expression in human tissues. Effects of obesity, weight loss, and regulation by insulin and glucocorticoids. J Clin Investig. 1997;99:2416–22.

41. Kersten S, Desvergne B, Wahli W. Roles of PPARs in health and disease. Nature. 2000;405:421–4.

42. Jiang X, Huang L, Xing D. Photoactivation of Dok1/ERK/PPAR gamma signaling axis inhibits excessive lipolysis in insulin-resistant adipocytes. Cell Signal. 2015;27:1265–75.

43. Christe M, Hirzel E, Lindinger A, Kern B, von Flüe M, Peterli R, et al. Obesity affects mitochondrial citrate synthase in human omental adipose tissue. ISRN Obes. 2013;2013:826027.

44. Cummins TD, Holden CR, Sansbury BE, Gibb AA, Shah J, Zafar N, et al. Metabolic remodeling of white adipose tissue in obesity. Am J Physiol Endocrinol Metab. 2014;307:E262–77.

45. Zadra G, Photopoulos C, Loda M. The fat side of prostate cancer. Biochim Biophys Acta. 2013;10:1518–32.

46. Ferramosca A, Conte A, Zara V. Krill oil ameliorates mitochondrial dysfunctions in rats treated with high-fat diet. Biomed Res Int. 2015;2015:645984.

7

Use of multi-trait and random regression models to identify genetic variation in tolerance to porcine reproductive and respiratory syndrome virus

Graham Lough[1†] [ID], Hamed Rashidi[2†], Ilias Kyriazakis[3], Jack C. M. Dekkers[4], Andrew Hess[4], Melanie Hess[4], Nader Deeb[5], Antti Kause[6], Joan K. Lunney[7], Raymond R. R. Rowland[8], Han A. Mulder[2†] and Andrea Doeschl-Wilson[1*†]

Abstract

Background: A host can adopt two response strategies to infection: resistance (reduce pathogen load) and tolerance (minimize impact of infection on performance). Both strategies may be under genetic control and could thus be targeted for genetic improvement. Although there is evidence that supports a genetic basis for resistance to porcine reproductive and respiratory syndrome (PRRS), it is not known whether pigs also differ genetically in tolerance. We determined to what extent pigs that have been shown to vary genetically in resistance to PRRS also exhibit genetic variation in tolerance. Multi-trait linear mixed models and random regression sire models were fitted to PRRS Host Genetics Consortium data from 1320 weaned pigs (offspring of 54 sires) that were experimentally infected with a virulent strain of PRRS virus to obtain genetic parameter estimates for resistance and tolerance. Resistance was defined as the inverse of within-host viral load (VL) from 0 to 21 (VL_{21}) or 0 to 42 (VL_{42}) days post-infection and tolerance as the slope of the reaction-norm of average daily gain (ADG_{21}, ADG_{42}) on VL_{21} or VL_{42}.

Results: Multi-trait analysis of ADG associated with either low or high VL was not indicative of genetic variation in tolerance. Similarly, random regression models for ADG_{21} and ADG_{42} with a tolerance slope fitted for each sire did not result in a better fit to the data than a model without genetic variation in tolerance. However, the distribution of data around average VL suggested possible confounding between level and slope estimates of the regression lines. Augmenting the data with simulated growth rates of non-infected half-sibs (ADG_0) helped resolve this statistical confounding and indicated that genetic variation in tolerance to PRRS may exist if genetic correlations between ADG_0 and ADG_{21} or ADG_{42} are low to moderate.

Conclusions: Evidence for genetic variation in tolerance of pigs to PRRS was weak when based on data from infected piglets only. However, simulations indicated that genetic variance in tolerance may exist and could be detected if comparable data on uninfected relatives were available. In conclusion, of the two defense strategies, genetics of tolerance is more difficult to elucidate than genetics of resistance.

*Correspondence: andrea.wilson@roslin.ed.ac.uk
†Graham Lough and Hamed Rashidi are equal first authors
‡Han A. Mulder and Andrea Doeschl-Wilson are equal last authors
[1] The Roslin Institute & R(D)SVS, University of Edinburgh, Edinburgh, Midlothian, UK
Full list of author information is available at the end of the article

Background

Infectious challenges in domestic livestock do not only raise health and welfare concerns, but also have detrimental effects on livestock production. The impact of infections on an animal's productive performance is controlled by two alternative (albeit not mutually exclusive) host traits that may be amenable to genetic improvement: resistance and tolerance. Resistance is defined as the ability of a host to prevent pathogen entry or inhibit replication of the pathogen, whereas tolerance refers to the ability of a host to limit the impact of infection on health or performance without interfering with the pathogen life-cycle per se [1]. Thus, animals with greater resistance are expected to harbor fewer pathogens that can lead to loss in performance. In contrast, animals with greater tolerance may harbor a high within-host pathogen load but are able to prevent or repair the damage of infection on health and performance [2, 3]. To date, most efforts to control infectious disease have targeted primarily improvement of host resistance. More recently, the focus has expanded towards boosting host tolerance as an alternative means to counteract the detrimental impact of infection on health and performance [4, 5]. However, little is known about the extent to which tolerance is genetically controlled and thus suitable for genetic improvement.

Porcine reproductive and respiratory syndrome (PRRS) is an endemic virus, which causes one of the most devastating swine diseases worldwide. PRRS causes considerable reduction in the growth rate of piglets, with estimates ranging from 10 to 20%, depending on pig breed and virus strain [6], and results in production losses amounting to an annual cost of $493.57 million to the U.S. swine industry alone [7]. Since vaccination has been largely unsuccessful [8], genetic solutions to PRRS have gained increased attention [9–11]. Recent large-scale PRRSV challenge studies carried out by the PRRS Host Genetics Consortium (PHGC) have demonstrated considerable genetic variation in resistance of pigs to PRRSV (virus) infection, as well as in weight gain of infected piglets [10, 12, 13]. Furthermore, genetic correlations between resistance and weight gain were shown to be positive and strong (ranging from 0.57 to 0.75 for two different PRRSV strains) [10], indicating that selection for improved resistance is expected to simultaneously improve growth under infection and vice versa. However, it is not currently known whether pigs also differ genetically in their tolerance to PRRSV infection, or whether pigs with greater genetic resistance to PRRSV are also genetically more tolerant to PRRS.

Resistance can be measured as the inverse of within-host pathogen load, whereas tolerance is related to the degree to which performance is reduced by infectious

pathogens. Tolerance is mathematically defined as a reaction-norm of performance with respect to pathogen load [2, 14]. Assuming a linear relationship, reaction-norms can be modelled by a linear regression of performance against pathogen load, where the regression slope provides a measure of tolerance (Fig. 1). Thus, a slope of 0 indicates complete tolerance, while a more negative slope indicates lower tolerance. Statistically significant differences in reaction-norm slopes associated with, e.g., different breeds or families are indicative of genetic variation in tolerance. For outbred populations, tolerance slopes for groups of related individuals can be estimated by random regression models, which provide estimates for genetic variance of tolerance and for genetic variance in host performance as a function of pathogen load when combined with pedigree or genomic information [15]. However, due to the large amount of data required to obtain unbiased variance estimates for reaction norm slopes [15–17], very few studies have applied this methodology to gain insight into the genetic basis of tolerance in outbred populations [18]. The PRRS Host Genetics Consortium (PHGC) data, which provide simultaneous measures of growth and viral load for over 1500 pedigreed pigs infected with the same PRRS virus load offer a unique opportunity to estimate genetic parameters for tolerance.

The main aim of this study was to determine whether pigs that were previously found to differ genetically in resistance to a virulent strain of PRRSV also differ genetically in tolerance. Furthermore, by augmenting the data with simulated data, novel insights into data requirements to accurately estimate genetic variance in tolerance using random regression models were obtained.

Methods
Infection experiment and data

Data were provided by the PRRS Host Genetics Consortium (PHGC) from nine different PRRSV challenge trials with an identical infection protocol [9, 10], which included 1569 pigs supplied by various commercial breeding companies, as outlined in Table 1.

All experimental protocols for these trials were approved by the Kansas State University Institutional Animal Care and Use Committee. In each trial, approximately 200 commercial crossbred piglets were transferred from high health farms at weaning age (mean age = 26 days, range = 17 to 32 days) to a research facility at Kansas State University. The source farms were controlled and found to be free of PRRSV, *Mycoplasma hyopneumoniae*, and swine influenza virus. Pigs were randomly placed in pens of 10 to 15 individuals. Following a 7-day acclimation period, pigs between 17 and 32 days of age were experimentally infected both

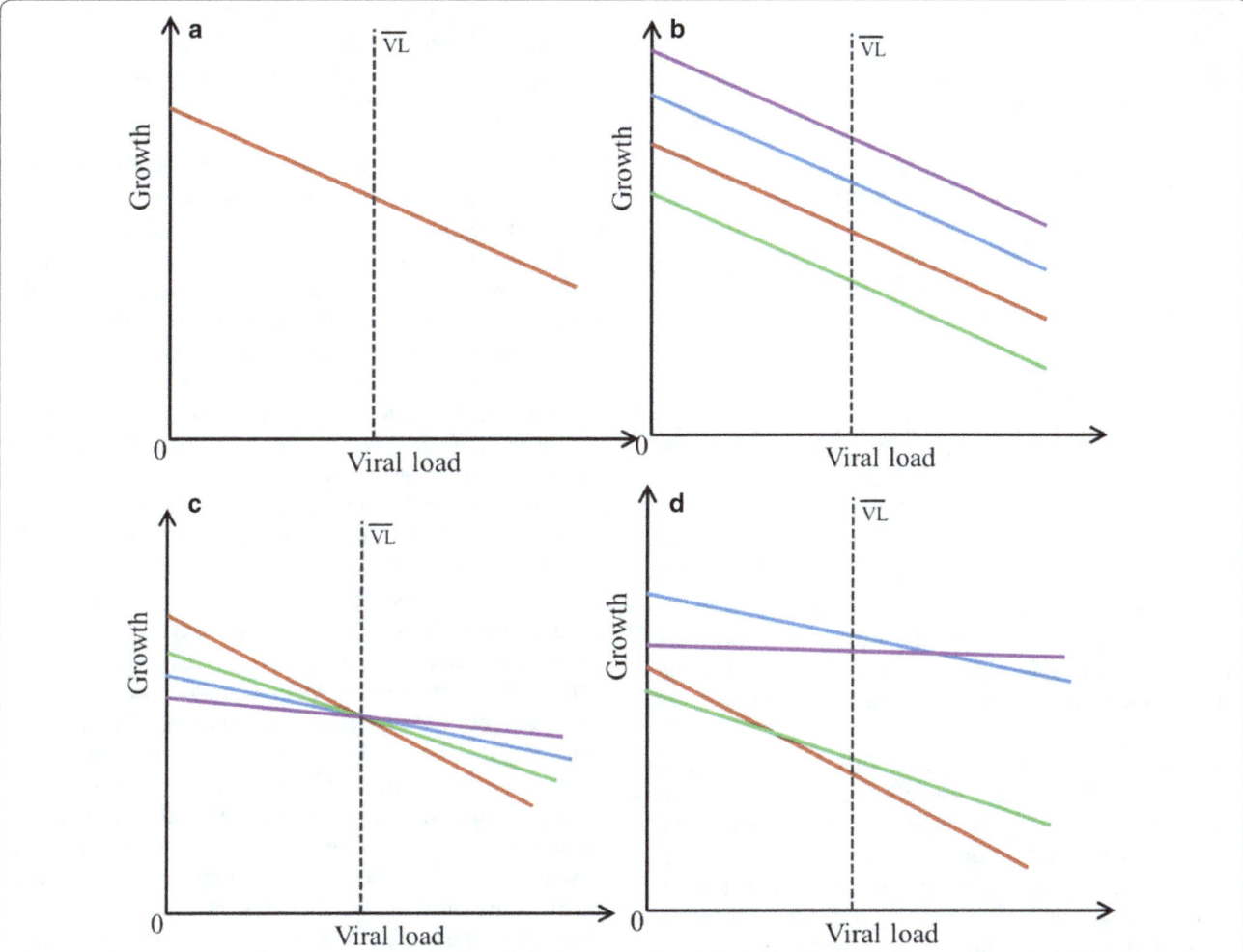

Fig. 1 Graphical illustration of reaction norms for analysis of tolerance. Mean VL is indicated by the *stippled line* in each graph. Each line corresponds to one of four hypothetical sires. **a** Null model, where all sires have equal tolerance and equal overall growth level. As such, there is only one (average) tolerance slope. **b** Reaction-norms of sires with equal tolerance. Sires differ in intercept (growth where VL = 0) and level (growth at mean VL), but have equal tolerance slopes. No re-ranking of sires occurs between growth associated with low and high VL, and genetic correlation between intercept and level is 1.00. **c** Reaction norms of sires with variation in intercept and tolerance slopes, but no variation in level. Re-ranking of sires occurs depending on whether offspring harbor low or high VL, respectively, as indicated by crossing over of lines before and after mean VL. **d** Reaction norms of sires where variation occurs at intercept, level and tolerance slope. Sire re-ranking occurs between low and high VL, and genetic correlation between intercept and level is below one

intramuscularly and intranasally with 10^5 (TCID50) of NVSL-97-7985, a highly virulent PRRSV isolate [19]. Body weight (BW) and blood samples were collected at 0, 7, 14, 21, 28, 35 and 42 days-post-infection (dpi). Pigs were then euthanized at 42 dpi and ear notches were collected for genotyping. Trials 7 and 8 were terminated at 35 dpi because of facility availability. Estimates for average daily gain (ADG) from 0 dpi until day of measurement were obtained by dividing the difference in body weight between the day of observation and 0 dpi by the corresponding time period. Note that neither measurements of ADG for these pigs prior to infection, nor ADG measurements for non-infected relatives were available.

Serum viremia, which was measured by using a semi-quantitative TaqMan PCR assay for PRRSV RNA, provided repeated (bi-weekly up to 14 dpi, then weekly) measures for $\log_{10}$-transformed qPCR viremia, as described in Boddicker et al. [12, 13, 20]. Mathematical functions were previously fitted to these $\log_{10}$-transformed viremia measures to smooth the data and to obtain continuous viremia estimates over the 42-day observation period [21]. As outlined in Islam et al. [21], the uni-modal Woods function and the extended bi-modal Woods function provided a good fit to the individual's data with either uni-modal $(y(t) = a_1 t^{b_1} e^{-c_1 t})$ (~67%) or bi-modal

Table 1 Animal, pedigree and breed composition of the PHGC trials

Trial	Number of animals	Number of sires	Number of dams	Breed cross
1	174	6	70	LW × LR
2	164	10	72	LW × LR
3	115	7	47	LW × LR
4	191	6	33	Duroc × LW/LR
5	182	10	38	Duroc × LR/LW
6	109	26	53	LR × LR
7	186	6	27	Pietrain × LW/LR
8	158	15	43	Duroc × LW/LR
15	166	11	49	Pietrain × LW

LW large white breed, *LR* landrace breed

$$\left(y(t) = a_1 t^{b_1} e^{-c_1 t} + \max\left(0, a_2(t - t_0)^{b_2} e^{-c_2}(t - t_0)\right)\right)$$

(~33%) viremia profiles, respectively, with strong correlations between model predictions of VL and actual viremia measures (genetic and phenotypic correlation estimates were 0.98 ± 0.03 and 0.90 ± 0.01, respectively) [10].

Across all trials, 198 pigs died before 42 dpi. PRRS was identified as the primary cause of mortality, except for trial 6, for which mortality was higher (46% by 42 dpi) and was potentially caused by secondary bacterial infections [13]. These pigs were included in the analyses until their time of death.

Only offspring from sires with more than 10 progeny with phenotypes were considered in this study to reduce the risk of bias in tolerance estimates [15]. As such, the number of animals included was 1320 from 0 to 21 dpi and 1001 from 0 to 42 dpi, all originating from 54 sires.

Pedigree information and genomic information using genotypes from Illumina's Porcine SNP60 Beadchip v.1 [22], was available for all pigs. The pedigree-based numerator relationship matrix (**A**) and genomic relationship **G**-matrix (**G**$_m$), were constructed in ASReml 3.0 [23] using the VanRaden method for all animals used in the analysis. For the **G**-matrix, single nucleotide polymorphisms (SNPs) that were fixed in a trial were removed. Trials 1, 2, and 3 had the most extensive pedigree information, with pedigree data up to two generations back, while the rest of the trials only had sire and dam recorded. As such, there were no relationships between animals in different trials, except for trials 1, 2, and 3, which consisted of animals from consecutive parities of the same breeding company (Table 1). Pedigree was corrected using parental genotypes for all trials, as described by Boddicker et al. [13] and Hess et al. [10]. The **G**-matrix was constructed using the VanRaden method [24], and

included relationships between animals across trials regardless of breed, as outlined by Hess et al. [10]. The **A**-matrix was used for all the following statistical models, unless otherwise noted.

Resistance, tolerance, and performance without infection

Resistance is often quantified by a measure of within-host pathogen load, whereby lower pathogen load reflects higher host resistance [2, 5, 16]. In this study, resistance to PRRS was defined as the inverse of serum viral load, whereby VL$_{42}$ represents the cumulative log-transformed viral load from 0 to 42 dpi from the Wood's curve. Since viremia had decreased to undetectable levels within 21 to 28 dpi for a large proportion of pigs, cumulative viral load (and thus resistance) was not only calculated for the entire observation period from 0 to 42 dpi, but also for the period from 0 to 21 dpi. This represents the acute phase of infection and yields two indicator traits for resistance (VL$_{21}$ and VL$_{42}$).

In this study, tolerance was assessed by regressing performance measures (i.e. ADG$_{21}$ or ADG$_{42}$ on the y-axis) on pathogen load (i.e. VL$_{21}$ or VL$_{42}$, respectively on the x-axis). The regression of ADG$_{42}$ on VL$_{21}$ was also evaluated to account for the possibility of a time-lag in growth response with respect to changes in pathogen load.

Growth performance of an infected individual is likely to depend on both their response to infection and performance in the absence of infection. Performance in absence of infection (i.e. when pathogen load is equal to zero), commonly denoted in the tolerance literature as vigor [25], constitutes the intercept of the linear reaction-norms (Fig. 1). Previous simulation studies indicated that performance measures in the absence of infection are important to obtain unbiased tolerance slope estimates [15]. However, information on performance of the PRRSV challenged pigs in absence of infection was not available in this study.

Two approaches were adopted to overcome this lack of performance measures without infection. (1) In line with the standard approach of quantitative genetic studies of reaction-norms, the origin of the explanatory variable VL was shifted to the mean VL; this 'shifted intercept' for ADG is referred to as the 'level', in contrast to vigor [17, 26, 27] (Fig. 1); note that this approach does not provide accurate information about the genetic relationship between tolerance and vigor, as the genetic correlation between level and slope is not equal to the genetic correlation between performance at VL = 0 and slope [28, 29]. Furthermore, individual body weight at the start of the infection (BW$_0$) was included as a fixed covariate in the corresponding statistical models to partially account for differences in vigor. (2) To gain better insight into data requirements for accurately estimating genetic parameters for tolerance, and about how these estimates depend on the genetic relationship between growth in absence or presence of infection, growth records of infected pigs were augmented with simulated growth records of non-infected half-siblings, as outlined in step 4 below.

Statistical analyses

All statistical analyses were carried out using ASReml 3.0 [23]. Random regression reaction-norm models have been found to provide biased estimates if data requirements to disentangle intercept from slope are not met [15, 17, 30], thus a stepwise approach was adopted: (Step 1) multi-trait animal models were used to estimate the genetic relationship between resistance and growth under infection; (Step 2) multi-trait models were used to provide evidence for genetic variation in tolerance of pigs to PRRS based on the genetic correlation between growth associated with low and high VL, respectively; (Step 3) a univariate random regression model was applied to obtain estimates for genetic variance in tolerance; and (Step 4) data were augmented using simulated performance in the absence of infection (ADG_{21}^0 or ADG_{42}^0), with increasing simulated genetic correlation from weak to strong between ADG_{21}^0 and ADG_{21} or ADG_{42}^0 and ADG_{42}, respectively. The random regression models from Step 3 were adapted to include variation in ADG_{21}^0 or ADG_{42}^0.

Step 1: multi-trait models to estimate the genetic relationship between resistance and performance prior to and post infection

Our first step in analyzing variation in growth under infection was to estimate heritabilities and correlations between VL and growth in absence of and post-infection with PRRSV using the following trivariate animal model:

$$
\begin{bmatrix} \mathbf{y}_1 \\ \mathbf{y}_2 \\ \mathbf{y}_3 \end{bmatrix} = \begin{bmatrix} \mathbf{X}_1 & 0 & 0 \\ 0 & \mathbf{X}_2 & 0 \\ 0 & 0 & \mathbf{X}_3 \end{bmatrix} \begin{bmatrix} \mathbf{b}_1 \\ \mathbf{b}_2 \\ \mathbf{b}_3 \end{bmatrix} + \begin{bmatrix} \mathbf{Z}_1 & 0 & 0 \\ 0 & \mathbf{Z}_2 & 0 \\ 0 & 0 & \mathbf{Z}_3 \end{bmatrix} \begin{bmatrix} \mathbf{a}_1 \\ \mathbf{a}_2 \\ \mathbf{a}_3 \end{bmatrix}
$$
$$
+ \begin{bmatrix} \mathbf{U}_1 & 0 & 0 \\ 0 & \mathbf{U}_2 & 0 \\ 0 & 0 & \mathbf{U}_3 \end{bmatrix} \begin{bmatrix} \mathbf{p}_1 \\ \mathbf{p}_2 \\ \mathbf{p}_3 \end{bmatrix}
$$
$$
+ \begin{bmatrix} \mathbf{M}_1 & 0 & 0 \\ 0 & \mathbf{M}_2 & 0 \\ 0 & 0 & \mathbf{M}_3 \end{bmatrix} \begin{bmatrix} \mathbf{l}_1 \\ \mathbf{l}_2 \\ \mathbf{l}_3 \end{bmatrix} + \begin{bmatrix} \mathbf{e}_1 \\ \mathbf{e}_2 \\ \mathbf{e}_3 \end{bmatrix}, \quad (1)
$$

where $\mathbf{y}_1$, $\mathbf{y}_2$ and $\mathbf{y}_3$ are vectors of phenotypes for body weight at the start of infection (BW_0) ($\mathbf{y}_1$), ADG_{21} or ADG_{42} ($\mathbf{y}_2$), and VL_{21} or VL_{42} ($\mathbf{y}_3$), respectively; $\mathbf{b}_1$, $\mathbf{b}_2$ and $\mathbf{b}_3$ are the vectors of the fixed effects for the interaction of experimental trial and parity of the dam when offspring were born (trial-by-parity), sex of the offspring, and age

at start of experimental infection, which was fitted as a fixed covariate. Note that no breed effect was included in the model since trial and breed effects were fully confounded in this experiment. To account for differences between viremia profiles and the two mathematical functions used to fit these, a binary variable associated with the viremia profile class (uni- or bi-modal) was also fitted as fixed effect; $\mathbf{a}_1$, $\mathbf{a}_2$ and $\mathbf{a}_3$ are vectors of additive genetic effects for each trait, with $\text{Var} \begin{bmatrix} \mathbf{a}_1 \\ \mathbf{a}_2 \\ \mathbf{a}_3 \end{bmatrix} = \mathbf{G} \otimes \mathbf{A}$,

where $\mathbf{G}$ is the genetic variance–covariance matrix and $\mathbf{A}$ the pedigree relationship matrix; $\mathbf{p}_1$, $\mathbf{p}_2$ and $\mathbf{p}_3$ are vectors of pen effects nested within a trial for each trait, with $\text{Var} \begin{bmatrix} \mathbf{p}_1 \\ \mathbf{p}_2 \\ \mathbf{p}_3 \end{bmatrix} = \mathbf{I} \otimes \mathbf{K}$, where $\mathbf{I}$ is the identity matrix and $\mathbf{K}$ is the corresponding variance–covariance matrix of pen effects for the different traits; $\mathbf{l}_1$, $\mathbf{l}_2$ and $\mathbf{l}_3$ are the vectors of litter effects for each trait, with $\text{Var} \begin{bmatrix} \mathbf{l}_1 \\ \mathbf{l}_2 \\ \mathbf{l}_3 \end{bmatrix} = \mathbf{I} \otimes \mathbf{L}$, with the corresponding variance–covariance matrix $\mathbf{L}$; $\mathbf{e}_1$, $\mathbf{e}_2$ and $\mathbf{e}_3$ are the vectors of error terms for each trait, with $\text{Var} \begin{bmatrix} \mathbf{e}_1 \\ \mathbf{e}_2 \\ \mathbf{e}_3 \end{bmatrix} = \mathbf{I} \otimes \mathbf{R}$, where $\mathbf{R}$ is the variance–covariance matrix for the residual effects for each trait; and $\mathbf{X}_1$, $\mathbf{X}_2$ and $\mathbf{X}_3$, $\mathbf{Z}_1$, $\mathbf{Z}_2$ and $\mathbf{Z}_3$, $\mathbf{U}_1$, $\mathbf{U}_2$ and $\mathbf{U}_3$, and $\mathbf{M}_1$, $\mathbf{M}_2$ and $\mathbf{M}_3$ are the incidence matrices for the fixed, animal, pen and litter effects, respectively. In addition to the trivariate animal model, corresponding bivariate and univariate models were also used to check the robustness of variance components. Since heritability estimates differed between models, heritability estimates were presented from the corresponding univariate models.

Step 2: multi-trait models to examine evidence for genetic variation in tolerance—growth associated with low versus high VL

The trivariate model (1) from step 1 does not show how growth changes with respect to viral load, and, therefore, does not account for genetic variance in tolerance. A multi-trait sire model for ADG of progeny with categorized VL was used to assess sire-by-VL interactions to get a first indication of whether sires varied genetically in tolerance to infection. If these genetic correlations are less than 1, this is indicative of sire rank changes when offspring are faced with low and high VL respectively, and provides evidence for genetic variation in tolerance slope. Hence, individuals were sorted according to their VL from 0 to 21 dpi or 0 to 42 dpi, and partitioned into VL groups, where the low and high VL groups (n = 330 each) consisted of individuals with VL values in the lower and upper quartiles, respectively, and the mid-range group consisted of the middle half of the data (n = 660). A trivariate sire model was then fitted to measures of ADG associated with low, mid and high VL from 0 to 21/0 to 42 dpi (ADG_{low}, ADG_{mid} and ADG_{high}), respectively. The fixed and random effects of this model were identical to those used in model (1), with exception of a, which now refers to sire effects on performance and explains one quarter of the additive genetic variance, and of e, where residual covariance was fixed at 0, because offspring have only a single record of ADG and therefore the residual covariance does not exist. Furthermore, the pedigree relationship A-matrix was replaced with the genomic relationship matrix (G-matrix) to improve convergence.

Step 3: univariate random regression sire models for estimating genetic variance in tolerance

The multi-trait models in the previous steps provide evidence for genetic variation in tolerance but do not yield direct estimates of genetic variance in tolerance. A random regression reaction norm model was applied, whereby the origin of the reaction-norms was centered at the mean viral load values, thus providing only variance component estimates for level (ADG at mean VL) rather than vigor (ADG at zero VL). The following linear random regression sire model (RRM) for ADG on centered values of VL, which will be referred to as the level-slope model (as shown in Fig. 1d), was used:

$$\mathbf{y} = \mathbf{Xb} + \mathbf{X}_{VL}\mathbf{b_s} + \mathbf{Za_i} + \mathbf{Z}_{VL}\mathbf{a_s} + \mathbf{Up} + \mathbf{Ml} + \mathbf{e}, \quad (2)$$

where $\mathbf{y}$ is the vector of ADG_{21} or ADG_{42}, respectively; $\mathbf{b}$ is the vector of fixed effects outlined in model (1), with age and BW_0 included as additional fixed covariates to account for variation in age and body weight at the start of infection; and $\mathbf{b}_s$ is the population average tolerance slope; $\mathbf{a}_i$ and $\mathbf{a}_s$ are the sire effects on level and on tolerance slope, respectively, assumed to follow a multi-variate normal distribution with mean zero and

$$\mathrm{Var}\begin{bmatrix} \mathbf{a_i} \\ \mathbf{a_s} \end{bmatrix} = \tfrac{1}{4}\mathbf{G}_{RN} \otimes \mathbf{A}, \text{ with } \mathbf{G}_{RN} = \begin{bmatrix} \sigma^2_{a_i} & \sigma_{a_i a_s} \\ \sigma_{a_i a_s} & \sigma^2_{a_s} \end{bmatrix}, \text{ where}$$

$\sigma^2_{a_i}$ and $\sigma^2_{a_s}$ are the variances of a_i, and a_s, respectively, $\sigma_{a_i a_s}$ is the covariance between sire effects for level and slope; other random effects $\mathbf{p}$, $\mathbf{l}$, and $\mathbf{e}$ were fitted as described in model (1); $\mathbf{X}_{VL}$ and $\mathbf{Z}_{VL}$ are the incidence matrices for population average tolerance slope and those associated with each sire, respectively, consisting of individual VL measures, and $\mathbf{X}$ is the incidence matrix for the fixed effects (including VL as fixed covariate) and $\mathbf{Z}$ is the incidence matrix for the random sire effect on level (Z).

To test the significance of sire effects on level and slope and to determine which of the models illustrated in Fig. 1

best described the data, the model fit of the level-slope model (2) was compared with that of hierarchical models: (a) without any additive genetic effects (Fig. 1a), (b) with only sire effects for level (Fig. 1b), and (c) containing only sire effects on slope (Fig. 1c). Significance of each random effect was assessed using the likelihood ratio test (LRT) [31], with the LRT test statistics below assumed to follow a χ^2 distribution, with 1 degree of freedom for inclusion of an additional sire effect (e.g. null to level model, including sire effect) and a mixture of 1 and 2 degrees of freedom for additional sire slope effects and covariance (for example, from level to level-slope model) [32, 33].

Step 4: random regression model using simulated performance in absence of infection for estimating genetic variance in tolerance

The random regression models fitted in Step 3 generated potential confounding between level and tolerance slope variance estimates i.e. genetic variance in slope was absorbed by genetic variance in level due to the limited distribution of VL around average VL required to estimate the genetic variance in level. To assess whether confounding could be resolved by inclusion of performance measures of non-infected relatives in the statistical models, growth in the absence of infection (ADG^0_{21} or ADG^0_{42}) was simulated for one hypothetical paternal half-sib for each individual with ADG_{21} and ADG_{42} records, respectively, thus doubling the size of the dataset. Data were simulated assuming a heritability of 0.4 for both ADG^0_{21} and ADG^0_{42} [34]. With the expectation that a higher r_g between the traits would imply less genetic variance in tolerance, low (0.05), moderate (0.30), strong (0.60) or high (0.90) genetic correlations (r_g) between ADG^0_{21} and ADG_{21}, or ADG^0_{42} and ADG_{42}, respectively, were simulated (see Additional file 1 for a detailed description of the simulations). Note that no assumptions were made with regards to genetic variance in tolerance. Ten thousand replicates of simulated half-sib records for ADG^0_{21} and ADG^0_{42} were generated.

The random regression models (2) were then applied to the extended datasets for each replicate, where the response vector $\mathbf{y}$ now comprised either simulated ADG^0_{21} and measured ADG_{21}, or ADG^0_{42} and ADG_{42}. VL was no longer centered at mean VL, but comprised VL equal to zero for the non-infected pigs and VL_{21} or VL_{42} for the infected pigs. The remaining fixed and random effects were identical to those in model (2), except that no fixed effects or random pen or litter effects were fitted for the simulated half-sibs. Thus, by including simulated data of non-infected pigs, model (2) was replaced by an intercept-slope model, with genetic variance estimated for growth in the absence of infection, and for tolerance slope.

As in Step 3, hierarchical models were fitted (a) without any additive genetic effects for intercept or slope (Fig. 1a, null model), and (b) with additive genetic effects for intercept only (Fig. 1b, intercept-only model) and (c) with additive genetic effects for intercept and slope (Fig. 1d, intercept-slope model). The model fit was assessed using the loglikelihood ratio test outlined in Step 3 above. Results were evaluated based on the mean and standard deviation of the estimates over replicates.

Results

Step 1: relationship between resistance and performance prior to and post infection

ADG_{21} and ADG_{42} ranged from a weight loss of 40 g/day to a weight gain of 720 and 680 g/day, respectively, with corresponding mean daily weight gains of 280 and 380 g/day (Table 2).

Table 2 Summary statistics of resistance and growth traits

Trait	Mean	SD	Min	Max	Number of records
BW_0 (kg)	7.30	1.39	3.45	12.88	1320
ADG_{21} (kg/day)	0.28	0.12	−0.04	0.72	1319
ADG_{42} (kg/day)	0.38	0.11	−0.04	0.68	1001
VL_{21} (AUC)	115.69	9.37	77.04	153.62	1320
VL_{42} (AUC)	159.90	23.42	88.00	236.35	1001

Body weight at 0 dpi (BW_0), average daily gain and viral load from 0 to 21 and 0 to 42 dpi (ADG_{21}, ADG_{42}, VL_{21} and VL_{42}), respectively

AUC is the area under the curve for the log-transformed estimates for viral load in blood as measured by RT-PCR

Figure 2 depicts the distributions of growth and VL for the two observation periods between 0 to 21 dpi and 0 to 42 dpi. The wide distribution of individuals with above average growth rate in spite of high VL (ADG^+VL^+), and with low growth rate in spite of low VL (ADG^-VL^-) may be indicative of phenotypic variation in tolerance.

Growth rate under infection and resistance were moderately heritable and had large standard errors (Table 3). Heritability estimates were similar for the two time periods considered.

Although standard errors were high, genetic correlations between VL and growth under infection were statistically significantly different from 1 ($p < 0.001$, based on the LRT that compares models with and without genetic correlations fixed to 1), indicating that not all genetic variation of growth under infection was explained by genetic differences in resistance (inverse of VL) (Table 3). Furthermore, genetic correlations between growth under infection and BW_0 were also significantly different from 1, implying that growth prior to and post infection were not under identical genetic regulation. Genetic correlations between growth under infection and VL were moderate to strong and negative whereas genetic correlations between growth under infection and BW_0 were moderately positive. Phenotypic correlations were of the same sign but generally weaker than the genetic correlations (Table 3). Phenotypically and genetically, these results indicate that pigs with greater resistance tend to grow faster.

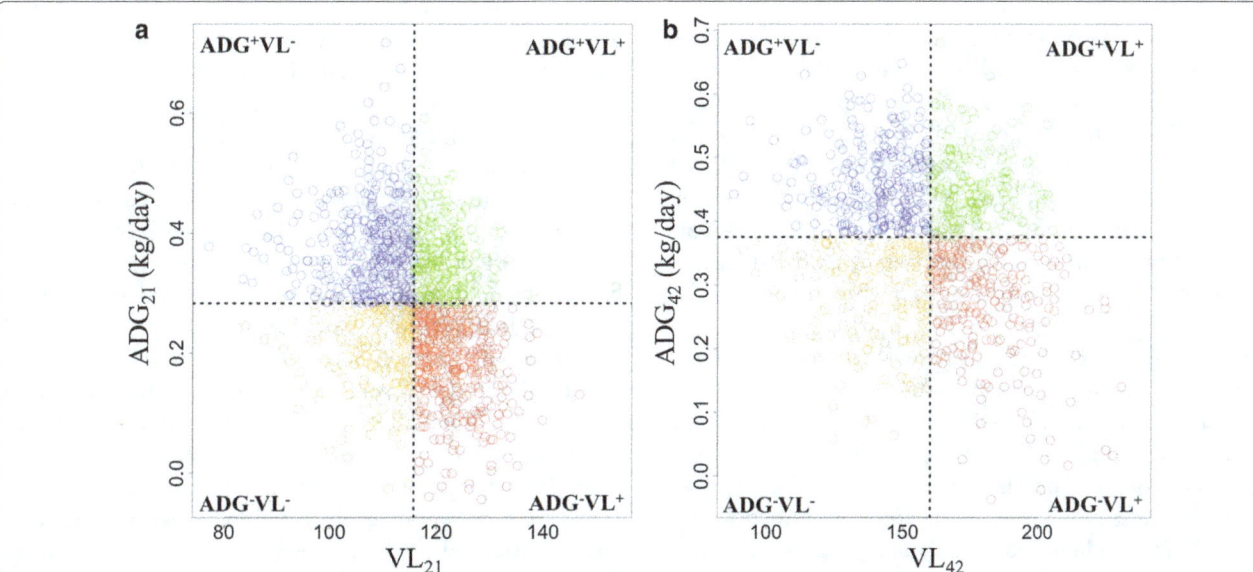

Fig. 2 Scatter plots of data for ADG and VL from **a** 0 to 21 and **b** 0 to 42 dpi. ADG and VL from 0 to 21 and 0 to 42 dpi (n = 1320 and 1001, respectively) were distributed into one of four quadrants according to their growth and VL after infection with PRRS virus (n = 330 and 250 in each quadrant for 0 to 21 and 0 to 42 dpi, respectively). The quadrants (ADG^+VL^- blue, ADG^+VL^+ green, ADG^-VL^- orange, and ADG^-VL^+ red) refer to high growth rate and high resistance (low VL), high growth rate and low resistance (high VL), low growth rate and high resistance and low growth rate and high low, respectively. Quadrants were centered at mean VL and at mean ADG

Table 3 **Estimates of heritability and correlations between resistance and growth traits**

Trait	Trait				
	BW_0	ADG_{21}	ADG_{42}	VL_{21}	VL_{42}
BW_0	*0.11 (0.10)*	0.35 (0.03)	0.40 (0.03)	−0.21 (0.07)	−0.20 (0.03)
ADG_{21}	0.48 (0.30)	*0.29 (0.11)*	0.80 (0.01)	−0.29 (0.03)	–
ADG_{42}	0.24 (0.45)	1.00 (0.04)	*0.34 (0.14)*	−0.33 (0.03)	−0.36 (0.03)
VL_{21}	−0.33 (0.45)	−0.53 (0.27)	−0.64 (0.26)	*0.19 (0.11)*	0.80 (0.01)
VL_{42}	−0.54 (0.37)	–	−0.82 (0.16)	0.79 (0.14)	*0.18 (0.10)*

Heritability estimates (diagonal) and phenotypic (upper triangle) and genetic correlations (lower triangle) with standard errors (SE) from the trivariate animal model for body weight at 0 dpi (BW_0), average daily gain and viral load from 0 to 21 and 0 to 42 dpi (ADG_{21}, ADG_{42}, VL_{21} and VL_{42}), respectively

Correlations between ADG_{21} and VL_{42} were not calculated, since VL is expected to impact ADG and not the other way around

Step 2: multi-trait models to examine evidence for genetic variation in tolerance

Trivariate models for growth at low, mid and high VL failed to converge for both time periods of infection. Using bivariate models for the upper and lower quartiles for VL, high genetic correlations of 0.94 (0.18) and 0.91 (0.13) between growth associated with low to high VL were identified for ADG_{21} and ADG_{42}, respectively. Genetic correlations significantly less than 1 would imply that growth rates associated with different degrees of infection severity, as indicated by low versus high VL, are genetically distinct traits and would thus be indicative of genetic variation in tolerance (Fig. 1). Genetic correlations close to 1 indicate limited reranking among sires between high and low levels of VL and, thus limited genetic variance in tolerance. Furthermore, there was no significant difference between genetic variances of ADG associated with low and high VL, for either the 0 to 21 and 0 to 42 day period (where genetic variances for ADG associated with low and high VL were $2.10E^{-03}$ ($1.22E^{-03}$) and $4.56E^{-03}$ ($1.81E^{03}$) for 0 to 21 dpi, and $3.46E^{-03}$ ($1.24E^{-03}$) and $6.89E^{-03}$ ($2.18E^{-03}$) for 0 to 42 dpi, respectively). Referring to the expectations outlined in Fig. 1, the results of this multi-trait model imply that random regression models of Step 3 with the same tolerance slope for each sire would provide a better fit to the data than models with different slopes for each sire (Fig. 1c, d).

Step 3: estimation of genetic variance in tolerance using univariate random regression models

Univariate random regression models without genetic effects, but including VL as a fixed linear (and higher order polynomial) covariate were used to test the average association between growth and VL (null model in Table 4). These identified a statistically significant linear association between growth and VL ($p < 0.0001$), with a population average tolerance slope estimate of $-2.78E^{-03}$ ($3.32E^{-04}$) and $-1.28E^{-03}$ ($1.51E^{-04}$) kg/day per unit of VL increase for ADG_{21} regressed on VL_{21} and ADG_{42} on VL_{42}, respectively. This corresponds to an average

growth rate difference of 213 and 190 g/day between pigs with the lowest and highest observed VL for the 21- and 42-day observation period, respectively, or differences in body weight of 4.5 and 8.0 kg over the 21- and 42-day observation periods, respectively. Similarly, body weight prior to infection had a significant association with ADG post infection (BW_0 $p < 0.0001$), with a positive regression coefficient of 0.025 (0.002) at 21 dpi and of 0.029 (0.003) at 42 dpi.

The log-likelihood of the model improved significantly when genetic effects (random sire effects) were included in the model (level model) ($p < 0.0001$) (Table 4). This indicates significant genetic variance in growth performance of pigs infected with PRRSV. However, including sire effects of slope only (Fig. 1c) did not improve model fit over the null model ($p > 0.60$) and resulted in negligibly small slope variance estimates.

Models with sire effects on both level and slope, as well as a genetic covariance between them, yielded a significantly better model fit than the null model ($p < 0.0001$). However, the level-slope model did not provide a significantly better fit than the level-only model for either 0 to 21 and 42 dpi ($p = 1.00$ and 0.66, respectively) (Table 4).

All four models provided similar estimates of variance components for non-genetic random effects (Table 4). Estimates of the sire variance in level were very similar between the level-only model and the level-slope model and very low, whereas estimates for sire variance in tolerance slope differed slightly between the slope-only and the level-slope model (Table 4). The fact that addition of the slope did not affect the variance estimate for level suggests potential confounding of level and slope (see statistical considerations). The estimate of the covariance between level and slope was close to zero, and constrained at the boundary for both time periods, indicating numerical difficulties in accurately estimating these variance components. However, shifting the covariate VL to ensure a zero covariance between the new level and slope has no effect on the model likelihoods, suggesting that the results are robust.

Table 4 Variance components for ADG (kg/d) from 0 to 21 dpi and 0 to 42 dpi

ADG period (dpi)	Null model Estimate (SE)	Level-only model Estimate (SE)	Slope-only model Estimate (SE)	Level-slope model Estimate (SE)
0 to 21				
Level		2.01E−03 (7.68E−04)		2.01E−03 (7.68E−04)
Covariance				2.21E−13 (1.04E−14)
Slope			4.37E−06 (2.06E−07)	1.00E−10 (4.71E−12)
Pen (trial)	4.12E−04 (1.45E−04)	3.97E−04 (1.42E−04)	4.12E−04 (1.45E−04)	3.97E−04 (1.42E−04)
Litter	9.25E−04 (2.26E−04)	4.72E−04 (2.04E−04)	9.25E−04 (2.26E−04)	4.72E−04 (2.04E−04)
Residual	6.18E−03 (2.91E−04)	6.18E−03 (2.91E−04)	6.18E−03 (2.91E−04)	6.18E−03 (2.91E−04)
LogLikelihood	2482.98	2495.03	2482.98	2495.2
0 to 42				
Level		2.32E−03 (1.02E−03)		2.33E−03 (1.03E−03)
Covariance				−3.95E−15 (2.04E−16)
Slope			8.60E−08 (1.47E−07)	3.41E−07 (5.94E−07)
Pen (trial)	2.43E−04 (1.30E−04)	2.82E−04 (1.36E−04)	2.39E−04 (1.29E−04)	2.78E−04 (1.35E−04)
Litter	1.76E−03 (3.27E−04)	1.23E−03 (2.98E−04)	1.75E−03 (3.27E−04)	1.22E−03 (2.98E−04)
Residual	5.39E−03 (3.03E−04)	5.33E−03 (2.99E−04)	5.36E−03 (3.05E−04)	5.30E−03 (3.02E−04)
LogLikelihood	1889.55	1911.18	1899.72	1911.35

Variance components estimated from random regression models: null model, containing no genetic effect; level-only model, containing only the overall sire effect on growth under infection; slope-only model, containing only sire effect on the slope of the regression line of growth over VL; and level-slope model, containing sire effects on level and slope, respectively

All other fixed effects/covariates and random effects were identical between models

Results for ADG_{42} on VL_{21} were similar to those for ADG_{42} on VL_{42} and are therefore not shown

In conclusion, the random regression models did not allow estimation of genetic variance in tolerance of pigs to PRRSV infection. Based on a statistical model fit alone, the level-only model accounting for genetic variance in growth rate at mean VL only constitutes a more appropriate model to describe genetic variation in growth response of infected pigs than the level-slope model accounting for genetic variance in both, growth rate at mean VL and tolerance. However, as outlined in more detail in the "statistical considerations" section below, it cannot be excluded that any genetic variance in tolerance that may exist is absorbed in the genetic variance for level because of the confounding between level and slope.

Step 4: random regression models including simulated performance in absence of infection for estimating genetic variance in tolerance

Models with genetic effects on both intercept and slope, as well as with a genetic covariance between them, consistently yielded a significantly better model fit than the null model ($p < 0.0001$ for both 0 to 21 and 0 to 42 dpi), regardless of the simulated genetic correlation between ADG_{21}^0 and ADG_{21} or ADG_{42}^0 and ADG_{42}. However, the intercept-slope model consistently provided a significantly superior fit over the intercept-only model only when the simulated genetic correlation between growth in absence of infection and growth under infection was low to moderate (Table 5). Generally, the ability to identify genetic variance in tolerance decreased with an increase in the simulated genetic correlation, as indicated by reduced improvement in log-likelihoods and a lower proportion of replicates with significant genetic variation in tolerance slope ($p < 0.05$) (Table 5). Somewhat surprisingly, for the 0 to 21 dpi observation period, the majority of replicates indicated significant genetic variation in tolerance, even for strong genetic correlations between ADG_{21}^0 and ADG_{21} (Table 5). In contrast, only low to moderate genetic correlations between ADG_{42}^0 and ADG_{42} resulted in significant genetic variance in tolerance for the majority of replicates for the 42 day observation period (Table 5).

Table 6 shows that random regression sire models when including records from both non-infected and infected siblings can generate robust genetic variance estimates for both intercept and slope. As expected, genetic variance estimates for tolerance slope tended to decrease with increasing genetic correlations between ADG_{21}^0 and ADG_{21} or ADG_{42}^0 and ADG_{42}, whereas the genetic variance estimates in the intercept tended to increase (see Additional file 1). Genetic correlations beween ADG in absence of infection and ADG under infection also affected the estimated genetic correlations between intercept and tolerance slope. Low (simulated) genetic correlations between ADG_{21}^0 and ADG_{21} or ADG_{42}^0 and

Table 5 Effect of the genetic correlation (r_g) between simulated ADG in the absence of infection and observed ADG under infection on evidence for genetic variance in tolerance

ADG period (dpi)	r_g	ΔLogLikelihood	p value	Proportion with significant genetic variance for tolerance ($p < 0.05$)
0 to 21	0.05	10.96 (4.19)	0.000	1.00
	0.30	6.18 (3.39)	0.005	0.98
	0.60	2.32 (1.49)	0.041	0.76
	0.90	1.00 (2.12)	0.067	0.55
0 to 42	0.05	8.67 (4.40)	0.003	0.99
	0.30	4.34 (3.16)	0.023	0.87
	0.60	1.31 (1.56)	0.107	0.41
	0.90	−0.80 (2.43)	0.187	0.06

Effect of the genetic correlation (r_g) of simulated ADG_{21}^0 with ADG_{21} and ADG_{42}^0 with ADG_{42} on the average change in log-likelihood of the intercept-slope model over the intercept-only model (ΔLogLikelihood), the average p-value of log likelihood improvement, provided by a log-likelihood ratio test, and the proportion of the 10,000 replicates with significant genetic variance in tolerance (i.e. p value of LRT was <0.05)

SD over 10,000 replicates are shown in brackets

Table 6 Variance components of intercept, slope and covariances from random regression models

ADG period (dpi)	r_g	Intercept-only model	Intercept–slope model		
		Intercept	Intercept	Covariance	Slope
0 to 21	0.05	7.65E−04 (2.24E−04)	9.93E−04 (2.98E−04)	−7.57E−06 (3.97E−06)	2.24E−07 (5.80E−08)
	0.3	9.20E−04 (2.53E−04)	9.95E−04 (2.99E−04)	−3.03E−06 (3.27E−06)	1.44E−07 (5.09E−08)
	0.6	1.13E−03 (2.71E−04)	1.03E−03 (2.84E−04)	1.54E−06 (2.13E−06)	5.54E−08 (3.24E−08)
	0.9	1.34E−03 (2.31E−04)	1.19E−03 (1.95E−04)	3.35E−06 (1.06E−06)	1.25E−08 (6.33E−09)
0 to 42	0.05	9.20E−04 (2.83E−04)	1.10E−03 (3.47E−04)	−5.80E−06 (3.59E−06)	1.18E−07 (3.87E−08)
	0.3	1.09E−03 (3.05E−04)	1.12E−03 (3.47E−04)	−1.90E−06 (2.85E−06)	6.85E−08 (3.23E−08)
	0.6	1.28E−03 (3.15E−04)	1.14E−03 (3.19E−04)	−5.57E−07 (1.75E−06)	2.37E−08 (1.65E−08)
	0.9	1.47E−03 (2.57E−04)	1.21E−03 (4.10E−04)	1.95E−06 (1.21E−06)	1.09E−08 (7.13E−09)

Variance components estimated from random regression models based on simulated ADG_{21}^0 and measured ADG_{21} (kg/d) or ADG_{42}^0 and ADG_{42}

Fitted models were the intercept-only model, containing only the overall sire effect on intercept; and the intercept-slope model, containing sire effect on intercept and slope for ADG_{21} or ADG_{42}, respectively

All other fixed effects/covariates and random effects were identical between models

SE (in brackets) were calculated as the SD over 10,000 replicates

r_g is the simulated genetic correlation between ADG_{21}^0 or ADG_{42}^0 and ADG_{21} or ADG_{42}

ADG_{42}, respectively, led to negative genetic correlations between performance in the absence of infection and tolerance, whereas strong positive genetic correlations between the growth traits suggested that pigs with greater genetic growth in the absence of infection were also genetically more tolerant to infection.

Discussion
Summary of findings
Performance of an infected individual is likely to depend on its ability to restrict pathogen load (resistance) and its ability to limit the impact of infection (tolerance). The extensive PHGC dataset has identified substantial genetic variation in resistance of growing pigs to PRRS and led to

the discovery of a major quantitative trait locus associated with both resistance and growth of pigs under infection [10, 12, 13, 20]. Surprisingly, the dataset provided little evidence that pigs also vary genetically in tolerance to this virus. However, the simulations revealed that genetic variation in tolerance to PRRS may exist, depending on the performance in the absence of infection (vigor). Furthermore, this analysis raised numerous statistical difficulties associated with genetic improvement of host tolerance, which could be overcome by including measures of performance of infected and non-infected relatives in the analysis.

Focusing on data from infected pigs alone, genetic correlations between body weight prior to infection, resistance (inverse of VL) and growth under infection were found to be moderately strong and positive, in line with previous studies [10, 20]. This indicates that heavier individuals prior to infection counteract an increase in pathogen load, and thus tend to have lower VL, and therefore lower infection-induced reductions in growth rate. Genetic correlations between VL and growth were strongly negative, implying that animals that were genetically more resistant also tended to grow faster under infection. However, correlations were significantly different from 1, indicating that genetic variation in growth of PRRSV infected pigs is not fully explained by heterogeneity in growth prior to infection and resistance. Therefore, genetic variation in tolerance may also play a part in host response to PRRSV infection. However, the multi-trait model provided little evidence of genetic variation in tolerance. This was further supported by the random regression models. These showed that, although growth rate declined, on average, linearly with increasing VL, there was no statistically significant difference in tolerance between the sires of the infected piglets.

However, closer inspection of the underlying data structure raised suspicion that genetic variance in the reaction norm level absorbed genetic variance in tolerance due to confounding between level and slope in these data (see Statistical considerations below). To disentangle the genetic variance in reaction-norm intercepts (i.e. growth rate in the absence of infection) and slopes (i.e. tolerance), the experimental data were augmented with simulated growth rates of non-infected relatives. Thus, the resulting data structure mimicked that of 'sib challenge tests' that are common practice in aquaculture and other livestock species [35–37]. The simulations demonstrated that inclusion of these additional data in the random regression models resolved the confounding between level and slope and resulted in more reliable genetic parameter estimates for tolerance. Most importantly, the simulations revealed that it would be wrong to conclude that pigs in this study lacked substantial genetic variation in tolerance to PRRS, as was suggested by the models based on the collected data alone. As demonstrated by the simulations, genetic variance estimates for tolerance strongly depend on the genetic correlations between growth in the absence of and growth under infection. Low to moderately strong genetic correlations between these two traits implied significant genetic variance in tolerance of the pigs in this study. Interestingly, estimated genetic correlations between body weight of pigs prior to infection and growth under infection were moderately strong. Thus, if body weight prior to infection was a reliable predictor for growth rate in the absence of infection, evidence for genetic variance in tolerance would emerge directly from the data.

Statistical considerations

Here, the conventional reaction-norm approach was adopted to model genetic variation in tolerance to infections [2, 38]. Using both simulated and real data, we demonstrated that random regression models embedded in the mixed model machinery are a powerful tool to estimate genetic variance in tolerance for outbred populations if the data structure is appropriate [15, 16, 18]. Random regression models are also known to be highly sensitive to the underlying data structure and prone to generate inaccurate variance estimates for slope, in particular, if sample size is limited or information on relatedness is poor, as was the case for the data in this study [15, 17, 30]. To prevent bias in the slope variance estimates [15, 30], only sires that had more than 10 offspring were included in this study. However, the associated reduction of the data to records from only 54 mostly unrelated sires may have caused a trade-off between reducing bias and reducing statistical power, as indicated by lower heritabilities for ADG and VL than found in previous analyses on the same data [10, 20]. Furthermore, to alleviate the potential impact of limited information of relatedness (as only sires and dams were known for the majority of pigs), the analyses were repeated including the genomic relationship matrix rather than the pedigree relationship matrix, which is not able to capture the difference between siblings due to Mendelian sampling. However, this had a negligible impact on the variance estimates and on the log-likelihoods of the reaction-norm models (results not shown).

As is common practice for quantitative genetics models using REML, the likelihood ratio test (LRT) was used to test the significance of random effects such as the sire tolerance slope estimates, and whether genetic correlations differed significantly from 1 [39]. For variance and co-variance components constrained to the positive parameter space, the conventional LRT that assumes the test-statistics to follow a Chi square distribution with degrees of freedom equal to the number of additional parameters to be estimated in the more complex model has been described to be overly conservative [23]. For this reason the widely used adjustment of Stram and Lee [32] based on mixture distributions was applied. However, in this proposed adjustment, individual subjects (in this case sires) were assumed independent. Due to lack of detailed pedigree information in the present study, the majority of sires were indeed assumed unrelated, with the exception of sires from trials 1 to 3. Repeating the analysis with the assumption that all sires were unrelated provided almost identical model results to those reported here. Thus, we believe that the LRT is a valid method for testing the null hypotheses of zero genetic variance in tolerance and genetic correlations equal to 0 or 1 in this study. Nevertheless, sires and sire by VL interactions were also fitted as fixed effects in the statistical models of Step 3. In accordance with the results of modelling sires as random effect, there were no significant differences between the tolerance slopes associated with different sires according to the Wald test ($p = 0.981$ and 0.081 for the 0 to 21 and 0 to 42 dpi time periods, respectively).

Perhaps most importantly, reaction-norms require considerable variation in the independent variable to generate unbiased tolerance slope estimates [1]. However, this study, in line with other infection challenge experiments, used an identical infection route, pathogen strain and dose for all individuals. Consequently, it provided a relatively narrow value range for pathogen load (VL_{42} values ranged between 88 and 236 AUC in our study), with no values close to 0. To better accommodate the distribution of the data in the models, the VL was centered at the mean VL value, in line with common practice in the animal breeding literature [17, 27, 30]. However, the relatively narrow range of the VL of offspring, combined with the relatively small numbers of offspring for some sires, may have hampered the ability of these models to disentangle sire effects on level and slope. This confounding is likely further aggravated by genetic variation in resistance to PRRS, which implies that VL is not homogeneously distributed among sires, with more resistant sires predominantly having progeny with low VL, and less resistant sires predominantly progeny with high VL.

Considering all these effects combined, the weak evidence for significant genetic variation in tolerance to PRRS from the random regression models in this study may simply reflect a lack of statistical power to disentangle sire effects on regression slope and level. The complementary simulation studies presented here, which assumed that additional performance measures of related uninfected individuals were available, demonstrated one way of increasing statistical power. Similarly, it might be possible to increase statistical power by harnessing information from repeated measures of growth and pathogen load for each individual over the course of infection in the statistical models. By increasing the range of distribution of VL for each individual, a more robust slope may be fitted through the centre of the data, alluding to an "overall" picture of tolerance across multiple time-points in infection.

Implications for genetic improvement of tolerance of pigs to PRRS and other diseases

Genetic improvement of tolerance may have several advantages over improving resistance. Firstly, host resistance limits pathogen replication within the host and, as a consequence, selection for host resistance may impose selection advantages on pathogen strains that can overcome host resistance mechanisms and eventually result in a loss of selection advantage of the host [40, 41]. Given the high mutation rate of RNA viruses such as PRRSV [42], this is a potential pitfall for a long-term breeding strategy focused on resistance. It has been proposed that, theoretically, tolerance might not impose such selection pressure on the pathogen [40].

Secondly, it has been suggested that improving host tolerance may offer cross-protection against other strains of the virus, or other prevalent infectious agents, as tolerance mechanisms primarily target host-intrinsic damage prevention or repair mechanisms, compared to resistance mechanisms, which interfere directly with the pathogen life-cycle [2, 5, 43]. This is particularly relevant for PRRS, which is often associated with co-infection with other respiratory viruses, such as PCV2 or the influenza virus, which can mimic the respiratory clinical signs associated with PRRS [44]. Furthermore, in a globalized animal breeding market, where PRRS is endemic and highly prevalent in farms, (estimated at 60 to 80% in the U.S, and up to 79% in mainland Europe), and where environmental conditions are difficult to improve, eradication of the virus has proven to be challenging [45–47]. Selective breeding for tolerance is considered desirable when pathogen prevalence is high, when pathogen elimination has proven difficult and when pathogens can evolve rapidly to evade control measures that aim at interfering with the pathogen life-cycle [48]. All these cases apply to PRRS. Therefore, improvement of tolerance of pigs to this ubiquitous virus may constitute a viable alternative to eradication programs, since it would allow pigs to maintain homeostasis despite infection [44]. However, tolerance would result in continued presence of the virus which could rebound and result in further pathogenesis in the host and threats to the herd. Thus, distinction between resistance and tolerance in genetic improvement programs is imperative if they have different effects on pathogen prevalence and evolution, as implied by theory [40, 49].

Obtaining reliable tolerance estimates from natural disease outbreaks is extremely difficult due to the myriad of confounding factors (e.g. difference in exposure and onset of infection, differences in the individual immune status, co-infections), which can severely bias tolerance estimates and mask the underlying genetic signal [16, 18]. For this reason, empirical evidence for genetic variation in host tolerance to infections stems primarily from challenge experiments in inbred lines of model species [2, 50, 51]. The PHGC challenge data constitute a unique data source for investigating the genetic basis and relative importance of host resistance and tolerance in outbred pigs' responses to virus infections, since it provides the required measures of both pathogen load and performance for large sample sizes, without the confounding factors inherent to field data. However, the analyses of these data demonstrated that the limited data range produced in challenge experiments, together with other factors that affect the distribution of the data, such as genetic variance in host resistance, can easily blur the tolerance signal in multi-trait and reaction-norm models, and highlight the importance of performance records of non-infected relatives for obtaining accurate tolerance estimates.

Collecting equivalent performance records of non-infected relatives of the challenged individuals would be extremely valuable to establish the relationship between tolerance and performance in the absence of infection, and identify shared or distinct genomic regions associated with these traits. A strong genetic correlation between these traits would imply that one could select for high performance at the nucleus to improve tolerance and performance in the more infectious commercial farms. In the current pig breeding structure, a direct data pipeline of performance measures between pigs in commercial farms experiencing disease outbreaks and those of related selection candidates in the almost pathogen free nucleus may be useful. Obtaining unbiased and comparable measures of within-host pathogen load from natural disease outbreaks constitutes the main challenge for producing reliable tolerance estimates from natural disease outbreaks [16]. A practically more feasible approach is to estimate genetic correlations between performance in clean and infectious environments and to include performance during disease outbreaks in the selection criterion [52, 53], although this approach does not allow distinction between resistance and tolerance.

Based on resource-allocation theory and earlier findings, resistance and tolerance are conventionally considered as alternative host defense mechanisms to infections, leading to the notion of a trade-off between improving resistance and tolerance. Indeed, a companion genome-wide association study on the same PHGC data found different regions that were associated with tolerance and with resistance [54]. Emerging evidence from different studies suggests that both resistance and tolerance mechanisms may be required for effective host protection to infection and that the optimal host response to infection likely depends on a carefully timed interaction between pathogen elimination (i.e. resistance) mechanisms and host mechanisms that promote tissue damage control and increase disease tolerance [51, 55]. The aforementioned companion study identified several overlapping genomic regions associated with resistance and tolerance of pigs to PRRS and found that the WUR10000125 SNP, previously associated to confer greater resistance to PRRS (lower VL_{21}), also confers

greater tolerance. Valuable insights about these interactions could be harnessed from the available longitudinal measures of pathogen burden and growth, e.g. by following the infection trajectories of individuals and target entire trajectories rather than resistance or tolerance for genetic improvement [51, 56].

In order to target both resistance and tolerance in a sustainable breeding program, the epidemiological and evolutionary consequences of genetic selection in either or both traits combined must be studied in more detail. In particular, it needs to be determined whether evolutionary theory predicts a lower risk of pathogen evolution from selection for improved host tolerance rather than resistance hold in the case of PRRS; and to what extent genetically more resistant or tolerant pigs are also less infectious [3, 57, 58]. It is probable that control of PRRS and other infectious diseases by genetic selection is a "balancing act" [9], which involves mechanisms associated with resistance and tolerance to provide the fittest pigs.

Conclusions

Using evidence from the available data alone suggests that growing piglets differ genetically in resistance but does not explicitly show evidence for genetic differences in tolerance to PRRSV infection. However, statistical constraints may have masked genetic variation in tolerance. Currently, unknown genetic correlations between performance under and in absence of PRRSV infection could reveal significant genetic variance in tolerance. Future studies are warranted to validate the results in this study for infections with the same and different strains of the PRRS virus, including vaccine strains. This study shows that genetics of tolerance is more difficult to analyze than genetics of resistance, and is therefore more difficult to target in genetic improvement.

Authors' contributions
GL and HR conducted the statistical analyses and interpretation of results, and wrote the manuscript. AH and MH aided statistical analyses. RRRR conceived the experimental trials and led the animal infection trials and sample collection. JKL conceived the experimental trials and coordinated the handling, storage, and sample preparation for DNA genotyping. JCMD helped conceive the study and collated the data. IK, JCMD, AK and ND all aided interpretation of results. ADW and HM helped to conceive the study, coordinated and oversaw statistical analysis of the data and contributed to the interpretation of results and writing the manuscript. All co-authors reviewed and contributed to development of the manuscript. All authors read and approved the final manuscript.

Author details
[1] The Roslin Institute & R(D)SVS, University of Edinburgh, Edinburgh, Midlothian, UK. [2] Animal Breeding and Genomics Centre, Wageningen University and Research, PO Box 338, 6700 AH Wageningen, The Netherlands. [3] School

of Agriculture Food and Rural Development, Newcastle University, Newcastle upon Tyne NE1 7RU, UK. [4] Department of Animal Science, Iowa State University, Ames, IA 50011, USA. [5] Genus plc, 100 Bluegrass Commons Blvd. Suite 2200, Hendersonville, TN 37075, USA. [6] Biometrical Genetics, Natural Resources Institute Finland, 00790 Jokioinen, Finland. [7] Animal Parasitic Diseases Laboratory, USDA, Beltsville, MD 20705, USA. [8] College of Veterinary Medicine, Kansas State University, Manhattan, KS 66506, USA.

Acknowledgements

The authors would like to thank the PRRS Host Genetic Consortium for access and use of the dataset. The PHGC was supported by US National Pork Board Grants, USDA NIFA Awards (2008-55620-19132, 2010-65205-20433, 2013-68004-20362), and pig breeding companies, consisting of PIC/Genus, Choice Genetics, Fast Genetics, Genesus, Inc., TopigsNorsvin, and PigGen Canada, Inc., that provided the pigs for the study.

Competing interests

The authors declare that they have no competing interests.

Funding

This study was funded by the BBSRC and Genus within the remit of a BBSRC Industrial Case Ph.D. studentship (GL) and BBSRC Institute Strategic Programme Grant to ABD-W (ISP1, BB/J004235/1, Theme 5 BBS/E/D/20211554). IK received funding from the Higher Education Funding Council for England (HEFCE). HR was funded by Marie Curie Initial Training Networks (FP7-People-2010-ITN) as part of the NematodeSystemHealth project, and co-financed by Topigs Norsvin, the Netherlands, and Dutch Ministry of Economic Affairs, Agriculture, and Innovation (Public–private partnership "Breed4Food" Code KB-12-006.03-004-ASG-LR and KB-12-006.03-005-ASG-LR).

References

1. Råberg L, Graham AL, Read AF, Raberg L, Graham AL, Read AF. Decomposing health: tolerance and resistance to parasites in animals. Philos Trans R Soc B Biol Sci. 2009;364:37–49.
2. Råberg L, Sim D, Read AF, Raberg L, Sim D, Read AF. Disentangling genetic variation for resistance and tolerance to infectious diseases in animals. Science. 2007;318:812–4.
3. Vale PF, McNally L, Doeschl-Wilson A, King KC, Popat R, Domingo-Sananes MR, et al. Beyond killing. Evol Med Public Health. 2016;2016:148–57.
4. Doeschl-Wilson AB, Kyriazakis I. Should we aim for genetic improvement in host resistance or tolerance to infectious pathogens? Front Genet. 2012;3:272.
5. Medzhitov R, Schneider DS, Soares MP. Disease tolerance as a defense strategy. Science. 2012;335:936–41.
6. Doeschl-Wilson AB, Kyriazakis I, Vincent A, Rothschild MF, Thacker E, Galina-Pantoja L. Clinical and pathological responses of pigs from two genetically diverse commercial lines to porcine reproductive and respiratory syndrome virus infection. J Anim Sci. 2009;87:1638–47.
7. Holtkamp DJ. Assessment of the economic impact of porcine reproductive and respiratory syndrome virus on United States pork producers. J Swine Health Prod. 2013;21:72–84.
8. Kimman TG, Cornelissen LA, Moormann RJ, Rebel JMJ, Stockhofe-Zurwieden N. Challenges for porcine reproductive and respiratory syndrome virus (PRRSV) vaccinology. Vaccine. 2009;27:3704–18.
9. Lunney JK, Chen H. Genetic control of host resistance to porcine reproductive and respiratory syndrome virus (PRRSV) infection. Virus Res. 2010;154:161–9.
10. Hess AS, Islam ZZ, Hess MK, Rowland RRRR, Lunney JJK, Doeschl-Wilson AA, et al. Comparison of host genetic factors influencing pig response to infection with two North American isolates of porcine reproductive and respiratory syndrome virus. Genet Sel Evol. 2016;48:43.

11. Lewis CRG, Ait-Ali T, Clapperton M, Archibald AL, Bishop S. Genetic perspectives on host responses to porcine reproductive and respiratory syndrome (PRRS). Viral Immunol. 2007;20:343–58.
12. Boddicker NJ, Garrick DJ, Rowland RRR, Lunney JK, Reecy JM, Dekkers JCM. Validation and further characterization of a major quantitative trait locus associated with host response to experimental infection with porcine reproductive and respiratory syndrome virus. Anim Genet. 2013;45:48–58.
13. Boddicker NJ. The genetic basis of host response to experimental infection with the porcine reproductive and respiratory syndrome virus in pigs [dissertation]. 2013;198
14. Simms EL, Triplett J. Costs and benefits of plant-responses to disease—resistance and tolerance. Evolution. 1994;48:1973–85.
15. Kause A. Genetic analysis of tolerance to infections using random regressions: a simulation study. Genet Res. 2011;93:291–302.
16. Doeschl-Wilson AB, Villanueva B, Kyriazakis I. The first step toward genetic selection for host tolerance to infectious pathogens: obtaining the tolerance phenotype through group estimates. Front Genet. 2012;3:265.
17. Knap PW, Su G. Genotype by environment interaction for litter size in pigs as quantified by reaction norms analysis. Animal. 2008;2:1742.
18. Hayward AD, Nussey DH, Wilson AJ, Berenos C, Pilkington JG, Watt KA, et al. Natural selection on individual variation in tolerance of gastrointestinal nematode infection. PLoS Biol. 2014;12(7):e1001917.
19. Truong HM, Lu Z, Kutish GF, Galeota J, Osorio FA, Pattnaik AK. A highly pathogenic porcine reproductive and respiratory syndrome virus generated from an infectious cDNA clone retains the in vivo virulence and transmissibility properties of the parental virus. Virology. 2004;325:308–19.
20. Boddicker N, Waide EH, Rowland RRR, Lunney JK, Garrick DJ, Reecy JM, et al. Evidence for a major QTL associated with host response to porcine reproductive and respiratory syndrome virus challenge. J Anim Sci. 2012;90:1733–46.
21. Islam ZU, Bishop SC, Savill NJ, Rowland RRR, Lunney JK, Trible B, et al. Quantitative analysis of porcine reproductive and respiratory syndrome (PRRS) viremia profiles from experimental infection: a statistical modelling approach. PLoS One. 2013;8(12):e83567.
22. Ramos AM, Crooijmans RPMA, Affara NA, Amaral AJ, Archibald AL, Beever JE, et al. Design of a high density SNP genotyping assay in the pig using SNPs identified and characterized by next generation sequencing technology. PLoS One. 2009;4:e6524.
23. Gilmour AR, Gogel BJ, Cullis BR, Thompson R. ASReml User Guide Release 3.0. Hemel Hempstead: VSN International Ltd; 2009.
24. VanRaden PM. Efficient methods to compute genomic predictions. J Dairy Sci. 2008;91:4414–23.
25. Stowe KA, Marquis RJ, Hochwender CG, Simms EL. The evolutionary ecology of tolerance to consumer damage. Annu Rev Ecol Syst. 2000;31:565–95.
26. Schaeffer LR. Application of random regression models in animal breeding. Livest Prod Sci. 2004;86:35–45.
27. Kolmodin R, Bijma P. Response to mass selection when the genotype by environment interaction is modelled as a linear reaction norm. Genet Sel Evol. 2004;36:435.
28. Van Tienderen PH, Koelewijn HP. Selection on reaction norms, genetic correlations and constraints. Genet Res. 1994;64:115–25.
29. Strandberg E. Analysis of genotype by environment interaction using random regression models. In: Proceedings of 8th world congress on genetics applied to livestock production, Belo Horizonte, Minas Gerais, Brazil, 13–18 August 2006; 2006. p. 25–05.
30. Calus MPL, Bijma P, Veerkamp RF. Effects of data structure on the estimation of covariance functions to describe genotype by environment interactions in a reaction norm model. Genet Sel Evol. 2004;36:489–507.
31. Lynch M, Walsh B. Genetics and analysis of quantitative traits. Sunderland: Sinauer Associates Inc.; 1998.
32. Stram DO, Lee JW. Variance components testing in the longitudinal mixed effects model. Biometrics. 1994;50:1171–7.
33. Visscher PM, Medland SE, Ferreira MAR, Morley KI, Zhu G, Cornes BK, et al. Assumption-free estimation of heritability from genome-wide identity-by-descent sharing between full siblings. PLoS Genet. 2006;2:e41.
34. Chen P. Genetic improvement of lean growth rate and reproductive traits in pigs. http://lib.dr.iastate.edu/rtd.

35. Ødegård J, Meuwissen TH, Meuwissen T, Hayes B, Goddard M, Luan T, et al. Identity-by-descent genomic selection using selective and sparse genotyping. Genet Sel Evol. 2014;46:3.

36. Kause A, van Dalen S, Bovenhuis H. Genetics of ascites resistance and tolerance in chicken: a random regression approach. G3 (Bethesda). 2012;2:527–35.

37. de Greef KH, Janss LL, Vereijken AL, Pit R, Gerritsen CL. Disease-induced variability of genetic correlations: ascites in broilers as a case study. J Anim Sci. 2001;79:1723–33.

38. Simms EL. Defining tolerance as a norm of reaction. Evol Ecol. 2000;14:563–70.

39. Wilson AJ, Réale D, Clements MN, Morrissey MM, Postma E, Walling CA, et al. An ecologist's guide to the animal model. J Anim Ecol. 2010;79:13–26.

40. Roy BA, Kirchner JW. Evolutionary dynamics of pathogen resistance and tolerance. Evolution. 2000;54:51–63.

41. Restif O, Koella JC. Concurrent evolution of resistance and tolerance to pathogens. Am Nat. 2004;164:E90–102.

42. Drake JW, Holland JJ. Mutation rates among RNA viruses. Proc Natl Acad Sci USA. 1999;96:13910–3.

43. Ayres JS, Schneider DS. Tolerance of Infections. In: Paul WE, editor. Annu Rev Immunol Vol 30. Palo Alto: Annual Reviews; 2012. p. 271–94.

44. Rowland RRR, Lunney J, Dekkers J. Control of porcine reproductive and respiratory syndrome (PRRS) through genetic improvements in disease resistance and tolerance. Front Genet. 2012;3:1–6.

45. Zimmerman JJ, Yoon KJ, Pirtle EC, Wills RW, Sanderson TJ, McGinley MJ. Studies of porcine reproductive and respiratory syndrome (PRRS) virus infection in avian species. Vet Microbiol. 1997;55:329–36.

46. Albina E. Epidemiology of porcine reproductive and respiratory syndrome (PRRS): an overview. Vet Microbiol. 1997;55:309–16.

47. de Pax X, Vega D, Duran C., Angulo J. PRRS prevalence in Europe: Perception of the pig veterinary practitioners—PRRS.com. ESPHM 2015. 2015. p. 1; Accessed on 22 Sep 2015.

48. Bishop SC, Woolliams JA. Genomics and disease resistance studies in livestock. Livest Sci. 2014;166:190–8.

49. Bishop SC. A consideration of resistance and tolerance for ruminant nematode infections. Front Genet. 2012;3:168.

50. Mauricio R, Rausher MD, Burdick DS. Variation in the defense strategies of plants: are resistance and tolerance mutually exclusive? Ecology. 1997;78:1301–11.

51. Lough G, Kyriazakis I, Bergmann S, Lengeling A, Doeschl-Wilson AB. Health trajectories reveal the dynamic contributions of host genetic resistance and tolerance to infection outcome. Proc Biol Sci. 2015;282:20152151.

52. Bisset SA, Morris CA. Feasibility and implications of breeding sheep for resilience to nematode challenge. Int J Parasitol. 1996;26:857–68.

53. Herrero-Medrano JM, Mathur PK, Napel J ten, Rashidi H, Alexandri P, Knol EF, et al. Estimation of genetic parameters and breeding values across challenged environments to select for robust pigs. J Anim Sci. 2015;93:1494–502.

54. Rashidi H. Breeding against infectious diseases in animals. Wageningen: Wageningen University; 2016.

55. Allen JE, Sutherland TE. Host protective roles of type 2 immunity: parasite killing and tissue repair, flip sides of the same coin. Semin Immunol. 2014;26:329–40.

56. Doeschl-Wilson AB, Bishop SC, Kyriazakis I, Villanueva B. Novel methods for quantifying individual host response to infectious pathogens for genetic analyses. Front Genet. 2012;3:266.

57. Gopinath S, Lichtman JS, Bouley DM, Elias JE, Monack DM. Role of disease-associated tolerance in infectious superspreaders. Proc Natl Acad Sci USA. 2014;111:15780–5.

58. Anacleto O, Garcia-Cortés LA, Lipschutz-Powell D, Woolliams JA, Doeschl-Wilson AB. A novel statistical model to estimate host genetic effects affecting disease transmission. Genetics. 2015;201:871–84.

8

Selecting sequence variants to improve genomic predictions for dairy cattle

Paul M. VanRaden[1]*, Melvin E. Tooker[1], Jeffrey R. O'Connell[2], John B. Cole[1] and Derek M. Bickhart[1]

Abstract

Background: Millions of genetic variants have been identified by population-scale sequencing projects, but subsets of these variants are needed for routine genomic predictions or genotyping arrays. Methods for selecting sequence variants were compared using simulated sequence genotypes and real July 2015 data from the 1000 Bull Genomes Project.

Methods: Candidate sequence variants for 444 Holstein animals were combined with high-density (HD) imputed genotypes for 26,970 progeny-tested Holstein bulls. Test 1 included single nucleotide polymorphisms (SNPs) for 481,904 candidate sequence variants. Test 2 also included 249,966 insertions-deletions (InDels). After merging sequence variants with 312,614 HD SNPs and editing steps, Tests 1 and 2 included 762,588 and 1,003,453 variants, respectively. Imputation quality from findhap software was assessed with 404 of the sequenced animals in the reference population and 40 randomly chosen animals for validation. Their sequence genotypes were reduced to the subset of genotypes that were in common with HD genotypes and then imputed back to sequence. Predictions were tested for 33 traits using 2015 data of 3983 US validation bulls with daughters that were first phenotyped after August 2011.

Results: The average percentage of correctly imputed variants across all chromosomes was 97.2 for Test 1 and 97.0 for Test 2. Total time required to prepare, edit, impute, and estimate the effects of sequence variants for 27,235 bulls was about 1 week using less than 33 threads. Many sequence variants had larger estimated effects than nearby HD SNPs, but prediction reliability improved only by 0.6 percentage points in Test 1 when sequence SNPs were added to HD SNPs and by 0.4 percentage points in Test 2 when sequence SNPs and InDels were included. However, selecting the 16,648 candidate SNPs with the largest estimated effects and adding them to the 60,671 SNPs used in routine evaluations improved reliabilities by 2.7 percentage points.

Conclusions: Reliabilities for genomic predictions improved when selected sequence variants were added; gains were similar for simulated and real data for the same population, and larger than previous gains obtained by adding HD SNPs. With many genotyped animals, many data sources, and millions of variants, computing strategies must efficiently balance costs of imputation, selection, and prediction to obtain subsets of markers that provide the highest accuracy.

Background

Accuracy of genomic predictions can be improved by using more variants, including variants that are preselected for their effect, located near genes or within genes, predicted to affect gene function, or known to be causal. Past analyses often gave equal weight to evenly spaced markers, whereas new analyses can focus on potential quantitative trait loci (QTL) or preselected variants that are more closely linked to QTL. Nearly 40 million variants have been identified from whole-genome sequence (WGS) data for over 1500 bulls, and several strategies to impute these variants to additional animals and use them in genetic evaluation for economic traits show potential [1–8]. For example, candidate variants

*Correspondence: Paul.VanRaden@ars.usda.gov
[1] Animal Genomics and Improvement Laboratory, Agricultural Research Service, USDA, Beltsville, MD, USA
Full list of author information is available at the end of the article

can be targeted to specific traits such as genes related to fertility, thereby slightly improving reliability for daughter pregnancy rate by 0.2 percentage points when 39 single nucleotide polymorphisms (SNPs) were added to the marker set used for genomic prediction [9]. The number of sequenced animals should continue to increase as researchers examine more families and the costs of generating data continue to decrease.

Imputing, selecting, and predicting effects for millions of variants and many thousands of individuals require efficient computation. Computational costs, which are proportional to the number of variants multiplied by the number of individuals, could exceed the marginal benefits from adding more variants. Variants within or near genes should improve the reliability of predictions, and direct use of causal variants is preferred to using linked markers. Strategies to choose variants for inclusion on genotyping arrays of different densities or in routine predictions were developed and compared using simulated data for Holstein bulls. Here, we first examined simulated data and then real sequence genotypes from the 1000 Bull Genomes Project [10].

The goals of this study were to (1) compare the reliability of prediction from sequence, array, and combined data as well as different types of variants, (2) test the methods first on simulated data before applying them to real sequence data imputed for a large reference population, and (3) investigate editing, imputation, and computing strategies that are efficient for even larger genotyped populations.

Methods

Simulated sequence data

Our simulation was designed to closely mimic an actual large-scale sequencing project for cattle, in which a subset of ancestor bulls had WGS data, another subset of ancestor bulls had high-density (HD) SNP-array genotypes, and most bulls had medium-density genotypes. Sequence variants were simulated for 26,984 Holstein bulls in the US reference population in December 2014 using a pedigree file that included 112,905 animals, and the sequences were then reduced to mimic the actual available array genotypes. Among these animals, the 1000 bulls that had the most daughters had genotypes observed for 30 million sequence variants, and 773, 24,863 and 343 other bulls that had fewer daughters were genotyped with 600,000 (600 k), 60,000 (60 k) and 12,000 SNPs, respectively. Each simulated chip was an evenly spaced subset of the previous chip and the sequence variants. The 30 million variant sites were randomly located across 30 chromosomes each 100 million bases long, and all variants had two alleles. The genotypes were simulated using genosim software [11], which generates founding

chromosomes with linkage disequilibrium (LD) and descendant chromosomes with recombination using the actual pedigree of the bulls. A parameter of 0.9998 was selected to generate average LD similar to that in the real sequence dataset, as in previous tests [12].

Editing reduced the list of variants to 8.4 million by removing SNPs with a minor allele frequency (MAF) lower than 0.01 and a level of LD less than 0.95 with any remaining neighbouring SNP, but all 0.5 million variants that were within or near the 10,000 (10 k) simulated QTL were retained. The QTL were located randomly across the genome, and the 25 variants on either side were retained. No actual genes were simulated, only the QTL and other variants. If any of the 350 variants on either side of a specific marker were correlated i.e. with an $|r|$ higher than 0.95, editing based on LD retained one variant and removed all others that had an $|r|$ higher than 0.95 with that variant. The 600 k SNPs were all retained to improve imputation, and the 505,210 SNPs that were within 2500 bases of a true QTL were retained to mimic bioinformatic selection using gene positions. The selected SNPs were imputed for all bulls. Strategies were compared to choose the most significant variants or those with the largest estimated variances or effect sizes for five independent traits using individual regressions on each variant or multiple regression on all variants.

Breeding values for five independent traits were simulated by summing across effects of the 10 k QTL. The five traits were not true replicates because the QTL locations did not vary, only the effects, mimicking quantitative inheritance where each QTL may affect most traits very little but some traits more. A heavy-tailed distribution was generated from normally-distributed effects (q) raised to the power of $2.7^{(|q|-2)}$ such that the largest effect contributed 3 to 13% of the genetic variance, the largest 10 effects contributed 20 to 34%, the largest 100 contributed 57 to 63%, and the largest 1000 contributed 90 to 93%. Actual traits may be controlled by QTL with smaller effects, however, most actual traits had at least one QTL as large as those simulated here [13]. Simulated phenotypes for five independent traits had reliabilities equal to those for milk evaluations of the actual bulls.

After imputing the 8.4 million edited variants for all bulls, the variants with the largest effect estimated by genomic prediction or the most significant variants from genome-wide association (GWA) analysis were selected. The oldest 17,896 bulls were used as the reference population, and true breeding values (TBV) of the 9088 younger bulls were used to validate predictions from the selected variants. In all tests, the phenotypes used for estimating effects and selecting variants were only from the truncated reference data so that validation phenotypes were independent and tests should be unbiased.

Many of the reference bulls and a few validation bulls had sequence data included in the 1000 Bull Genomes Project and used for variant discovery, which might bias estimates of allele frequency, but should not bias the phenotypic effects.

Variants can be selected based on the highest significance test, largest absolute effect, or largest genetic variance contributed by the locus, which is computed as $2p(1-p)\alpha^2$, where p is the allele frequency and α is the allele substitution effect. All three methods were compared. Selecting the variants that contribute the most variance has more theoretical appeal and results in variants with higher MAF, which could also contribute to improve imputation accuracy. Using the nonlinear Bayes A algorithm of VanRaden et al. [12], the highest ranking markers were selected based on their largest effect or largest variance regardless of their location. Using GWA, the significance of each variant was tested conditional on neighbouring variants already included, and the tests were then combined for each of the five independent traits into an overall measure of significance. The single regression model in GWA was processed using MMAP [14, 15] and included SNP as a fixed effect and breeding values as random effects modelled with pedigree relationships. Pedigree information was used rather than genomic relationships based on sequence data to separate the individual effect of SNPs from the random, polygenic effect. Multiple regression requires hundreds of iterations to converge, whereas GWA can test many variants without iteration.

Genomic predictions from 60 or 600 k SNPs were compared with predictions from additional markers selected also using Bayes A multiple regression. To mimic the selection process used to design the GeneSeek HD version 1 chip [16], the top 5000 HD SNPs for each of the five traits were selected, and the combined set of 23,600 (24 k) selected SNPs after removing 1400 duplicates were added to the 60 k SNPs. To mimic selection on net merit [17], another test selected 24 k SNPs with the largest variance averaged across the five traits instead of selecting the top SNPs for each trait and then combining them.

Selection based on sequence variants should improve accuracy more than selection on HD SNPs, but the previously genotyped SNPs must be retained during imputation because sequence variants are not available for most animals. Genomic predictions included the 600 k SNPs plus 500 k sequence variants near QTL totalling 1.1 million variants, which was similar to the analysis of real data by Hayes et al. [10]. The variants that were chosen in close proximity to QTL are referred to as the genic subset of WGS variants although gene locations were not simulated, only QTL locations were. Final tests of the simulated data added the 10 k true QTL to the 60 k SNPs,

and an upper limit on reliability was obtained using only the imputed QTL in prediction with no prior variance assigned to the markers, the parameter of the heavy-tailed distribution set to the true parameter, and polygenic variance set to 0% instead of the 10% in other tests.

Real variants derived from population-scale WGS data

SNP and insertion-deletion (InDel) calls (sequence variants) from run 5 of the 1000 Bull Genomes Project [18] were released in July 2015. Sequence variants for 444 Holstein animals and HD imputed genotypes for 26,970 progeny-tested Holstein bulls were combined by imputation using findhap software (version 3) [19]. The total number of variants identified in run 5 was equal to 38 million SNPs and 1.7 million InDels, but many of those variants are monomorphic within the Holstein breed. InDels were on average 3 bp long and no more than 86 bp. Imputed sequence genotypes from the 1000 Bull Genomes Project data were set to missing if none of the three genotype probabilities (AA, AB, or BB) were higher than 0.98 as estimated by Beagle [20].

The HD genotypes of 2394 Holsteins mainly from North America, Italy, and Great Britain were used to impute genotypes of 590,363 other Holsteins that had genotypes obtained mainly by using SNP chips with 50,000 or fewer SNPs. The imputed HD genotypes of bulls used in this study were a subset of those animals. The original 777,962 HD SNPs were reduced to 312,614 by removing highly correlated markers with an |r| higher than 0.95 and by further editing before imputation with findhap (version 3) [12]. To verify direction and consistency of allele codes, genotypes called from sequences were matched to corresponding chip SNPs for 179 Holstein or red Holstein animals that had SNP genotypes imputed in the US database and sequences in the 1000 Bull Genomes Project database.

Variants with a MAF lower than 0.01, incorrect map locations, an excess of heterozygotes, or low correlations (|r| < 0.95) between sequence and HD genotypes for the same variant were removed. A few hundred sequence variants were removed in specific regions that were known to be mapped incorrectly in the UMD3.1 bovine reference assembly. Most map issues had been previously detected by using small sets of SNPs that were lowly correlated to adjacent sets within windows that had excessive total numbers of haplotypes [12].

After merging sequence and HD data, Mendelian conflicts between parents and progeny were set to missing for 0.01% of the genotypes. The percentage of conflicts was expected to be small because both the HD and sequence genotypes had been previously edited. About 1% of the HD imputed genotypes were unknown in the findhap output, and their allele frequencies were substituted when used in genomic prediction. All HD SNPs that were also in the sequence data were retained except in cases when the absolute correlation between HD SNPs was lower than 0.95. This editing step removed less than 1000 (0.3%) of the HD SNPs because a similar edit had previously been applied before imputation [12].

Three different sets of variants were imputed to test the use of candidate SNPs (Test 1), candidate SNPs and InDels (Test 2), and candidate SNPs, InDels, and intergenic and intronic variants (Test 3). Predictions and QTL discovery using Test 3 data will be reported separately. The initial edits for sequence genotypes used in Tests 1 and 2 were revised in Test 3 because imputation accuracy decreased when millions of intergenic and intronic variants were included. The new edits for Test 3 computed statistics across all samples to improve imputation accuracy instead of editing each animal individually. The VCF file contains three genotype probabilities from Beagle, and the editing done for Tests 1 and 2 simply retained any genotype with a probability higher than 0.98. The new edits were based on an individual probability higher than 0.95, and after processing all animals, a second edit deleted any variant that had more than 5% missing genotypes for low frequency variants (MAF < 0.10) or more than MAF/2 missing genotypes for more common variants. Thus, variants with MAF = 0.50 were not used if more than 25% of the called genotypes had a probability below 95%. The third new edit for Test 3 checked for Hardy–Weinberg equilibrium and deleted variants that had 1.5 times more heterozygotes than the expected fraction of $2p(1 - p)$. After these edits, only 3,148,506 variants remained.

Quality and orientation of calls were examined using 179 bulls that had both sequence and HD genotypes. After reversing the orientation of the HD SNPs to match sequence data and keeping the sequence instead of the HD genotype for animals that had both, the two datasets were combined, resulting in 27,235 animals. Quality of imputation was assessed by keeping 404 of the sequenced animals in the reference population and randomly choosing 40 animals as a test set. Their sequence genotypes were reduced to the subset of genotypes that were in common with HD genotypes and then imputed back to sequence. The percentage of imputed genotypes that matched the original genotypes was the simple measure of sequence imputation accuracy.

Genomic predictions were computed using deregressed evaluations from August 2011 for 33 traits and 19,575 bulls. Predictions were tested using 2015 data of 3983 bulls with daughters that were first phenotyped after August 2011. Reliabilities were estimated from the squared correlations of predictions with the deregressed evaluations, divided by their reliabilities to account

for error variance, and adding the difference between observed and expected reliability of parent average to account for selection [21]. Regressions of 2015 data on 2011 predictions were compared to the expected value of 1.0.

Test 1 combined 481,904 candidate sequence SNPs with HD genotypes for 312,614 markers and a total of 762,588 variants. The candidate variants included 107,471 variants in exons, 9422 in splice sites, 35,242 in untranslated regions at the beginning and end of genes, 254,907 within a 2-kb region upstream, and 74,862 within a 1-kb region downstream, for a total of 481,904 candidate variants based on the Ensembl gene annotation [22] database version 79 released in 2015 (ftp://ftp.ensembl.org/pub/release-79/gtf/bos_taurus). Test 2 also included any InDels that were located within genes or within the regions 2 kb upstream and 1 kb downstream of genes. Imputed data of Test 3 were used only for GWA because genomic predictions converged too slowly with more than 3 million variants, and the GWA results from real data will be reported separately. Additional file 1: Table S1 lists the variants included in each test.

A subset of variants was selected for potential use in routine genomic prediction by applying methods similar to those used previously to select the HD SNPs with the largest effects in the national evaluation [16] except that only Holstein data were used in the current test. The top 1000 SNPs by absolute effect size for each of the 33 traits were selected from Test 1 and merged to eliminate duplicates. These 16,648 sequence variants with the largest effects were selected from the analysis of 762,588 markers and added to the 60,671 markers used previously. However, 6584 or about 10% of those previously used markers were not called as variable and thus not reported in the sequence data and were not used in the final test set of 70,735 markers.

Results
Simulated sequence

Edits for MAF and LD removed 3.4 and 18.4 million variants, respectively, from the simulated WGS variants from our 1000 bull founder population, which reduced the variant list from 30 million initial simulated variants to 8.4 million that included the 600 k array SNPs and the 505,210 genic variants. For the 26.6 million variants with a MAF higher than 0.01, the maximum absolute correlation with any of the 350 variants on either side was on average equal to 0.96. High correlations improve imputation and also indicate that most QTL can be efficiently traced by nearby markers.

Average reliability of prediction was equal to 28.4% based on the simulated parent average, 77.8 and 80.1% based on the 60 and 600 k chips, respectively, 79.2%

based on the markers selected by GWA from the 600 k chip, and 87.2% based on only the 10 k imputed true QTL with no weight on the markers (Table 1). The reliability gain of 2.3 percentage points obtained for the 600 k compared with the 60 k SNPs is larger than reported earlier from either simulated (0.9) or actual (0.4) genomic predictions [12]. The previous results led to the conclusion that simply adding more markers resulted only in small improvements because prior variance for each marker was smaller, causing more shrinkage for all marker effects. Also, the additional markers were imputed rather than directly observed.

In Table 1, the other variant subsets were selected using effects from multiple regression instead of GWA. Adding 24 k SNPs from the 600 k with the largest effects to the 60 k SNPs resulted in higher reliability by 2.2 percentage points than adding 24 k SNPs selected by GWA and also in 1.3 percentage points higher than using all 600 k SNPs, which was consistent with previous results from real data [16]. Selecting SNPs on effect variance was expected to be more efficient than selecting on effect size, but effect size resulted in slightly higher reliability (81.5 vs. 81.2%). The increased MAF should have improved imputation accuracy, but only 19% of the SNPs differed between the two selection strategies. Selecting 24 k SNPs based on an average of the five traits to mimic index selection (results not shown in Table 1) led to about only 50% of the markers being in common with the other two strategies and resulted in slightly lower reliability than selecting for each trait and then combining them (81.1 vs. 81.2%).

The genic subset of 1.1 million simulated sequence variants resulted in a reliability of 86.4%, which was much higher than the 81.5% obtained from the best analysis from selecting 600 k SNPs and only about 1 percentage point less than the 87.2% maximum obtained by using just the 10 k true QTL. This confirms that selection of variants near genes improves accuracy if all genes are known and all variation is associated with genes, which is in agreement with Pérez-Enciso et al. [6]. Including 1.1 million

variants in routine evaluations or on chips is difficult, but 60 k SNPs plus the top 24 k SNPs that are chosen from the 1.1 million by multiple regression resulted in a reliability of 85.0%. If the 10 k true QTL were added to the 60 k SNPs but were not given extra prior variance, the reliability was then only 84.5% because too much prior variance was assigned to the 60 k SNPs compared to the 10 k QTL. All tests of simulated data had regressions of TBV on genomic predictions that averaged 1.02 to 1.05 across five traits, which is slightly higher than the expected value of 1.0; regressions on parent average averaged 0.98.

Computing resources are in Table 2 for each step run on an IBM X3850 X5 with 4 Intel X7560 CPUs (32 cores, 64 threads @ 2.27 GHz), and 512 GB of memory. Genotype simulation required 56 h with one thread and 210 GB of memory and the output was a 32-GB file. Calculation of linkage correlations between neighbouring sequence variants and pruning those that were highly correlated took 1 h with 10 threads and 27 GB of memory. Imputation of 8.4 million variants for 26,984 bulls required 38 h with 20 threads and 13 GB of memory and the output was a 220-GB file. Selection of variants by GWA required only 30 min with 30 threads and very little memory. Genomic prediction for 1.1 million variants and five traits required 22 h with five threads and 20 GB of memory. Thus, GWA was faster for selecting variants, but multiple regression selected marker sets that gave more reliable predictions.

Real variants

Edits for real as well as simulated sequence variants are documented in Table 3. In the real data, 20 million of the initial 39 million variants were removed because of low MAF, and another 13 million were removed because of high linkage with neighbouring variants. Further edits in Tests 1 and 2 retained only the HD markers, candidate SNPs, and candidate InDels. In Test 3, 3 million of the remaining variants with lower genotype probabilities were removed to improve imputation accuracy.

Table 1 Reliabilities for five simulated traits from ten sources of genetic information

Trait	Parent average	60 k	60 k + 24 k$_{GWA}$	60 k + 24 k$_{ES}$	60 k + 24 k$_{EV}$	60 k + 24 k$_{G}$	60 k + 10 k QTL	Only 10 k QTL	600 k	1.1 m genic
1	24.4	77.9	79.2	81.6	81.3	85.4	84.6	87.2	80.3	86.7
2	31.2	77.9	79.3	81.4	81.2	85.3	84.9	87.7	80.1	86.7
3	32.7	78.3	79.5	81.7	81.5	84.9	85.0	87.8	80.4	86.1
4	23.3	76.6	77.7	80.2	79.8	83.5	82.9	85.9	78.6	84.8
5	30.4	78.3	80.0	82.5	82.2	86.0	85.2	87.5	81.2	87.6
Average	28.4	77.8	79.2	81.5	81.2	85.0	84.5	87.2	80.1	86.4

Reliabilities expressed as percentages; 24 k markers selected from 600 k SNPs by GWA p value, multiple regression effect size (ES) or effect variance (EV); 24 k markers selected from sequence SNPs in or near genes (G) by effect size; 600 k markers plus 500 k SNPs in or near genes (1.1 m genic) by effect size

Table 2 Computer resources needed to select markers from 30 million simulated variants

Variant selection step	Number of threads	Computational time (h)	GB of memory	GB of disk space
Simulate 30 million	1	56	210	32
Prune linkage	10	1	27	10
Impute 8.4 million	20	38	13	220
Select 25,000	30	0.5	<1	<1
Predict 1 million	5	22	20	<1

1000 sequenced and 25,984 genotyped bulls

Table 3 Edits applied to simulated data and real data from Test 3

SNP edit	Simulated data	Real data
Original number of SNPs called	30 million	39 million
Removed for MAF of <0.01	3 million	20 million
Removed for linkage of >0.95	18 million	13 million
Removed for imputation inaccuracy	0	3 million
Remained after edits	8 million	3 million

Test 3 included candidate SNPs, InDels, and intergenic and intronic variants

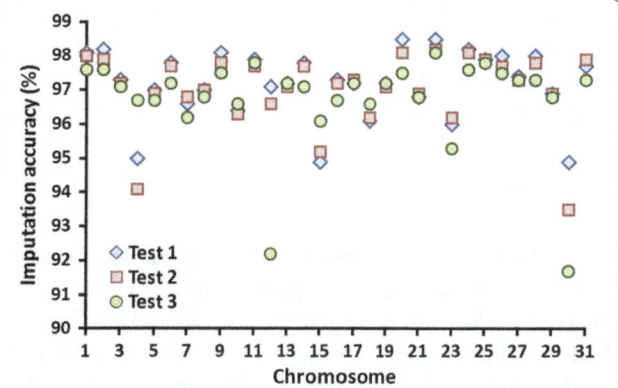

Fig. 1 Accuracy of imputing sequence variants. Test 1 included 762,588 candidate SNPs. Test 2 included candidate SNPs plus 249,966 InDels for a total of 1,003,453 variants. Test 3 included candidate SNPs, InDels, and intergenic and intronic variants for a total of 3,148,506 variants. Chromosome 30 refers to the pseudo-autosomal region of chromosome X, and chromosome 31 refers to X-specific loci

Only 91% of the 60,671 chip SNPs currently used in official US evaluations were included in the sequence data. It is expected that some markers with a low MAF will be missing, but the average MAF of the 9% that were missing and the 91% that matched were both equal to about 0.28 in Holsteins. The missing markers are evenly scattered across the chromosomes; therefore, they probably do not indicate reference genome misassemblies but likely result from edits during variant identification [18]. The individual correlations of HD genotypes with sequence genotypes were mostly near +1 or −1, which indicates good quality for the 91% of HD SNPs present in the sequence data. About half of the genotypes had reversed allele coding compared to the sequence variant calls because sequence alternate alleles are coded as differences from a Hereford cow-derived reference genome, whereas the array alleles were in Illumina TOP encoding.

Average imputation accuracy was equal to 97.2% of correct genotypes for the 762,588 variants in Test 1 across all chromosomes, with a maximum of 98.5% for bovine chromosome BTA20 (BTA for *Bos taurus* chromosome) and BTA22 and a minimum of 94.9% for BTA15 and 95.0% for BTA4 (Fig. 1). The X chromosome was split into the pseudo-autosomal region, which was labelled as BTA30 with poor imputation and the X-specific loci labelled as BTA31; no Y loci were present. Imputation accuracy was equal to 97.0% for the 1,003,453 variants that included InDels in Test 2 and 96.7% for the 3,148,506 variants that also included intronic and intergenic variants in Test 3. The percentages are inflated because they

include the HD SNPs that were already present. If HD SNPs are not counted, accuracies of 95.3, 95.6, and 96.4% for just the new variants were found for Tests 1, 2, and 3, respectively. The lower imputation accuracy for BTA12 in Test 3 was mainly caused by a gap between 72.4 and 75.2 Mb for which no SNPs were available on the HD array.

The total time required to prepare, edit, and impute the 762,588 variants for 27,235 animals ranged from 1 to 5 h per chromosome (Table 4) and was about 5 days for all 30 chromosomes. Data manipulation steps such as transposing the sequence data and merging with HD SNPs used one thread and took more time than the imputation, which used 20 threads and took less than 1 day.

Reliability of predictions improved by only 0.6 percentage points on average using 762,588 variants (481,904 candidate sequence variants and HD SNPs) compared with using HD SNPs only (Table 5). Inclusion of InDels decreased the advantage over HD SNPs to only 0.4 percentage points. Reliability improved by about 2.7 percentage points compared with 60 k SNPs only for the final set of 70,735 variants (60 k SNPs minus 6584 markers

Table 4 Computation time[a] required with real sequence data for the longest (BTA1) and shortest (BTA29) chromosomes

Computational step	BTA1	BTA29
Unzip VCF files	6	2
Read and transpose sequence	95	36
Subset sequenced animals	1	1
Subset matching HD markers	8	10
Merge sequence and HD data	143	6
Compute sequence linkage	3	1
Subset edited variants	3	1
Fix Mendelian conflicts	3	1
Impute with edited data	16	10
Reduce some sequence to HD data	1	1
Impute with reduced data	17	9
Total	296	78

[a] Time in minutes

that were not included in the sequence data plus 16,648 sequence variants with the largest effects). Reliability was equal to 35.2% based on parent average, 64.7% for predictions from 60 k SNPs only, 67.4% from 762,588 SNPs, 64.0% from HD SNPs only, 64.6% for HD plus genic SNPs, and 64.4% from HD plus genic SNPs and InDels. The 60 k SNPs already included the best SNPs selected from the HD chip [16], which may explain why 60 k predictions slightly outperformed HD predictions. For most traits, regressions of validation data on genomic predictions were near the expected value of 1.0 and changed little with the selected subset of variants used (Table 6).

For use with lower-density genotyping arrays, the list of 16,648 sequence variants was further restricted to 4822. Hand-made edits were applied to prevent too many candidate SNPs from all tagging the same QTL. Figure 2 provides an example for BTA5 of the SNPs that were retained or removed. The same list of 4822 SNPs was provided to Zoetis (Florham Park, NJ), GeneSeek (Lincoln, NE), and Genetic Visions (Middleton, WI) for potential inclusion on revised arrays. Benefits of adding the sequence SNPs directly to lower-density rather than only to medium- or higher-density arrays are that more young animals can be genotyped quickly and imputation loss can be avoided when including sequence SNPs in routine predictions. Re-genotyping or sequencing more reference animals could also help avoid imputation loss when estimating SNP effects for newly discovered variants.

Discussion

Comparison with previous studies

Previous studies used 5000 bulls with HD genotypes and 10 million variants from run 3 sequence data [8] or 4 million variants from run 4 [3], but sequence predictions in those studies had slightly lower reliabilities than predictions from BovineHD or BovineSNP50 genotypes. The HD genotypes in those studies were all observed, but HD genotypes used in our study were mostly imputed. Use of run 3 or run 4 instead of run 5 sequence data could explain their slightly negative instead of slightly positive gains. The results from those studies and ours suggest that errors in the sequence data or remaining reference assembly mistakes that altered the order of variant sites could account for the small changes in prediction reliability when hundreds of thousands or millions of sequence variants were added.

Our results indicate that adding smaller numbers of selected sequence variants can be useful in routine prediction even if the analysis of all variants is not more accurate or feasible, which is consistent with previous conclusions for sequence [2] or HD data [16, 23]. Brøndum et al. [2] added 1623 sequence variants selected by GWA from multiple breeds to a custom chip and reported gains in reliability that averaged about 2 percentage points. Small improvements (0.2 percentage points) from adding SNPs that are located in genes associated with fertility were observed by Ortega et al. [9], which is consistent with gains reported in this and earlier studies [12]. Using selected sequence variants and giving extra weight to candidate variants or QTL can improve predictions across breeds [5, 24–27], but advantages of focusing on candidate variants decrease if not all QTL are in the variant set [6]. Multi-trait methods can detect QTL that single-trait methods might miss [28], and even uncorrelated traits can help separate QTL from markers if many independent traits are controlled by a limited number of QTL.

Comparison of simulated and real selection

Properties of the real sequence data from the 1000 Bull Genomes Project were similar to those of the simulated data by VanRaden and O'Connell [29]. LD and MAF distributions in the real and simulated data are compared in Figs. 3 and 4, respectively. Overall, results were similar for real and simulated data, but more of the variants in the real data have a very low MAF or are in very low LD with neighbouring variants. Average MAF was the same (0.20) for the HD and genic SNPs in Test 1 but was lower (0.15) for the InDels added in Test 2, which could have affected imputation accuracy. Edits for MAF and for high LD reduced the 30 million simulated SNPs to 8.4 million, whereas the same edits reduced the 39 million real variants to 6.3 million (Table 3). Our edits for Test 3 were similar to those of Calus et al. [3], who obtained 4.1 million variants from Holstein data in run 4. The simulated variants were for one breed with a common pedigree, whereas the real variants were discovered in a wide

Table 5 Reliability gains when adding real sequence variants to HD or 60 K

Trait	Reliability for PA (%)	Gain for HD SNPs only	Gain for HD SNPs + 481,904 candidate SNPs[a]	Gain for HD SNPs + 481,904 candidate SNPs + indels	Gain for 60 k SNPs only	Gain for 60 k SNPs + 16,648 candidate SNPs[b,c]
Milk	37.9	34.1	33.9 (−0.2)	33.9	34.3	35.7 (1.4)
Fat	37.9	33.7	34.0 (0.3)	33.4	34.3	35.1 (0.8)
Protein	37.9	27.9	27.0 (−0.9)	26.7	27.5	28.2 (0.7)
Fat percentage	37.9	49.2	52.7 (3.5)	52.4	52.9	54.8 (1.9)
Protein percentage	37.9	42.1	41.6 (0.5)	43.0	41.6	44.3 (2.7)
Productive life	32.0	36.1	35.8 (−0.3)	36.4	35.6	38.2 (2.6)
Somatic cell score	34.7	35.9	36.1 (0.2)	37.1	35.1	37.0 (1.9)
Daughter pregnancy rate	31.5	30.8	30.0 (−0.8)	31.2	29.0	33.0 (4.0)
Cow conception rate	29.8	28.7	28.1 (−0.6)	28.8	28.9	31.8 (2.9)
Heifer conception rate	30.0	19.0	20.3 (1.3)	19.7	20.5	21.5 (1.0)
Sire calving ease	29.9	27.8	27.7 (−0.1)	25.2	24.5	28.5 (4.0)
Daughter calving ease	25.3	32.5	30.8 (−1.7)	29.9	31.5	31.4 (−0.1)
Sire stillbirth	29.0	7.6	7.3 (−0.3)	7.1	7.6	7.8 (0.2)
Daughter stillbirth	23.8	37.4	37.0 (−0.4)	35.8	35.4	38.0 (2.6)
Final score	36.2	24.7	25.5 (0.8)	25.8	24.6	27.8 (3.2)
Stature	38.2	30.4	32.4 (2.0)	32.8	30.3	34.7 (4.3)
Strength	37.4	29.9	31.8 (1.9)	31.8	29.9	34.5 (4.6)
Dairy form	37.4	33.8	35.3 (1.5)	35.8	35.0	38.2 (3.2)
Foot angle	36.7	17.3	17.6 (0.3)	18.2	17.2	19.6 (2.4)
Rear legs (side view)	37.3	21.9	22.7 (0.8)	22.0	22.1	24.1 (2.0)
Body depth	37.6	31.0	33.1 (2.1)	33.7	31.2	36.0 (4.8)
Rump angle	37.8	32.7	34.0 (1.3)	33.5	32.9	36.1 (3.2)
Rump width	37.1	29.2	30.4 (1.2)	30.2	29.1	32.5 (3.4)
Fore udder attachment	37.5	35.1	36.4 (1.3)	36.1	35.0	39.0 (4.0)
Rear udder height	37.3	24.7	25.7 (1.0)	25.8	24.1	27.3 (3.2)
Udder depth	38.0	40.2	42.6 (2.4)	42.8	40.6	44.6 (4.0)
Udder cleft	37.1	23.7	24.5 (0.8)	24.0	23.6	25.5 (1.9)
Front teat placement	37.6	32.6	33.4 (0.8)	32.3	30.9	35.0 (4.1)
Teat length	37.7	29.0	30.3 (1.3)	29.9	28.0	32.7 (4.7)
Rear legs (rear view)	36.0	20.7	20.3 (−0.4)	20.1	20.4	22.8 (2.4)
Feet and leg score	36.4	16.9	16.5 (−0.4)	16.6	15.9	18.3 (2.4)
Rear teat placement	37.4	33.1	33.6 (0.5)	32.1	32.9	35.2 (2.3)
Net merit	34.4	23.8	24.3 (0.5)	24.4	23.4	24.7 (1.3)
Average	35.2	28.8	29.4 (0.6)	29.2	29.5	32.2 (2.7)

Reliability gains in percentage points over parent average reliability

PA parent average

[a] Difference from reliability gain for HD SNPS only in parentheses

[b] Difference from reliability gain for 60 k SNPS only in parentheses

[c] Does not include 6584 60 k markers that were not available in sequence data

variety of breeds and only the variants that were polymorphic in Holsteins were retained. Also, the real data contain some false positive variants because of sequencing, alignment, and calling errors that are not modelled in the simulated data. Many variants had to be excluded from the Test 3 data because of low previous imputation

accuracy, whereas the simulated data was of high quality for all variants.

Gains in reliability from the use of real sequence data were smaller than from simulated data but higher than previous gains reported from HD data. Larger gains may be possible if the selected SNPs are added to arrays

Table 6 Coefficients for regression of validation data on genomic predictions when adding real sequence variants to HD or 60 k

Trait	PA	HD SNPs only	HD SNPs + 481,904 candidate SNPs	HD SNPs + 481,904 candidate SNPs + InDels	60 k SNPs only	60 k SNPs + 16,648 candidate SNPs[a]
Milk	0.81	1.03	1.06	1.06	1.04	1.05
Fat	0.68	0.92	0.95	0.94	0.94	0.93
Protein	0.75	0.93	0.96	0.95	0.94	0.95
Fat percentage	0.97	1.14	1.13	1.12	1.12	1.09
Protein percentage	0.77	0.96	0.98	0.97	0.95	0.96
Productive life	1.24	1.30	1.32	1.25	1.27	1.25
Somatic cell score	0.89	1.09	1.10	1.06	1.08	1.06
Daughter pregnancy rate	1.20	1.47	1.49	1.48	1.43	1.43
Cow conception rate	0.72	0.94	0.95	0.92	0.91	0.91
Heifer conception rate	0.75	0.97	1.03	0.98	0.94	0.92
Sire calving ease	0.65	0.83	0.83	0.81	0.82	0.84
Daughter calving ease	0.80	1.04	1.03	1.02	1.04	1.02
Sire stillbirth	0.84	0.75	0.76	0.78	0.77	0.76
Daughter stillbirth	0.77	1.15	1.16	1.15	1.12	1.16
Final score	0.71	0.93	0.92	0.92	0.91	0.88
Stature	0.84	1.04	1.02	1.01	1.01	1.00
Strength	0.80	1.05	1.03	1.02	1.01	0.99
Dairy form	0.82	1.10	1.08	1.08	1.07	1.05
Foot angle	0.71	0.84	0.82	0.82	0.81	0.79
Rear legs (side view)	0.87	1.01	0.99	0.99	0.98	0.96
Body depth	0.76	1.01	0.99	0.99	0.97	0.96
Rump angle	0.80	1.08	1.07	1.05	1.06	1.05
Rump width	0.78	1.01	0.99	0.98	0.98	0.96
Fore udder attachment	0.80	1.06	1.04	1.03	1.03	1.01
Rear udder height	0.78	0.97	0.96	0.96	0.94	0.93
Udder depth	0.76	1.11	1.09	1.08	1.07	1.06
Udder cleft	0.87	1.00	0.99	0.99	0.98	0.95
Front teat placement	0.80	1.05	1.03	1.01	1.02	0.99
Teat length	0.91	1.06	1.06	1.04	1.04	1.03
Rear legs (rear view)	0.58	0.86	0.85	0.83	0.83	0.80
Feet and leg score	0.54	0.74	0.72	0.72	0.71	0.68
Rear teat placement	0.90	1.13	1.10	1.09	1.09	1.04
Net merit	0.85	0.82	0.84	0.81	0.83	0.81
Average	0.81	1.01	1.01	1.00	0.99	0.98

PA parent average

[a] Does not include 6584 60 k markers that were not available in sequence data

and genotyped directly with high accuracy instead of imputed from less accurate sequence data. Accuracies of genotypes from sequence variant calling can vary [30], whereas the error rate of Illumina BeadChip arrays is less than 1% for nearly all SNPs.

Computation

Most computing steps in Table 4 were programmed in Fortran for efficiency, but several steps were in SAS for convenience. The SAS program used to merge sequence and HD data took only 6 min for the shortest chromosome but 143 min for the longest one; it could be rewritten because it became a limiting step. Total times required for Tests 2 and 3 were only a little longer than those shown for Test 1 because imputation took a small fraction of the total time. Imputation of 8 million simulated variants took only 38 h with 20 threads for 25,984 reference bulls. Larger populations or variant sets can be imputed, but genomic predictions then become the limiting step. More research is needed on how to accurately and efficiently select the best subset of variants for routine use.

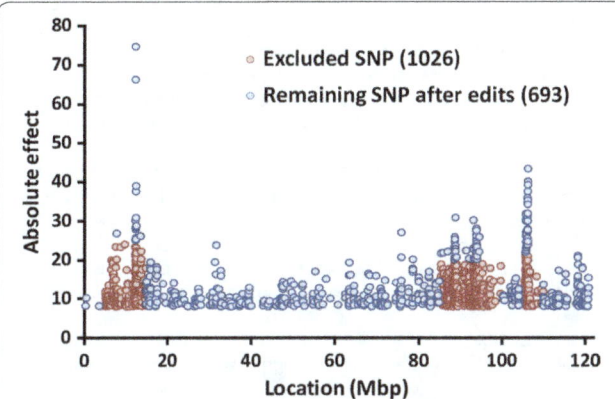

Fig. 2 Example of variant selection on chromosome 5. For 1719 SNPs, windows were designated for SNPs with the largest effects. Then, only SNPs with larger effects were retained in those windows (1026 SNPs excluded)

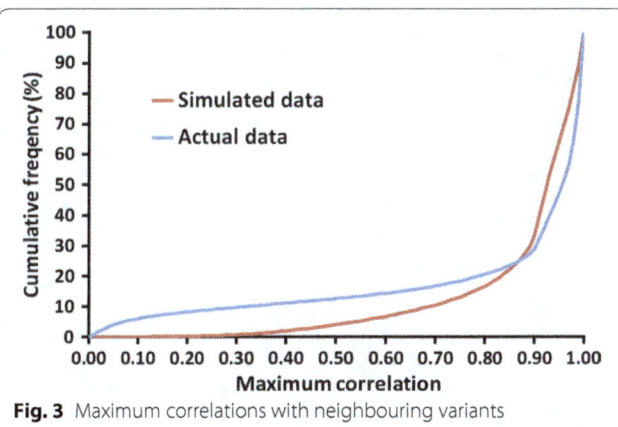

Fig. 3 Maximum correlations with neighbouring variants

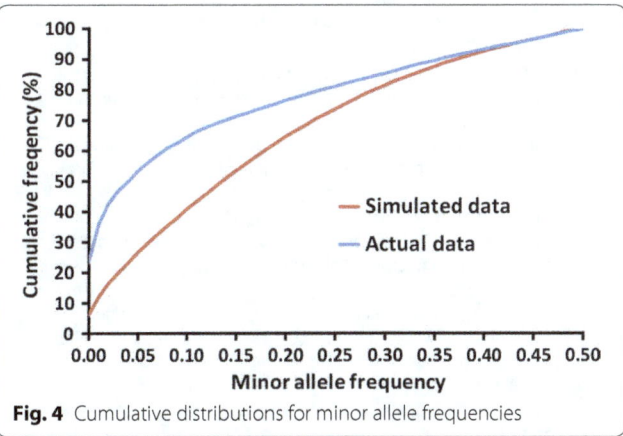

Fig. 4 Cumulative distributions for minor allele frequencies

Economic benefit

Increasing the reliability of selection by 2.7 percentage points from 64.7 to 67.4% would add about $3 million per year to national genetic progress. Additional

progress would be realized globally for foreign breeders that directly use the new genotyping arrays or that indirectly benefit by selecting breeding stock from the improved US population. Annual domestic progress is now about $50 per cow and would increase to $51 after multiplying by the accuracy ratio of 1.02, which is the square root of the reliability ratio (67.4/64.7). This higher accuracy has an annual national value of about $3 million because each year 3.3 million of the 9.2 million US dairy cows are replaced. These annual gains are permanent and will accumulate. The initial cost of generating the US sequence data for the 88 dairy bulls contributed to the 1000 Bull Genomes Project was $132,000 at current estimates of reagent costs (assuming a cost of ~$1500 per sample). The return on investment from this research is high and greatly increased because of data sharing.

New animals will be directly genotyped for the selected variants and thus could have slightly higher reliability gains than in these tests that use imputed data, but most reference animals will still have imputed data. Re-genotyping old animals with the new arrays might be less expensive than additional sequencing to improve accuracy of imputation.

Conclusions

Variant selection is needed because routine genomic predictions cannot impute and include all of the millions of sequence variants for all animals. Significant gains in reliability are possible if the true QTL can be identified or if bioinformatic methods can choose the regions that are more likely to contain causative variants. Because individual QTL have such small effects, large reference populations are needed with phenotypes for the relevant traits and observed or imputed genotypes for the QTL or closely linked variants. Testing many individual traits gives more power because the effect of each QTL may be detectable only for a few traits, but these same QTL may have smaller effects on several correlated traits. Assigning more prior variance to the QTL or to the newly selected variants can improve reliability when estimating effects, but the SNPs from previous arrays must be retained during imputation because genotypes of previous animals include only the SNPs and not the new variants.

Computation becomes a limiting factor as reference populations and target populations grow in size. Total computing time was only a few days with up to 1000 sequences and 30,000 reference bulls, but more than 150,000 reference cows and 800,000 young animals were not included. Multiple regressions used for genomic prediction were more accurate than GWA for selecting variants but required much more computation time. Imputation allows many more sequence variants to be tested, selected, and included in routine predictions to increase their reliability. For both the simulated and real data, gains from selecting and including candidate sequence variants were larger than from selecting HD SNPs.

Additional file

Additional file 1. List of variants from Run 5 of the 1000 Bull Genomes Project used in Tests 1, 2 and 3. All edited variants are listed with 1 or 0 in the final three columns indicating if the variant was used in Test 1, 2 or 3. Fields included are VariantName, Chromosome, Location, VariantType, Test_1, Test_2, and Test_3 in a space delimited file. Variant types use the 3-character codes EXN = exonic, SPL = splice site, UTR = untranslated region, UPS = upstream, DNS = downstream, SNP = other intronic or intergenic SNP, and IND = InDel.

Authors' contributions
PMV, JRO, and DMB developed the experimental designs. MET and PMV performed many of the computations. PMV, JBC, and JRO drafted the paper. All authors read and approved the final manuscript.

Author details
[1] Animal Genomics and Improvement Laboratory, Agricultural Research Service, USDA, Beltsville, MD, USA. [2] University of Maryland Baltimore, Baltimore, MD, USA.

Acknowledgements
The authors thank Suzanne Hubbard for technical editing and manuscript improvement, George Liu and Steve Schroeder for assistance in generating the US sequence data, the 1000 Bull Genomes Project for global sequence data, the Council on Dairy Cattle Breeding for genotype, phenotype, and pedigree data, Interbull for global trait evaluations, and the anonymous reviewers for many helpful comments. Mention of trade names or commercial products in this article is solely for the purpose of providing specific information and does not imply recommendation or endorsement by the US Department of Agriculture.

Competing interests
The authors declare that they have no competing interests.

Funding
PMV, MET, DMB, and JBC were supported by appropriated project 8042-31000-101-00 (Improving Genetic Predictions in Dairy Animals Using Phenotypic and Genomic Information) of the Agricultural Research Service, USDA. JRO was supported by a Specific Cooperative Agreement with the Agricultural Research Service, USDA.

References
1. Brøndum RF, Guldbrandtsen B, Sahana G, Lund MS, Su G. Strategies for imputation to whole genome sequence using a single or multi-breed reference population in cattle. BMC Genomics. 2014;15:728.
2. Brøndum RF, Su G, Janss L, Sahana G, Guldbrandtsen B, Boichard D, et al. Quantitative trait loci markers derived from whole genome sequence data increases the reliability of genomic prediction. J Dairy Sci. 2015;98:4107–16.
3. Calus MPL, Bouwman AC, Schrooten C, Veerkamp RF. Efficient genomic prediction based on whole-genome sequence data using split-and-merge Bayesian variable selection. Genet Sel Evol. 2016;48:49.
4. Druet T, MacLeod IM, Hayes BJ. Toward genomic prediction from whole-genome sequence data: impact of sequencing design on genotype imputation and accuracy of predictions. Heredity (Edinb). 2014;112:39–47.
5. MacLeod IM, Bowman PJ, Vander Jagt CJ, Haile-Mariam M, Kemper KE, Chamberlain AJ, et al. Exploiting biological priors and sequence variants enhances QTL discovery and genomic prediction of complex traits. BMC Genomics. 2016;17:144.
6. Pérez-Enciso M, Rincón JC, Legarra A. Sequence- vs. chip-assisted genomic selection: accurate biological information is advised. Genet Sel Evol. 2015;47:43.
7. van Binsbergen R, Bink MCAM, Calus MPL, van Eeuwijk FA, Hayes BJ, Hulsegge I, et al. Accuracy of imputation to whole-genome sequence data in Holstein Friesian cattle. Genet Sel Evol. 2014;46:41.
8. van Binsbergen R, Calus MPL, Bink MCAM, van Eeuwijk FA, Schrooten C, Veerkamp RF. Genomic prediction using imputed whole-genome sequence data in Holstein Friesian cattle. Genet Sel Evol. 2015;47:71.
9. Ortega MS, Denicol AC, Cole JB, Null DJ, Hansen PJ. Use of single nucleotide polymorphisms in candidate genes associated with daughter pregnancy rate for prediction of genetic merit for reproduction in Holstein cows. Anim Genet. 2016;47:288–97.
10. Hayes BJ, MacLeod IM, Daetwyler HD, Bowman PJ, Chamberlain AJ, Vander Jagt CJ, et al. Genomic prediction from whole genome sequence in livestock: the 1000 Bull Genomes Project. In: Proceedings of the 10th world congress on genetics applied to livestock production: 17–22 August 2014; Vancouver. 2014. https://asas.org/docs/default-source/wcgalp-proceedings-oral/183_paper_10441_manuscript_1644_0.pdf. Accessed 27 Dec 2016.
11. VanRaden P, Sun C. genosim: Simulate genotypes, breeding values, and phenotypes; simulate DNA sequence read depth (numbers of A and B alleles); and resolve SNP conflicts between parent and offspring genotypes. In: Animal improvement program. Animal Genomics and Improvement Laboratory, ARS, USDA. 2014. https://aipl.arsusda.gov/software/genosim. Accessed 27 Dec 2016.
12. VanRaden PM, Null DJ, Sargolzaei M, Wiggans GR, Tooker ME, Cole JB, et al. Genomic imputation and evaluation using high-density Holstein genotypes. J Dairy Sci. 2013;96:668–78.
13. Cole JB, VanRaden PM, O'Connell JR, Van Tassell CP, Sonstegard TS, Schnabel RD, et al. Distribution and location of genetic effects for dairy traits. J Dairy Sci. 2009;92:2931–46.
14. O'Connell J. MMAP: a comprehensive mixed model program for analysis of pedigree and population data. In: Proceedings of the 63rd annual meeting of the American society for human genetics: 22–26 October 2013; Boston. 2013. http://www.ashg.org/2013meeting/abstracts/fulltext/f130123097.htm. Accessed 27 Dec 2016.
15. O'Connell JR. MMAP user guide. 2016. http://edn.som.umaryland.edu/mmap/index.php. Accessed 27 Dec 2016.
16. Wiggans GR, Cooper TA, VanRaden PM, Van Tassell CP, Bickhart DM, Sonstegard TS. Increasing the number of single nucleotide polymorphisms used in genomic evaluation of dairy cattle. J Dairy Sci. 2016;99:4504–11.
17. VanRaden PM, Cole JB. AIP research report NM$5: net merit as a measure of lifetime profit: 2014 revision. In: Animal improvement program. Animal Genomics and Improvement Laboratory, ARS, USDA. 2014. https://aipl.arsusda.gov/reference/nmcalc-2014.htm. Accessed 27 Dec 2016.
18. Daetwyler HD, Capitan A, Pausch H, Stothard P, van Binsbergen R, Brøndum RF, et al. Whole-genome sequencing of 234 bulls facilitates mapping of monogenic and complex traits in cattle. Nat Genet. 2014;46:858–65.
19. VanRaden PM. findhap.f90: Find haplotypes and impute genotypes using multiple chip sets and sequence data. In: Animal improvement program. Animal Genomics and Improvement Laboratory, ARS, USDA. 2016. https://aipl.arsusda.gov/software/findhap. Accessed 27 Dec 2016.
20. Browning SR, Browning BL. Rapid and accurate haplotype phasing and missing-data inference for whole-genome association studies by use of localized haplotype clustering. Am J Hum Genet. 2007;81:1084–97.
21. VanRaden PM, Van Tassell CP, Wiggans GR, Sonstegard TS, Schnabel RD, Taylor JF, et al. Invited review: reliability of genomic predictions for North American Holstein bulls. J Dairy Sci. 2009;92:16–24.

22. Cunningham F, Amode MR, Barrell D, Beal K, Billis K, Brent S, et al. Ensembl 2015. Nucleic Acids Res. 2015;43:D662–9.

23. Saatchi M, Garrick DJ. Improving accuracies of genomic predictions by enriching 50K genotypes with markers from 770K genotypes at QTL regions. J Dairy Sci. 2014;97(Suppl 1):6.

24. Kizilkaya K, Fernando RL, Garrick DJ. Genomic prediction of simulated multibreed and purebred performance using observed fifty thousand single nucleotide polymorphism genotypes. J Anim Sci. 2010;88:544–51.

25. Iheshiulor OOM, Woolliams JA, Yu X, Wellmann R, Meuwissen THE. Within- and across-breed genomic prediction using whole-genome sequence and single nucleotide polymorphism panels. Genet Sel Evol. 2016;48:15.

26. van den Berg I, Boichard D, Guldbrandtsen B, Lund MS. Using sequence variants in linkage disequilibrium with causative mutations to improve across-breed prediction in dairy cattle: a simulation study. G3 (Bethesda). 2016;6:2553–61.

27. van den Berg I, Boichard D, Lund MS. Comparing power and precision of within-breed and multibreed genome-wide association studies of production traits using whole-genome sequence data for 5 French and Danish dairy cattle breeds. J Dairy Sci. 2016;99:8932–45.

28. Pausch H, Emmerling R, Schwarzenbacher H, Fries R. A multi-trait meta-analysis with imputed sequence variants reveals twelve QTL for mammary gland morphology in Fleckvieh cattle. Genet Sel Evol. 2016;48:14.

29. VanRaden PM, O'Connell JR. Strategies to choose from millions of imputed sequence variants. Interbull Bull. 2015;49:10–3.

30. Baes CF, Bapst B, Seefried FR, Flury C, Signer-Hasler H, Garrick DJ, et al. Across-breed imputation with whole genome sequence data in dairy cattle. In: Proceedings of plant & animal genome XXIII: 10–14 January 2015; San Diego. 2015. https://pag.confex.com/pag/xxiii/webprogram/Paper16562.html. Accessed 27 Dec 2016.

9

Deciphering mechanisms underlying the genetic variation of general production and liver quality traits in the overfed mule duck by pQTL analyses

Yoannah François[1], Alain Vignal[1], Caroline Molette[1], Nathalie Marty-Gasset[1], Stéphane Davail[2], Laurence Liaubet[1] and Christel Marie-Etancelin[1*] ⓘ

Abstract

Background: The aim of this study was to analyse the mechanisms that underlie phenotypic quantitative trait loci (QTL) in overfed mule ducks by identifying co-localized proteomic QTL (pQTL). The QTL design consisted of three families of common ducks that were progeny-tested by using 294 male mule ducks. This population of common ducks was genotyped using a genetic map that included 334 genetic markers located across 28 APL chromosomes (APL for *Anas platyrhynchos*). Mule ducks were phenotyped for 49 traits related to growth, metabolism, overfeeding ability and meat and fatty liver quality, and 326 soluble fatty liver proteins were quantified.

Results: One hundred and seventy-six pQTL and 80 phenotypic QTL were detected at the 5% chromosome-wide significance threshold. The great majority of the identified pQTL were trans-acting and localized on a chromosome other than that carrying the coding gene. The most significant pQTL (1% genome-wide significance) were found for alpha-enolase on APL18 and fatty acid synthase on APL24. Some proteins were associated with numerous pQTL (for example, 17 and 14 pQTL were detected for alpha-enolase and apolipoprotein A1, respectively) and pQTL hotspots were observed on some chromosomes (APL18, 24, 25 and 29). We detected 66 co-localized phenotypic QTL and pQTL for which the significance of the two-trait QTL (2t-QTL) analysis was higher than that of the strongest QTL using a single-trait approach. Among these, 16 2t-QTL were pleiotropic. For example, on APL15, melting rate and abundance of two alpha-enolase spots appeared to be impacted by a single locus that is involved in the glycolytic process. On APLZ, we identified a pleiotropic QTL that modified both the blood level of glucose at the beginning of the force-feeding period and the concentration of glutamate dehydrogenase, which, in humans, is involved in increased glucose absorption by the liver when the *glutamate dehydrogenase 1* gene is mutated.

Conclusions: We identified pleiotropic loci that affect metabolic pathways linked to glycolysis or lipogenesis, and in the end to fatty liver quality. Further investigation, via transcriptomics and metabolomics approaches, is required to confirm the biomarkers that were found to impact the genetic variability of these phenotypic traits.

Background

To date, approaches based on transcript abundance quantitative trait loci (QTL), better known as expression QTL (eQTL) have been the primary method used to understand the genetic architecture that underlies physiological traits controlled by QTL and the relationships between the genome and the phenome. However, the measure of transcript abundance used for eQTL analysis does not necessarily reflect the real abundance of the proteins coded by the genes. Indeed, mRNA levels can be influenced by multiple and complex regulation

*Correspondence: christel.marie-etancelin@inra.fr
[1] GenPhySE, INRA, INPT, INP-ENVT, Université de Toulouse, 31326 Castanet Tolosan, France
Full list of author information is available at the end of the article

processes, which, for instance, affect transcription levels or mRNA stability, whereas protein abundance depends also on other levels of regulation, such as translation, maturation, post-translational modification or protein degradation. Proteomic analyses can be performed to determine whether the protein is an inactive propeptide or in a modified active state. A study by Darmeval et al. [1] showed that there is a link between protein abundance and genome variability, which suggests that quantitative proteomic analyses are a better indicator of genetic distances between maize lines than qualitative analyses. These authors later introduced the concept of PQL (protein quantitative loci), hereafter designated pQTL for consistency with the current nomenclature of eQTL, when they successfully mapped loci that influence protein abundance [2]. One key benefit of the identification of eQTL and pQTL lies in their possible co-location with phenotypic QTL, thus highlighting the importance of specific proteins or candidate genes, as was shown in a study on pea [3]. In the animal kingdom, research on pQTL is more recent, but has proven effective in finding genes that cause variation in plasmatic protein abundance in mice, and one of these genes was linked to both a pQTL and a QTL for HDL cholesterol levels [4]. To our knowledge, no pQTL analyses have been performed on animals of agricultural interest. Although various large-scale studies on eQTL have already been implemented owing to the availability of adequate techniques, they need to be complemented by pQTL analyses, which are effective for a deeper understanding of phenotypes. Indeed, since proteins are the actual cellular effectors of many physiological processes, identification of the loci

that control their availability and abundance is an essential step in understanding the links between the genome and the phenome.

In a previous study, we identified QTL that are related to force-feeding traits [5] and are of great interest to the duck industry. In the current study, we quantified the proteins that are present in the fatty liver of the same ducks by quantitative 2D-gel electrophoresis [6] in order to perform pQTL analyses. The co-localized QTL and pQTL were investigated in an attempt to make connections between the phenotype and the proteome, and thus identify the biological mechanisms that underlie the genetic variability of these traits. Here, we present the results of QTL analyses on fatty liver proteomic data by focusing on the proteomic and phenotypic QTL that co-localized, and identified those that appear to have pleiotropic effects.

Methods

Experimental procedures were performed in accordance with the French National Guidelines for the care and use of animals for research purposes (Certificate of Authorization to Experiment on Living Animals no 7740, Ministry of Agriculture and Fish Products).

Experimental design and animal husbandry

Due to the complexity of generating the proteomic dataset on a large scale, the experimental design used here (Fig. 1b) is a subset of the complete design (Fig. 1a) used by Kileh-Wais et al. [5]. Briefly, it consists of a backcross (BC) design in which an additional generation (G) of overfed male mule ducks (G3) was phenotyped to

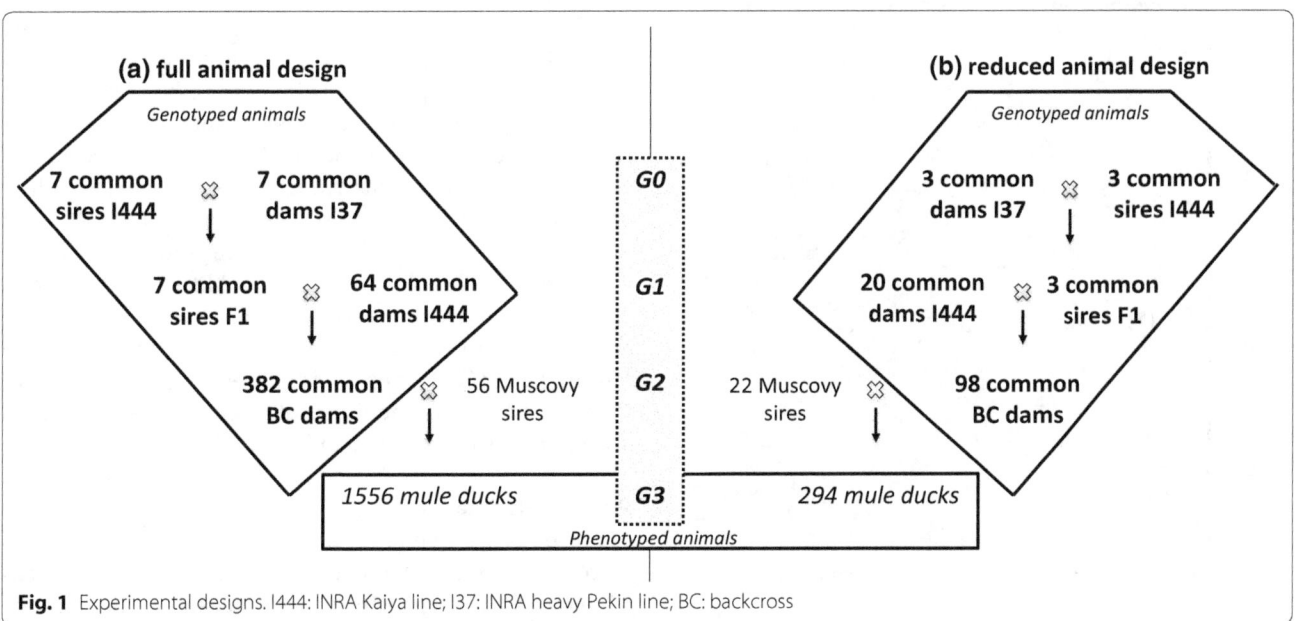

Fig. 1 Experimental designs. I444: INRA Kaiya line; I37: INRA heavy Pekin line; BC: backcross

estimate the value of their G2 common duck mothers. G0 animals were recruited in two experimental common duck lines: I444, a light Kaiya line (the crossbred product of a Tsaiya duck and an Asian Pekin duck) and I37, a heavy Pekin line (a synthetic strain created from three heavy European Pekin lines) [5]. The design was reduced by (1) selecting three F1 families from the initial seven, in which QTL for fatty liver quality traits segregated and (2) reducing the number of mule duck offspring per BC female down to three.

Breeding of the G3 mule ducklings is described in [5] and [7]. The 294 mule ducks of the subset used here, were hatched in two batches, with a 3-week gap between hatches. From 0 to 12 weeks of age, they were bred in growing batches and then were overfed for 12 days by three different handlers. At the end of the overfeeding period, animals were slaughtered, and liver tissue was sampled 20 min *post-mortem* via a small slit in the abdomen and frozen in liquid nitrogen for proteomics analyses. Carcasses were refrigerated for 24 h at 4 °C, prior to evisceration.

Proteomic 2D electrophoresis and identification of spots
Bi-dimensional gel electrophoreses of protein extracts (Fig. 2) were performed for all 294 mule duck livers as reported by François et al. [6], according to the method described in [8]. Briefly, soluble protein fractions were extracted by grounding the frozen liver samples in liquid nitrogen, mixing them with a low ionic strength

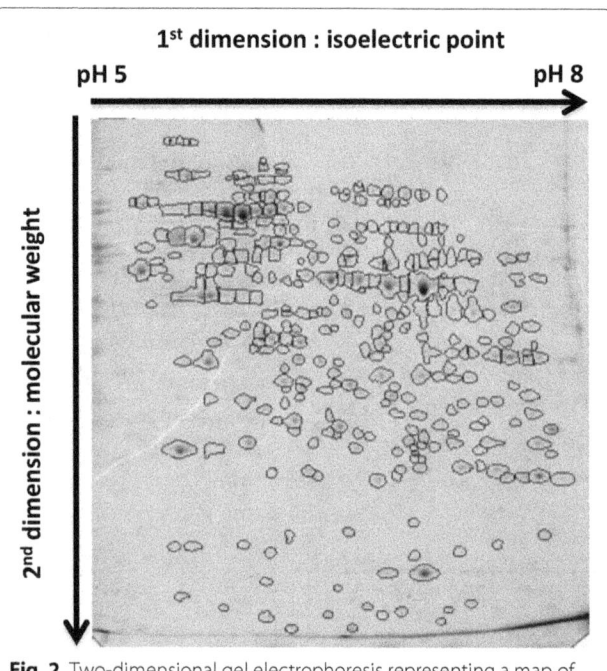

Fig. 2 Two-dimensional gel electrophoresis representing a map of duck fatty liver soluble proteins

buffer, centrifuging the homogenates and collecting the supernatants. Protein concentrations were determined using the Bradford assay (Bio-Rad, Hercules, USA). For the first-dimensional electrophoresis, samples were loaded onto pH gradient strips (pH 5–8; Bio-Rad) and isoelectric focusing (IEF) was performed using a Protean IEF cell system (Bio Rad, Hercules, USA). The second dimension consisted of sodium dodecyl sulfate–polyacrylamide gel electrophoresis (SDS-PAGE) using a Protean II XL system (Bio Rad). IEF were processed in 30 series of 12 samples, and for each IEF series, SDS-PAGE were done in two series of six samples. SDS-PAGE gels were stained overnight with Coomassie Blue G250 (Fermentas Page Blue), scanned and analyzed with the Progenesis SameSpots software® (TotalLab Ltd, Newcastle-upon-Tyne, UK). When spots seemed to be affected by the background, their outer edges were manually defined. As the general aspect of a gel had an impact on image analysis, gels were assigned to three categories: broken, blurred or correct. Spot matching was performed for all 294 samples and the software calculated the intensity that was corrected for background, of all of the spots detected for each of the 294 samples.

Detected spots were manually excised from the gels and sent to the proteomics platform in Clermont-Ferrand for protein identification (PFEMcp, INRA, Clermont-Ferrand Theix, France). In short, after protein digestion, peptide mixtures were analyzed by online nanoflow liquid chromatography using an Ultimate 3000 RSLC system (Dionex, Voisins le Bretonneux, France). Raw data were processed with Proteome Discoverer 1.4 (Thermo Fisher Scientific Inc., USA) and database searching with MASCOT v. 2.3 (Matrix Science Ltd., USA), using the UniP_tax_Aves database for protein identification. The genes that coded for the identified proteins were mapped on the chicken genome with Ensembl (http://www.ensembl.org). Since considerable synteny has been demonstrated between duck and chicken genomes, except for GGA4 (GGA for *Gallus gallus* chromosome), which is separated into two chromosomes in ducks, i.e. APL4 and 10 (APL for *Anas platyrhynchos* chromosome) [9], we considered that duck chromosomes APL1 to APL9 correspond to chicken chromosomes GGA1 to GGA9, APL10 corresponds to GGA4p and finally, that the rest of the karyotype is offset by one, with GGA10 corresponding to APL11 and so on. The list of all identified protein spots with pQTL is in Additional file 1: Table S1.

Phenotypic data
Six groups of phenotypes corresponding to 49 traits were measured and recorded for the 294 mule ducks (Table 1). For growth traits measured before the

Table 1 Trait descriptions

Abbreviation	Unit	Meaning
Growth measurements		
BW12, BW28, BW42, BW70	kg	Body weights at 12, 28, 42, 70 days of age
BWG12-28, BWG12-42, BWG12-70, BWG28-42, BWG28-70, BWG42-70	g/d	Body weight gains (all combinations between 12, 28, 42 and 70 days of age)
Corticosterone traits		
CortL, CortH	ng/ml	Corticosterone level before and after stress
DeltaC	ng/ml	Difference in corticosterone level before and after stress
Body weights and metabolic traits during overfeeding period		
TG 2nd M, TG 10th M, TG 20th M	g/l	Plasma triglyceride level after 2nd, 10th and 20th meal
CHO 2nd M, CHO 10th M, CHO 20th M	g/l	Plasma cholesterol level after 2nd, 10th and 20th meal
GLU 2nd M, GLU 10th M, GLU 20th M	g/l	Plasma glucose level after 2nd, 10th and 20th meal
DFI	kg/d	Daily feed intake
BWbeg, BWend	kg	Body weight at beginning and end of overfeeding period
OWG	kg	Weight gain during the overfeeding period
Overfeeding ability traits		
CW	kg	Bled-plucked carcass weight
FLW	kg	Fatty liver weight
pmMW	kg	*Pectoralis major* muscle weight
pmSFW	kg	Breast skin + subcutaneous fat weight
TSW	kg	Thigh + shank weight
AFW	kg	Abdominal fat weight
Liver quality traits		
MR	%	Liver melting rate
LLipC, LProtC	%	Liver lipid and protein content
LColC	mg/g	Liver collagen content
LL*, La*, Lb*		Liver lightness, redness and yellowness
Muscle quality traits		
MpH20, MpHu		Muscle pH 20 min *post mortem* and muscle ultimate pH 24 h *post mortem*
MCookL, MvacL	%	Muscle cooking losses and muscle drip losses
MLipC	%	Muscle lipid contents
ML*, Ma*, Mb*		Muscle lightness, redness and yellowness
Menergy	mJ	Energy needed to cut the muscle
MFmax		Maximal shear force

overfeeding period, animal body weights were recorded at 12, 28, 42, and 70 days of age and the combinations of six body weight gains between these ages were estimated.

Corticosterone levels under stress were recorded at 6 weeks of age: ducks were hung by the legs on a string for 10 min in order to measure the animal's response to stress and blood samples were taken before and after the test in order to measure corticosterone levels and to assess the response of the HPA (hypothalamic–pituitary–adrenal) axis to this stress. Differences in corticosterone levels before and after stress were computed. During the overfeeding period, plasma metabolic indicators such as glucose, triglyceride and cholesterol levels were measured at the beginning (after the second meal), the middle (after the 10th meal) and the end (after the 20th meal) of the 12-day overfeeding period. Body weight at the beginning and the end of the overfeeding period, the corresponding body weight gain and the food consumption during the whole overfeeding period were recorded. To appreciate the overfeeding ability of the ducks, the carcass and component pieces (fatty liver, thigh, breast skin, breast muscle and abdominal fat) were dissected and weighed. Measurements related to liver quality such as melting rate (percentage of fat loss during cooking, obtained by sterilizing 60 g of liver for 50 min at 105 °C), lipid, protein and collagen contents, and liver color (L*, a*, b* coordinates in the CIELAB system) were recorded. Finally, breast muscle quality (*pectoralis major* muscle) was estimated by measuring the pH 20 min and 24 h (ultimate pH) *post-mortem*, cooking and drip losses under vacuum, the descriptive color L*, a*, b* values and by recording the lipid content. Raw meat tenderness was measured using the maximal shear force and energy levels using the Warner–Bratzler test. Mean and standard error values for all these traits are described in [5] and estimated genetic parameters are in [7].

Marker development, genotyping and map construction

The same BC design that was used here was previously used to detect phenotypic QTL based on a first set of 91 microsatellite markers, which led to the construction of 16 linkage groups that covered 778 cM [5]. In order to extend this rudimentary map, we developed additional single nucleotide polymorphisms (SNPs) [10]. Briefly, the seven G1 sires of the QTL design (Fig. 1a) were sequenced with 100 bp paired-end reads at a depth of 35X with the Illumina HiSeq. Sequence quality was verified and correct paired-end alignments were generated by alignment to the duck genome reference [11] using the Burrows-Wheeler Aligner (BWA) program [12], then SNPs were detected using the GATK software [13]. Over 11 million SNPs were detected, of which 90% were heterozygous in only one G1 sire. To guide our choice of SNPs, while allowing for the largest possible duck genome coverage, we took advantage of the known synteny conservation between the duck and chicken genomes [9, 14] and chose a final set of 384

SNPs among the 157,436 that were bi-allelic in at least five sires and had known positions on the chicken genome. These SNPs were used to genotype the 382 G2 female ducks, their G1 parents (seven F1 sires and 64 I444 dams) and their 14 G0 paternal grand-parents (Fig. 1a) using the Illumina® Veracode technology. Analysis of genotype clusters and selection of high-quality SNPs, based on call rates and correct Mendelian inheritance, were performed with the Genome Studio™ software (Illumina).

Genetic maps were constructed with CRI-MAP 2.4 [15] by including the SNP genotypes generated here and previous microsatellite data. The new genetic map contains 334 markers (278 SNPs and 56 microsatellites) aggregated into 28 linkage groups corresponding to 28 APL chromosomes (Fig. 3).

Statistical methods

Prior to QTL detection, all mule duck traits (proteomic or phenotypic) were corrected for environmental fixed effects using the GLM procedure in SAS [16]. For all phenotypic traits, the "hatching batch" effect (two levels) was taken into account (Model 1), and the "handler" effect (three levels) was added for traits related to overfeeding or product quality (Model 2). For proteomic traits, these zootechnical effects were cumulated with the technological effects of the bi-dimensional electrophoresis. Then, the sum of the spot intensities of each gel was treated as a covariate and six fixed effects were defined (Model 3): the "handler" effect (three levels), the "hatching batch" effect (two levels), the general aspect of the gels (three levels), the first electrophoresis dimension effect (30 levels), the second electrophoresis dimension effect (two levels per first electrophoresis series) and the interaction of both dimensions (60 levels). The residual effects of the three previous linear models were conserved for each mule duck, and the performance of each G2 female was computed as the average of the residual effects of her three male mule duck offspring.

QTL detection was carried out using the QTLMap software [17–19] in order to implement linkage analysis according to the interval mapping method [20]. For each chromosome, first the probabilities of each possible phase of the G1 male founders were estimated using marker information from their progenies (the G2 dams). The sire phases with the highest probabilities were assumed to be the correct ones: for a set of tested positions (practically at each 1 cM), the probabilities that the corresponding chromosomal segments were transmitted to the offspring were estimated. Then, QTL detection was carried out by within-sire linear regression [21]. The model was the following:

$$Y_{ij} = s_i + (2p_{ij} - 1)a_i + e_{ij},$$

where the dependent variable Y_{ij} is the average performance (previously corrected for fixed effects) of the three male mule duck offspring of G2 dam j and sire i. For each location on the genome, s_i is the male founder i effect, a_i is equal to half the substitution effect of the putative QTL carried by the sire i, and p_{ij} is the probability that the daughter (BC) j might inherit one arbitrarily defined QTL allele from her sire i, given the marker information. The residual variance e_{ij} was defined within sire families to improve robustness to unlinked QTL segregation between families [22]. In our design, phenotypes were recorded only at G3, but since the number of mule ducks per G2 dam was strictly equal to 3, it was not necessary to take the variance of the phenotypes assigned to the G2 generation into account, in contrast with our previous study in which the number of G3 mule ducks per G2 dam was variable [5].

For each trait and each linkage group, 1000 within-family permutations were performed to estimate the empirical chromosome-wide significance level of the test statistics [23]. The conservative genome-wide thresholds were derived from chromosome-wide significance levels, using an approximate Bonferroni correction:

$$P_{genome-wide} = 1 - (1 - P_{chromosome-wide})^{1/r},$$

where r is the ratio between the length of a specific linkage group and the length of the genome considered for QTL detection (1728 cM). The 95% confidence intervals of the QTL locations were estimated by LOD drop-off. In practice, the bounds of each interval were the two locations at which the likelihood was equal to the maximum likelihood minus 3.84 ($=\chi^2(1, 0.05)$) [24]. The QTL effect (α) was expressed in phenotypic standard deviation units (SD), and estimated as: $\alpha = \frac{1}{SD} \times \frac{1}{n} \sum_{i=1}^{n} |\alpha_i|$, where SD is the phenotypic standard deviation, n the number of sires and α_i the effect of the within-sire ith QTL allele [25].

QTL detections were first carried out for phenotypic traits (QTL) and proteomic traits (pQTL) on a single-trait basis. For all confidence intervals of single phenotypic QTL and pQTL that overlapped, multi-trait QTL analyses, usually via a two-trait approach (2t-QTL), were performed [26] in order to identify possible pleiotropic effects between the phenotypes and liver protein variations. In addition, when a protein was identified for several spots each having a QTL on the same linkage group, the two-trait approach was also implemented to check whether the overall change in this protein improved the QTL.

To distinguish between pleiotropy and close linkage in 2t-QTL results, we performed the CLIP (Close LInkage versus Pleiotropy) test proposed by David et al. [27]. The

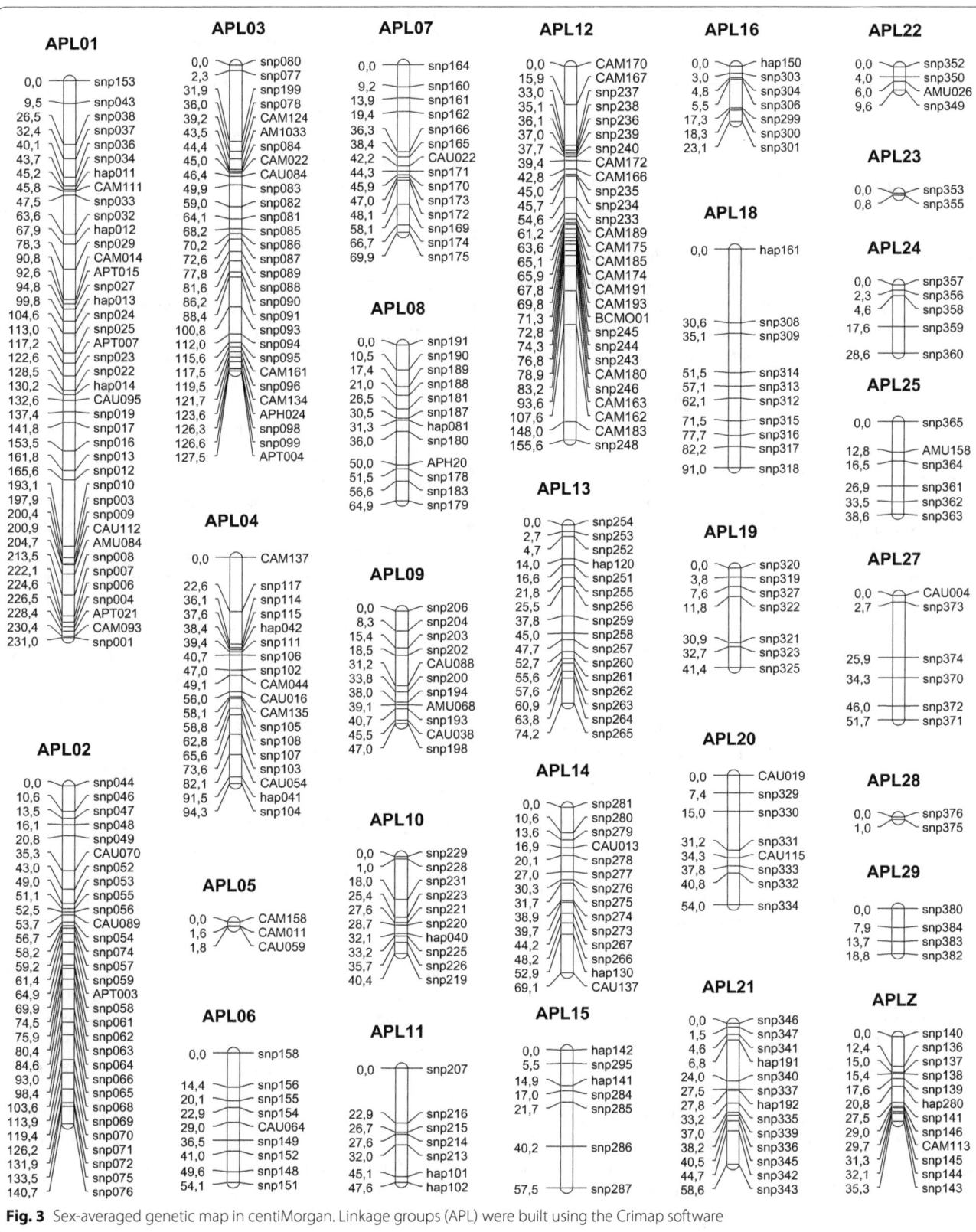

Fig. 3 Sex-averaged genetic map in centiMorgan. Linkage groups (APL) were built using the Crimap software

CLIP test considers that under the assumption of pleiotropy (H0), the pattern of the SNP effects when moving along the tested genomic region should be similar for both traits, whereas under the close-linked QTL assumption (H1) it should be different.

Graph inference

To aid interpretation, data from the CLIP test showing pleiotropy were transformed into graphs using the Gephi 0.9.1 software [28]. Gephi is an open-source and free visualization and exploration platform for all kinds of graphs. Weight was added to links for which pleiotropy was not rejected, and spatial statistics were used to identify nodes of importance in the graph. For example, nodes with a strong betweenness related to centrality were essential for the stability of the graph, and without such nodes the graph is disrupted [29].

Functional annotation

To determine the biological relevance of the results, the Ingenuity Pathway Analysis (IPA, QIAGEN, Redwood City, www.qiagen.com/ingenuity) software was used to perform enrichment analysis (biological functions and canonical pathways), to construct bibliographic networks and regulation networks based on the identification of potential upstream regulators. Since IPA uses gene names, protein names were changed for gene names when necessary. Briefly, IPA constructed networks based on bibliographic data in which the edges were obtained from biological links such as receptor-ligand interactions, enzyme activity on another protein, or a transcriptional factor that activates the expression of targeted genes. IPA proposed the most probable network with an associated score. The final graph was reconstructed from the proposed IPA network with the best score using the PathDesigner function and also included information on some of the most significant canonical pathways and biological functions, as well as information from an interesting pleiotropic QTL.

Results

Single-trait QTL analysis

A total of 10,500 single-trait QTL analyses (28 chromosomes with 326 protein quantification traits and 49 phenotypic traits) were performed. We detected 287 significant pQTL at the 5% chromosome-wide threshold and in 176 cases, the protein was successfully identified (see Additional file 2: Table S2). We also detected 80 significant QTL at the 5% chromosome-wide threshold for the phenotypic traits (see Additional file 3: Table S3). Of these QTL and pQTL, 45 and 21 were significant at the 1% chromosome-wide threshold for the proteomic and phenotypic traits, respectively. At the genome-wide level,

six phenotypic and five proteomic traits reached the 5% threshold and one phenotypic and two proteomic traits reached the 1% threshold.

The 176 pQTL were located across the 28 linkage groups of the genetic map (see Additional file 2: Table S2). On average, we detected 6.3 (SD = 3.2) pQTL per chromosome. Surprisingly, the number of pQTL tended to be smaller on the macro-chromosomes (APL1 to APL10 and APLZ) than on the micro-chromosomes, with mean numbers of 5.7 ± 2.3 and 6.8 ± 3.7, respectively. In general, the allelic substitution effect for these 176 pQTL was low (on average 0.42 ± 0.17 of the standard deviation for the considered trait and ranged from 0.25 to 1.53) and the confidence intervals of the QTL were relatively large, with an average of 20 cM. Some chromosomes were considered particularly noteworthy because they harbored very significant pQTL. On APL18 and 24, we observed two pQTL significant at the 1% genome-wide significance level, respectively for alpha-enolase (ENO1) and fatty acid synthase (FASN) (see Additional file 2: Table S2). Moreover, the allele substitution effect at the QTL for ENO1 reached 1.5 standard deviations, which was one of the most important effects among all the pQTL detected. At the 5% genome-wide threshold, we observed two pQTL on APL10 for 3-hydroxyisobutyryl-CoA hydrolase (HIBCH) and persulfite dioxygenase ETHE1 (ETHE1), and a single pQTL on APL1 for peroxiredoxin 3 (PRDX3), on APL7 for apolipoprotein A1 (APOA1) and on APL21 for carbonic anhydrase 2 (CA2). Other chromosomes displayed a large number of pQTL at the 5% chromosome-wide threshold, i.e. APL24, 25 and 29 harboured more than 10 pQTL, and APL18 carried 15 pQTL. In a few cases, single protein spots mapped to several pQTL, i.e. spots 116 (proteasome 26S subunit ATPase 3—PSMC3), 124 (ENO1), 230 (phosphoglycerate mutase 1—PGAM1) and 301 (guanosine diphosphate dissociation inhibitor 2—GDI2) mapped to four pQTL each at the 5% chromosome-wide threshold. In addition, several spots can correspond to different co-existing forms of the same protein, due to variations of the electric charge and/or molecular weight resulting from post-translational modifications. Each of the spots for a given protein may map to one or several pQTL, which may or may not co-localize. For example, this was the case for ENO1, for which 14 protein spots were identified on the gels (Fig. 4), among which 12 mapped to up to 17 pQTL.

Likewise, 14 pQTL were detected for APOA1, which displayed nine protein spots on the gel (Fig. 5). Five to seven pQTL were observed for phosphoglycerate mutase 1 (PGAM1), the putative Parkinson disease autosomal recessive early onset 7 variant 1 (PARK7), triose phosphate isomerase (TPI1), peroxiredoxin 4 (PRDX4), malate dehydrogenase 1 (MDH1) and 3-hydroxyanthranilate

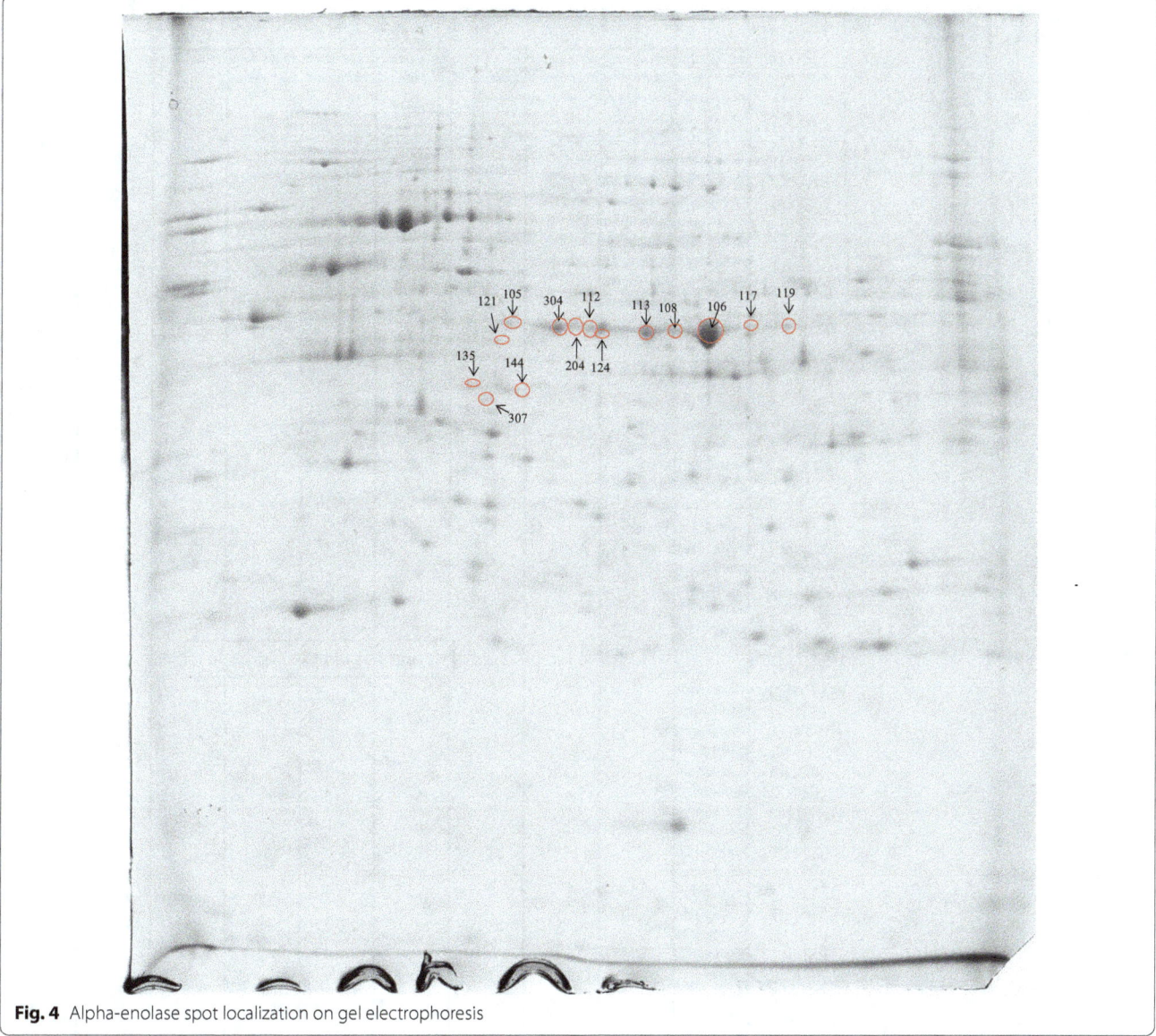

Fig. 4 Alpha-enolase spot localization on gel electrophoresis

3,4-dioxygenase (HAAO). For 86% of the 176 pQTL, the gene corresponding to the identified protein was mapped to the chicken genome, which allowed us to assign it to a duck chromosome. In 148 cases, the gene was localized on a chromosome other than that carrying the pQTL, which allowed us to unambiguously define it as a trans-pQTL [30]. In six cases, the gene was localized on the same chromosome than that carrying the pQTL, i.e. for S-formylglutathione hydrolase (ESD) on APL1, MDH1 on APL3, glutamate deshydrogenase (GLUD1) and PGAM1 on APL6, annexin A5 (ANXA5) on APL11 and alpha-aminoadipic semialdehyde dehydrogenase (ALDH7A1) on APLZ.

Regarding the 80 phenotypic QTL, the average allele substitution effect was equal to 0.42 ± 0.12 standard deviations (ranging from 0.26 to 1.04), with a confidence interval of about 17 cM (see Additional file 3: Table S3). These QTL are located on 24 of the 28 linkage groups of the genetic map. Some linkage groups seemed to be specific to a type of trait, with QTL for similar traits mapping very close to one another. Thus, five QTL related to growth mapped to APL3 at position 0.44 M, whereas the QTL detected on APL2 and 23 were more specific to liver composition and its melting rate, at 0.64 and 0 M on APL2 and APL23, respectively. Moreover, on APL2 we detected a QTL for melting rate

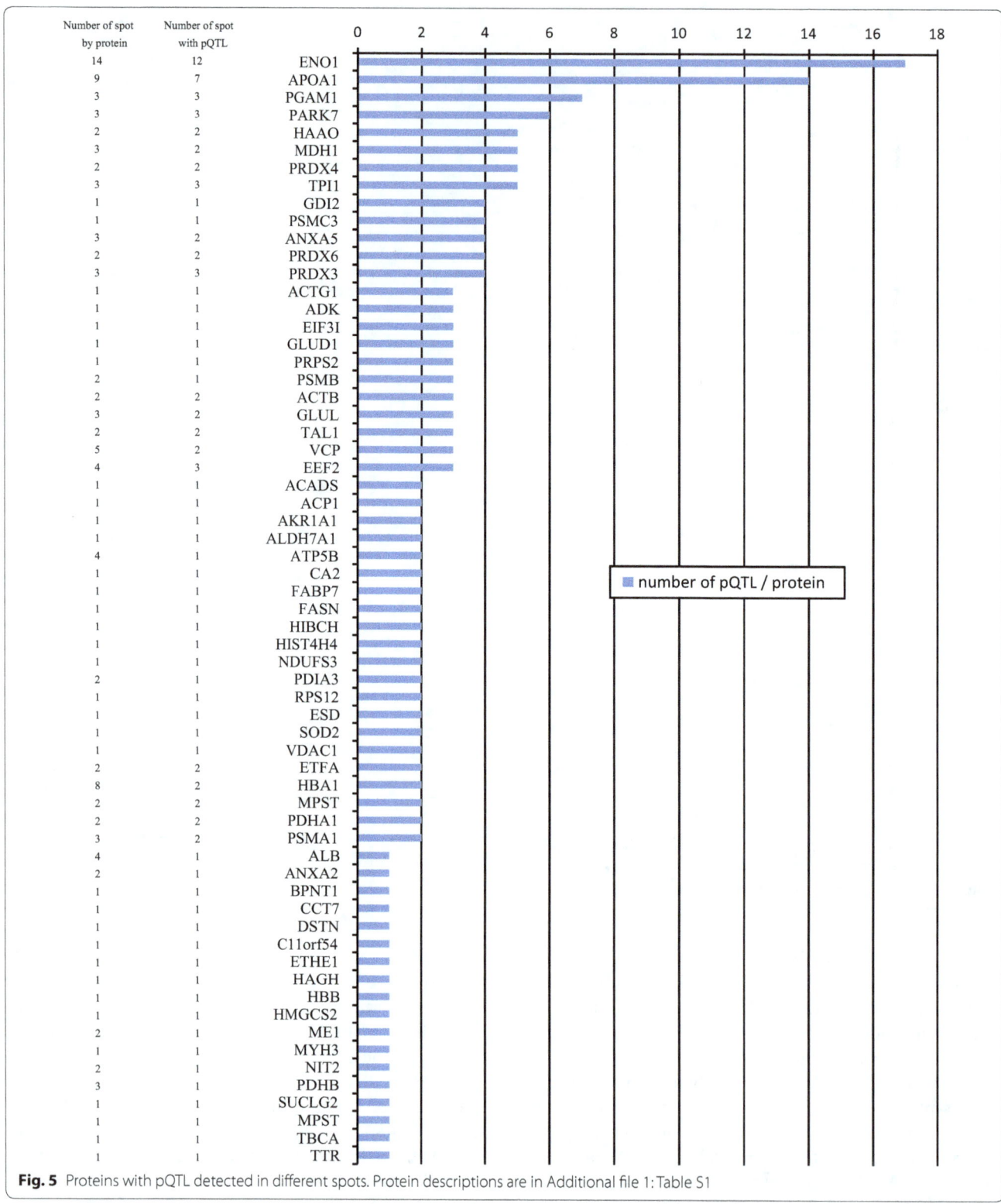

Fig. 5 Proteins with pQTL detected in different spots. Protein descriptions are in Additional file 1: Table S1

that reached the 1% genome-wide threshold. At the 5% genome-wide threshold, six QTL were noteworthy: for liver protein content and liver weight on APL2, for bodyweight at ages 28 and 42 days on APL3, for weight gain during the overfeeding period on APL9 and for liver yellowness on APL18.

Two-trait QTL analysis

Following single-trait QTL analyses, we conducted 290 protein-phenotype two-trait analyses (2t-QTL) when the confidence intervals for pQTL and phenotypic QTL overlapped. Among these, the P values for 66 2t-QTL were more significant than the P value of the strongest QTL using the single-trait approach (Table 2). The CLIP test was performed for all 66 2t-QTL and provided results for 37 of them, whereas for the 29 other 2t-QTL, the CLIP test did not converge mainly due to the lack of variability for traits such as plasma level of cholesterol, and to a lesser extent plasma level of triglycerides at the beginning of the overfeeding period, and corticosterone levels before stress.

Among the 37 CLIP tests that provided results, the hypothesis of pleiotropy was not rejected for 16 2t-QTL. In particular, this was the case for: liver lightness and GLUD1 on APL6; thigh/shank weight and APOA1 on APL7; bodyweight at 12 days and fatty acid binding protein 7 (FABP7) on APL9; blood glucose at the beginning of the force-feeding period and HIBCH on APL10; blood cholesterol level at the beginning of the force-feeding period and 3-mercaptopyruvate sulfurtransferase (MPST) on APL15; melting rate and two spots for ENO1 on APL15; bodyweight at 28 days and eukaryotic translation initiation factor 3 subunit 1 (EIF3I), acid phosphatase 1 (ACP1), eukaryotic elongation factor 2 (EEF2) and bodyweight gain between 12 and 28 days of age and EIF3I and ACP1 on APL19; liver yellowness and PRDX4 on APL22; and ultimate muscle pH and ATP synthase subunit beta (ATP5B) and TPI1 and blood glucose at the beginning of the force-feeding period and GLUD1 on APLZ.

For 21 of the 37 two-trait analyses, we concluded that both QTL were in close linkage and rejected the hypothesis of pleiotropy. For example, although the P value of the 2t-QTL identified on APL21 for muscle maximal shear force and albumin protein (ALB) was clearly higher than those obtained in the single-trait QTL analysis, we concluded that these two QTL were linked but not pleiotropic. The same applied to thigh/shank weight and alcohol dehydrogenase (AKR1A1) on APL7, bodyweight gain between 12 and 42 days and valosin containing protein (VCP) on APL5, breast skin and subcutaneous fat weight and histone H4 (HIST4H4) on APL9, and bodyweight at 28 days and PARK7 on APL19.

Graph inference using data from Table 2 resulted in nine graphs (Fig. 6) where pleiotropy is highlighted by weighted links (in bold on Fig. 6). This graphical representation of the data helps to detect pleiotropic traits and even possible epistatic events. It is interesting to observe how genomic regions that control many traits are represented as organized networks. For example, the QTL on APL10 (12 cM) and APLZ (7 cM) may both control plasma glucose levels (Fig. 6f). The ultimate pH of the *pectoralis major* muscle seems to be regulated by a QTL on APLZ (between 23 and 32 cM; Fig. 6a), which is associated with the abundance of ATP5B and TPI1, and to a lesser extent, with the abundance of ENO1, PSMA1 and ALDH7A1. Moreover, expression of ALDH7A1 is also controlled by another QTL on APL5 (0 cM). Likewise, even if no pleiotropy was detected, a region between 0 and 18 cM on APL18 seems to control the plasma levels of cortisol before stress, together with the abundance of PGAM1, PRDX3, MDH1, GLUD1, VCP and GDI2 (Fig. 6e).

Sixteen two-trait analyses were conducted for proteins that displayed several spots on 2D electrophoresis gels and for which QTL were detected on the same chromosome: eight for ENO1, four for APOA1, and one each for hemoglobin alpha (HBA1), PGAM1, glutamine synthetase (GLUL) and PRDX4. Among these analyses, the P values for six of the 2t-QTL were more significant than those for the strongest underlying single-trait QTL (Table 3), of which four involved ENO1. The CLIP test was performed for these six 2t-QTL and the pleiotropic hypothesis was not rejected in two cases: for ENO1, with spot numbers 124 and 307 on APL29 and spot numbers 112 and 124 on APL15. The phenotypic correlations between these ENO1 spots were quite low, about +0.24 for both spot pairs 112 and 124, and 124 and 307. Conversely, for APOA1 on APL24, we concluded that the QTL for spot numbers 174 and 262 were closely linked.

Biological analysis

Among the 326 quantified spots, 190 were identified as corresponding to 97 unique proteins. Sixty-six proteins were regulated by at least one QTL (Fig. 5), i.e. two-thirds of the proteome were detected as being genetically regulated. We used the Ingenuity Pathway Analysis software to detect differences between the full proteome (all identified proteins) and the genetically-regulated proteome. Since not all proteins are recognized by IPA, 91 of the 97 unique proteins and 63 of the 66 regulated proteins were analysed. However, as expected, the processes were globally the same for the two proteome groups because proteins with pQTL form a subgroup of the complete proteome. For example, glycolysis and gluconeogenesis pathways were clearly enriched since all the proteins involved (ENO1, MDH1, ME1, PGAM1 and TPI1) were genetically regulated (Table 4 and Fig. 7). Likewise, the most significant pathway enriched in the genetically-regulated proteome is mitochondrial dysfunction for which seven of the nine identified proteins (PDHA1, PRDX3, SOD2, ATP5B, PARK7, VDAC1 and NDUFS3) had pQTL (Table 4 and Fig. 7).

The most significant biological function is the synthesis of purine nucleotides with nine of the 11 identified

Table 2 Sixty-six significant two-trait QTL for protein quantification and zootechnical traits

APL[a]	Traits Protein[b]	Phenotype	Location (cM)[c]	LRTx	Confidence interval[d]	Threshold biQTL P value (%)	UniQTL1 P value (%)	UniQTL2 P value (%)	CLIP test Number of markers	Hyp[e]
3	MDH1 (179)	BW12	61	27.155	48–69	0.66	2.09	3.44	29	CL
5	ALDH7A1 (300)	BWG12-42	0	23.653	0–2	0.14	0.68	4.18	1	CL
5	ACTB (159)	BWG12-42	1	18.018	0–2	1.05	3.06	4.18	1	CL
5	VCP (283)	BWG12-42	1	20.996	0–2	0.38	3.30	4.18	1	CL
5	VCP (283)	AFW	1	20.125	0–2	0.61	3.30	4.84	1	CL
6	PRDX6 (231)	LColC	1	25.817	0–18	0.44	4.41	2.18	8	–
6	MDH1 (169)	LColC	14	27.870	0–22	0.15	0.33	2.18	8	–
6	GLUD1 (319)	LL*	36	20.153	10–48	2.02	3.80	2.54	8	PL
7	PGAM1 (230)	TSW	37	33.005	32–66	0.03	4.33	0.80	12	–
7	AKR1A1 (149)	TSW	42	38.135	33–45	0.03	0.98	0.80	12	CL
7	PGAM1 (230)	BWbeg	61	26.099	44–70	0.61	4.33	4.54	12	–
7	GLUD1 (319)	TSW	63	32.601	53–70	0.11	4.16	0.80	12	–
7	GLUD1 (319)	BWbeg	65	27.396	58–70	0.40	4.16	4.54	12	–
7	APOA1 (270)	TSW	69	38.558	61–70	0.01	0.06	0.80	12	PL
7	APOA1 (270)	BWbeg	69	38.103	62–70	0.04	0.06	4.54	12	CL
8	PRPS2 (192)	Menergy	0	23.879	0–9	1.20	1.25	2.72	10	CL
8	PRDX4 (237)	Menergy	5	22.179	0–13	1.84	4.65	2.72	10	CL
9	FABP7 (318)	BW12	21	22.066	11–35	1.66	3.97	2.45	11	PL
9	HISTH4 (315)	pmSFW	80	23.876	49–83	0.81	3.84	4.06	11	CL
10	HIBCH (151)	GLU 2nd M	12	31.044	4–21	0.03	0.03	0.81	9	PL
12	PRDX6 (226)	CHO 2nd M	61	23.217	37–66	1.00	3.04	3.33	26	CL
14	PDHA1 (133)	Mb*	0	19.704	0–9	2.33	3.75	3.67	14	–
14	ADK (136)	Mb*	0	19.395	0–8	2.71	3.15	3.67	14	–
14	HIBCH (151)	TG 2nd M	40	21.241	27–69	1.34	2.93	2.44	14	–
14	HIBCH (151)	CHO 20th M	69	27.010	45–69	0.17	2.93	4.90	14	–
15	PSMC3 (116)	CHO 2nd M	29	19.869	11–40	2.63	4.38	4.94	6	CL
15	MPST (188)	CHO 2nd M	33	19.938	22–48	2.58	4.16	4.94	6	PL
15	ENO1 (124)	CHO 2nd M	35	24.632	26–50	0.63	0.73	4.94	6	CL
15	ANXA5 (207)	CHO 2nd M	35	21.660	25–48	1.52	3.25	4.94	6	–
15	CCT7 (294)	MR	40	26.662	30–48	0.29	0.56	0.77	6	CL
15	ENO1 (124)	MR	43	28.102	30–52	0.19	0.73	0.77	6	PL
15	ENO1 (112)	MR	53	24.743	44–57	0.49	1.20	0.77	6	PL
18	PGAM1(325)	CortL	0	26.128	0–37	0.53	2.27	4.86	10	–
18	PGAM1 (232)	CortL	0	27.844	0–12	0.26	1.01	4.86	10	–
18	PRDX3 (257)	CortL	5	30.485	0–12	0.15	0.43	4.86	10	CL
18	MDH1 (179)	CortL	11	28.325	0–15	0.16	1.40	4.86	10	–
18	GLUL (131)	CortL	13	28.171	8–16	0.32	1.07	4.86	10	–

Table 2 continued

APL[a]	Traits					Threshold	UniQTL1	UniQTL2	CLIP test	
	Protein[b]	Phenotype	Location (cM)[c]	LRTx	Confidence interval[d]	biQTL P value (%)	P value (%)	P value (%)	Number of markers	Hyp[e]
18	VCP (285)	CortL	17	22.468	0–37	1.85	4.52	4.86	10	–
18	GDI2 (301)	CortL	18	27.892	15–27	0.35	1.34	4.86	10	–
19	PARK7 (263)	LProtC	0	19.718	0–21	1.95	2.45	4.37	6	CL
19	EIF3I (180)	LProtC	3	20.937	0–7	1.29	1.95	4.37	6	CL
19	EIF3I (180)	CHO 2nd M	4	26.900	0–7	0.19	1.95	3.31	6	–
19	PARK7 (263)	CHO 2nd M	4	24.653	0–8	0.37	2.45	3.31	6	–
19	ACP1 (274)	CHO 2nd M	4	25.729	0–6	0.29	2.00	3.31	6	–
19	EEF2 (306)	CHO 2nd M	4	20.905	0–20	1.12	4.69	3.31	6	–
19	EIF3I (180)	BW28	4	24.539	0–12	0.38	1.95	2.71	6	PL
19	ACP1 (274)	BW28	4	22.269	0–8	0.73	2.00	2.71	6	PL
19	EIF3I (180)	BWG12-28	4	22.948	0–16	0.62	1.95	3.39	6	PL
19	ACP1 (274)	BWG12-28	4	22.473	0–8	0.82	2.00	3.39	6	PL
19	PARK7 (263)	BWG12-28	6	23.640	0–20	0.46	2.45	3.39	6	–
19	PARK7 (263)	BW28	6	23.817	0–20	0.49	2.45	2.71	6	CL
19	EEF2 (306)	BWG12-28	16	22.160	0–20	0.83	4.69	3.39	6	–
19	EEF2 (306)	BW28	33	22.876	23–41	0.64	4.69	2.71	6	PL
21	ENO1 (112)	MFmax	46	18.664	41–57	3.72	5.00	4.84	12	CL
21	HAAO (196)	MFmax	46	20.570	41–55	2.04	2.12	4.84	12	CL
21	ALB (290)	MFmax	55	20.368	44–58	0.11	4.63	4.84	12	CL
22	BPNT1 (156)	BWG28-42	0	19.784	0–10	1.17	2.67	3.87	4	–
22	PRDX4 (309)	Lb*	0	23.820	0–4	0.28	0.83	0.98	4	PL
22	CA2 (227)	BWG28-42	9	19.204	0–10	1.63	3.26	3.87	4	–
22	CA2 (227)	Lb*	9	22.351	0–10	0.51	3.26	0.98	4	–
Z	GLUD1 (319)	GLU 2nd M	7	25.930	5–11	0.29	1.13	1.22	6	PL
Z	TPI1 (236)	MpHu	23	30.798	18–34	0.01	0.63	0.29	6	PL
Z	ENO1 (144)	MpHu	23	28.755	17–35	0.06	4.84	0.29	6	CL
Z	ALDH7A1 (300)	MpHu	30	28.204	22–35	0.11	4.99	0.29	6	–
Z	PSMA1 (212)	MpHu	32	30.809	31–35	0.05	1.14	0.29	6	–
Z	ATP5B (103)	MpHu	32	27.477	31–35	0.14	2.51	0.29	6	PL

Only 2t-QTL for which the P value is more significant than that of the stronger of the two QTL detected using the single-trait approach are reported in this table. These results were used to identify 16 assumed pleiotropic QTL

[a] Duck (*Anas platyrhynchos*) APL chromosome or linkage group

[b] Protein descriptions: see supplementary data

[c] Position on the genetic map in centiMorgans

[d] Confidence interval in centiMorgans

[e] CLIPtest: CL, close linkage; PL, pleiotropism; –, not tested

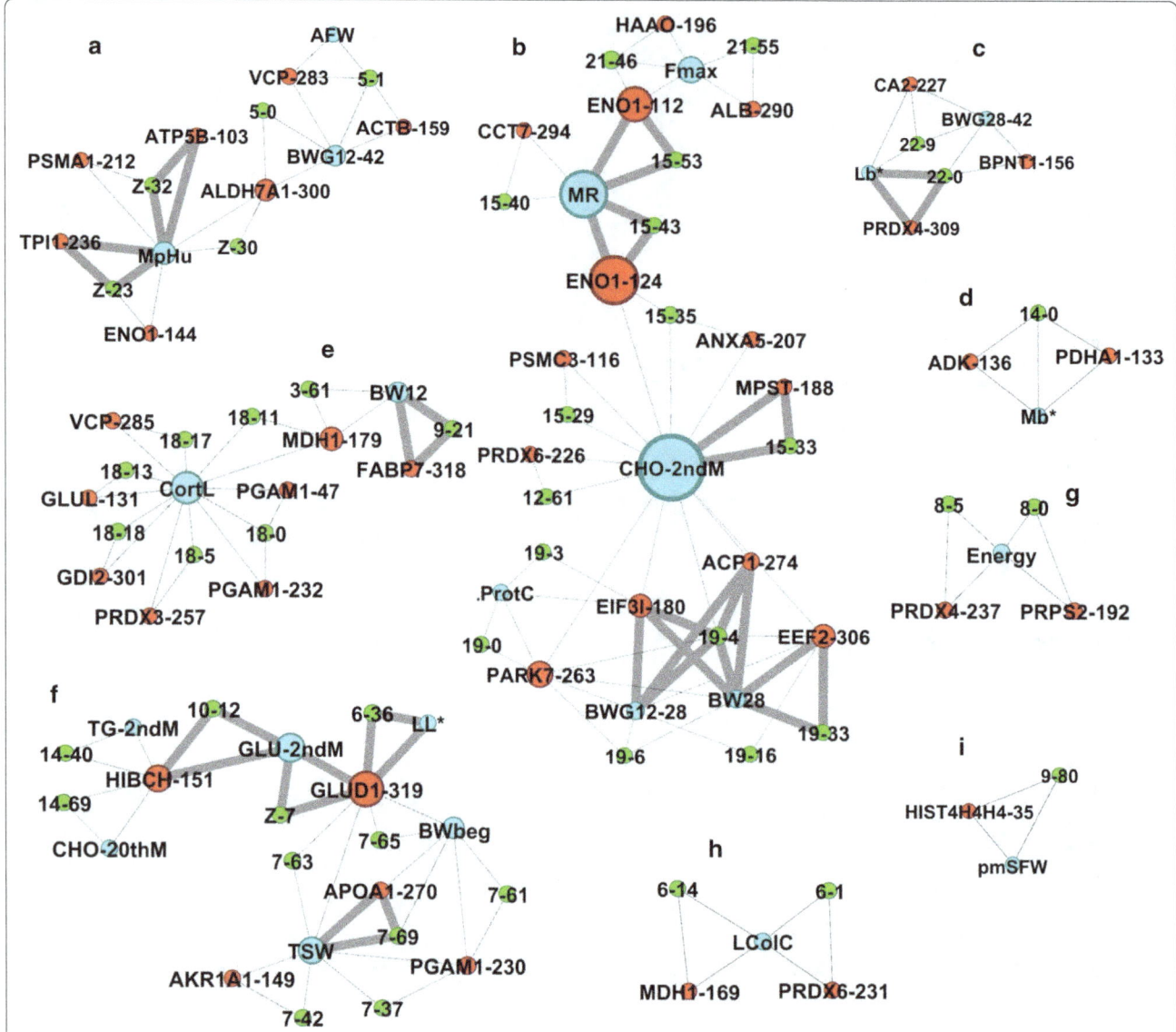

Fig. 6 Graphs inferred from two-trait QTL detection with pleiotropy. These graphs are a representation of the data from Table 2. The chromosome locations are illustrated in green with the APL chromosome number and the location in cM. The phenotypic traits are in *blue* and the proteins are in *red* associated with the spot number. A weight is given for links (*in bold*) when a pleiotropic QTL was detected. The size of the nodes (proteins or phenotypes) is related to the betweenness (calculated by Gephi), i.e. an indicator of centrality that identifies the most important nodes within a graph

proteins regulated by a pQTL (Table 5). An interesting change between the full proteome versus the pQTL regulated proteome was observed for the function related to cell viability, which was found at the 26th and 41th positions for the complete proteome and at the 6th and 8th positions for the pQTL-regulated proteome. Finally, we implemented an integrative approach to reconstruct a biological network (Fig. 7) with PathDesigner (from Ingenuity) to highlight key results for the proteins with pQTL, for relevant pathways that are a priori regulated

in our study, and for the liver melting rate trait, which is most important for producers since it is related to *foie gras* production.

Discussion

Sixty-eight percent of the proteins analyzed are partially controlled by QTL

Our group recently published the complete results of proteomic analyses carried out on 294 mule ducks [6] and showed that the abundance of 23 proteins was

Table 3 Two-trait QTL detections of different spots of the same protein traits reveal two pleiotropic QTL

APL[a]	Protein[b]	Spot number[c]	Location (cM)[d]	LRTx	Confidence interval[e]	biQTL threshold (%)	UniQTL threshold (%)		CLIPTest[f]	
15	ENO1	112–124	51	26.220	41–57	0.41	0.73	1.20	6[g]	PL
18	PGAM1	232–325	0	31.645	0–11	0.12	1.01	2.27	10	–
24	APOA1	174–262	22	29.271	10–29	0.05	0.78	1.95	5	CL
25	ENO1	108–124	37	24.025	27–39	0.35	2.29	3.32	6	–
25	ENO1	108–304	38	28.653	34–39	0.14	2.29	0.40	6	–
29	ENO1	124–307	14	16.435	4–19	3.69	3.94	5.02	4	PL

[a] Duck (*Anas platyrhynchos*) APL chromosome or linkage group

[b] Protein descriptions: see supplementary data

[c] Spot number on the 2D gels

[d] Position on the genetic map in centiMorgans

[e] Confidence interval in centiMorgans

[f] CLIP test: CL, close linkage; PL, pleiotropy;–, nontested

[g] number of markers

associated to three quality traits: liver weight, melting rate, and dry protein content. In the current study, our objective was to highlight the proteins for which abundance is partly genetically regulated. QTL detection was performed for all identified proteins and the issue of false positive results was raised. After Benjamini–Hochberg correction, even the most significant pQTL (for FASN on APL24) did not reach the 5% significance level since the adjusted *P* value was approximately 18%. However, regarding the power of our design and given the large number of QTL detections performed, we considered that the Benjamini–Hochberg correction was too drastic and decided to focus only on the more significant pQTL reaching the genome-wide significance threshold before correction. In this context, 66 out of the 97 unique proteins identified (68%) were regulated by at least one QTL.

Most of the detected pQTL are trans-QTL

Amongst the 176 pQTL identified, the most significant were for APOA1 on APL7, ENO1 on APL18 and FASN on APL24. These three pQTL, together with more than 96% of the pQTL identified in this study, are located on

Table 4 Functional enrichment analysis of canonical pathways between proteins with pQTL and the complete list of proteins

Ingenuity canonical pathways	Complete		pQTL		Proteins with pQTL in italic
	Regulated	Score[a]	Regulated	Score[a]	
Mitochondrial dysfunction	9/171 (5%)	7.22	7/171 (4%)	6.18	*PDHA1*, *PRDX3*, NDUFS1, *SOD2*, ATP5B, *PARK7*, GPX4, *VDAC1*, NDUFS3
Gluconeogenesis I	4/25 (16%)	5.40	4/25 (16%)	6.10	*ENO1*, *PGAM1*, *ME1*, *MDH1*
NRF2-mediated oxidative stress response	7/180 (4%)	4.85	6/180 (3%)	4.84	*AKR1A1*, *SOD2*, PRDX1, *ACTB*, VCP, CCT7, *ACTG1*
Glycolysis I	3/25 (12%)	3.76	3/25 (12%)	4.28	*ENO1*, *TPI1*, *PGAM1*
Acetyl-CoA biosynthesis I	3/7 (43%)	5.56	2/7 (29%)	3.76	*PDHA1*, DLAT, *PDHB*
LXR/RXR activation	5/121 (4%)	3.72	4/121 (3%)	3.36	*TTR*, *ALB*, *APOA1*, TF, *FASN*
FXR/RXR activation	5/126 (4%)	3.64	4/126 (3%)	3.29	
Caveolar-mediated endocytosis signaling	3/71 (4%)	2.43	3/71 (4%)	2.93	*ALB*, *ACTB*, *ACTG1*
Acute phase response signaling	5/169 (3%)	3.06	4/169 (2%)	2.82	*TTR*, *ALB*, *SOD2*, *APOA1*, TF
TR/RXR activation	3/85 (4%)	2.21	3/85 (4%)	2.70	*ENO1*, *FASN*, *ME1*
Tryptophan degradation X	4/23 (17%)	5.55	2/23 (9%)	2.69	ALDH2, *AKR1A1*, ALDH9A1, *ALDH7A1*
Ethanol degradation II	4/35 (11%)	4.79	2/35 (6%)	2.33	
Noradrenaline and adrenaline degradation	4/38 (11%)	4.65	2/38 (5%)	2.26	
Clathrin-mediated Endocytosis signaling	5/185 (3%)	2.88	4/185 (2%)	2.67	*ALB*, *APOA1*, TF, *ACTB*, *ACTG1*

Only the top 14 canonical pathways are in this table

Proteins regulated by a pQTL are in italics; pQTL may concern only a sub-list of the complete list of proteins identified by proteomic analysis

[a] Score corresponds to −log(*P* value)

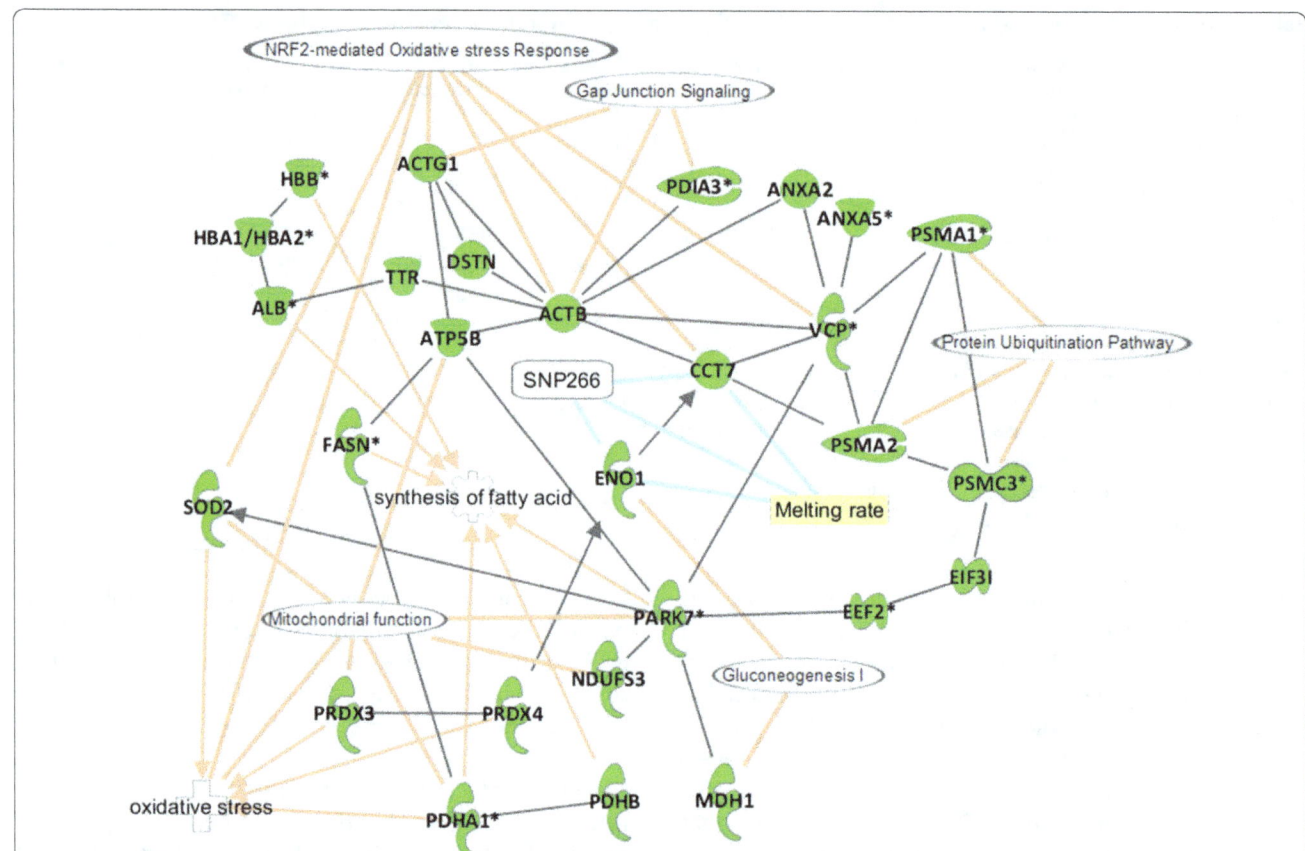

Fig. 7 Biological network. This biological network was constructed with the proteins that are regulated by a QTL and associated with a significant enrichment score using Ingenuity Pathway Analysis software. Other information was added, such as some significant biological functions and canonical pathways (*links in orange*), proteins involved in cell viability are indicated with an *asterisk*. One trait related to liver function, i.e. melting rate, which is controlled by a pleiotropic QTL on APL15 (*links in blue*) was added

Table 5 **Functional enrichment analysis of biological functions between proteins with pQTL and the complete list of proteins**

Diseases or function annotation (Ingenuity)	Complete			pQTL		
	P value	Number of molecules	Rank	P value	Number of molecules	Rank
Synthesis of purine nucleotide	9.97E−10	11	6	5.69E−09	9	1
Metabolism of nucleic acid component or derivative	7.89E−12	20	1	6.02E−09	14	2
Metabolism of dicarboxylic acid	2.21E−07	5	16	2.91E−08	5	3
Metabolism of nucleotide	2.07E−09	16	7	5.88E−08	12	4
Metabolism of hydrogen peroxide	2.63E−10	10	2	1.03E−07	7	5
Cell viability	6.29E−07	24	26	1.13E−07	20	6
Metabolism of nucleoside triphosphate	2.3E−08	9	11	3.14E−07	7	7
Cell viability of tumor cell lines	1.57E−05	16	41	3.45E−07	15	8
Catabolism of hydrogen peroxide	3.02E−10	6	4	3.83E−07	4	9
Biosynthesis of purine ribonucleotide	3.85E−07	7	21	6.28E−07	6	10
Synthesis of nucleotide	6.13E−07	12	25	6.86E−07	10	11
Biosynthesis of nucleoside triphosphate	5.98E−07	7	24	9.19E−07	6	12
Polymerization of protein	6.77E−06	11	35	1.06E−06	10	13
Fatty acid metabolism	1.46E−06	15	28	2.39E−06	12	14
Synthesis of acetyl-coenzyme A	1.64E−07	4	13	5.15E−06	3	15

Only the top 15 biological functions are shown according to Ingenuity analysis a chromosome other than that carrying the gene coding for the protein analysed. This very high proportion of trans-acting pQTL suggests that the detected variations in protein quantity are generally not due to variations within their coding genes and the associated regulatory regions, such as promoters or enhancers. Such a high proportion of trans-acting eQTL was previously reported in humans, pigs [31] and rats, but cis-QTL usually have stronger effects [32]. Only six of the detected pQTL were putatively found on the same chromosome as that carrying the gene encoding the protein. However, at this point given the wide confidence intervals of these six pQTL, it is difficult to determine whether they are actually true cis-acting QTL. Until now, only three of the six genes coding for the six putative cis-pQTL are located on the duck genome assembly (*MDH1* on APL3, *ANXA5* on APL4 and *ALDH7A1* on APLZ). Only the pQTL for ALDH7A1 on APLZ is close to the gene coding for this protein, near the microsatellite marker CAM113 (Faraut T, personal communication). To explore this question further, a higher density genetic map and probably also addition of more families in the proteomics study are required to be able to observe a larger number of meiotic recombination events. The very high proportion of trans-acting QTL found in the current study could be due to the fact that protein levels are regulated by many more factors in addition to gene transcription. This is supported by the results of analysing separately spots corresponding to different forms of the same protein, which are very likely due to post-translational modifications.

The most significant pQTL are related to fatty acid and amino acid metabolism, and glycolysis

Chromosome APL7, which harbours a pQTL for APOA1 that is significant at the 5% genome-wide level, seems to play an important role in regulating liver metabolism. APL7 also harbours phenotypic QTL for plasma glucose and cholesterol levels (Table 3) and for some weight traits (bodyweight before the overfeeding period, thigh and shank weight at slaughter). Indeed, APOA1 is involved in the transport of triglycerides from liver cells to adipose tissues by taking part in the formation of HDL (high density lipoprotein). Lagarrigue et al. [33] reported that the amounts of APOA1 mRNA were significantly larger in chickens from fat lines than from lean lines, which supported the hypothesis that it has a role in lipid transport and storage in birds. Szapacs et al. [34] showed that when APOA1 was exposed to oxidative changes, the formation of HDL and its exportation to the liver were altered. In chicken, GGA7, which is homoeologous to APL7, carries numerous QTL related to abdominal fat [35, 36]. Taken together, these results strengthen the hypothesis that chromosome APL7 is important in "fat" metabolism and

further studies will be required to identify the genes that underlie the QTL and pQTL mapped to this chromosome. However, the only protein that we detected by 2D gel electrophoresis with a gene located on APL7 is HIBCH, which is involved in amino acid metabolism, but for which no QTL were mapped to APL7. The pleiotropic analysis with graphs (Fig. 6f) proposed interesting possible interactions between HIBCH, which is controlled by QTL on APL10 and APL14, and other QTL controlled by APL7.

Another strong pQTL was detected for ENO1 and mapped to APL18. Chromosome GGA17 is homoeologous to APL18 and harbours a QTL related to insulin levels in chickens [37]. This is interesting because both ENO1 levels and insulin levels are linked. Indeed, ENO1 is an enzyme of the glycolysis pathway where an increase in blood glucose level results in increased insulin synthesis and secretion by the pancreas leading to absorption of the glucose by the liver. Thus, glucose enters the glycolysis pathway to be transformed into pyruvate prior to fatty acid synthesis [38].

The strongest pQTL identified in this study was for FASN. In the liver, this enzyme plays a major role in lipid metabolism and lipid synthesis. Functional enrichment analysis identified FASN as playing a significant role in a pathway related to RXR activation (Table 4). RXR is a member of the nuclear receptor family of transcription factors and is closely related to nuclear receptors such as PPAR and FXR. The liver X receptors (LXR) are known to be important regulators of cholesterol, fatty acid, and glucose homeostasis. The pQTL related to FASN on APL24 co-localized with a QTL that affects plasma cholesterol levels but the significance of the 2t-QTL was lower, even if it is difficult to exceed the 1% genome-wide threshold in our design. It is interesting to note that other proteins for which the *P* value of the related QTL is between 1 and 5% on APL24, such as APOA1, PGAM1 or pyruvate dehydrogenase, are involved in lipid metabolism, which suggests that the locus on APL24 plays an important role in this metabolic pathway.

Exploring the pleiotropic QTL

Previously, Gilbert and Leroy [26] demonstrated that, in the case of linked or pleiotropic QTL, combining phenotypic information from different traits could increase the precision of QTL mapping and possibly the power of single-trait analysis to detect QTL. Among the 66 CLIP tests that we performed (22% of the 2t-QTL), the pleiotropy hypothesis was not rejected for 16 of them, i.e. 5% of the initially performed two-trait analyses. This approach proved very effective for identifying likely pleiotropic QTL, and some of the 2t-QTL identified in this study are particularly interesting. Owing to the complexity of the data output, graphical representations were constructed (Fig. 6) to better illustrate the results and aid interpretation.

On chromosome APL15 (Fig. 6b), we were able to map several QTL and pQTL that were significant at the 1% chromosome-wide threshold around SNP266 among which one QTL was related to melting rate and two pQTL were related to CCT7 and ENO1 (spot 124), respectively. Two-trait analysis of CCT7 and liver melting rate revealed the presence of two closely-linked QTL, whereas two-trait analysis of ENO1 and melting rate revealed the presence of a QTL with a pleiotropic effect. Moreover, a second spot for ENO1 (spot 112) also appeared to act pleiotropically with melting rate, which means that a single locus affects both liver melting quality and ENO1 levels in spots 112 and 124, suggesting that the locus is involved in regulating glycolytic processes. Mapping duck SNP266 on the chicken genome showed that it is located in an intron of the *LMF1* (*lipoprotein maturation factor 1*) gene, which codes for a protein that is involved in the maturation of the lipoproteins before they leave liver cells [39]. These findings argue in favour of future studies on this region of APL15, to test this candidate gene and other nearby genes and identify the polymorphism that underlies the pleiotropic QTL.

On APLZ, a 2t-QTL was detected for GLUD1 and plasma glucose levels at the beginning of the force-feeding period, for which the pleiotropy hypothesis was not rejected. GLUD1 is a mitochondrial glutamate dehydrogenase 1 which plays a role in glutamine metabolism by converting L-glutamate into α-ketoglutarate. Although this enzyme is not directly involved in the lipid metabolism pathway, α-ketoglutarate is involved in the mitochondrial Krebs cycle by taking part in citrate synthesis, which is necessary for lipid synthesis in the liver. In humans, a syndrome called hyperinsulinism/hyperammonemia (HI/HA) could be due in part to mutations in the *GLUD1* gene [40] that increase the synthesis of α-ketoglutarate leading to an increase of insulin exocytosis in the pancreatic β-cells and consequently to an increase of glucose absorption by the liver. Since this mechanism occurs naturally after each meal, a pleiotropic QTL that, in ducks, affects both the abundance of GLUD1 and plasma glucose levels after feeding appears quite plausible. Since *GLUD1* is located on APL6, we can only speculate on the gene that is involved in this transacting two-trait QTL on APLZ.

A pleiotropic 2t-QTL for APOA1 and thigh weight mapped to APL7. Such an association of traits is unusual since the main peripheral tissue studied and linked with APOA1 is abdominal fat as explained previously. Although no association between abdominal fat and APOA1 could be tested since there is no known QTL

for abdominal fat on APL7, our results are consistent with the fact that APOA1 has an important role in lipid exportation.

On APL19, the pleiotropic hypothesis was not rejected for the strong 2t-QTL between BW28 and EIF3I, ACP1 and EEF2, and between BWG12-28 and EIF3I and ACP1. EIF3I and EEF2 are proteins that act simultaneously on the ribosome to translate mRNA into protein. ACP1 is an enzyme that hydrolyses protein tyrosine phosphate. The association of such proteins with growth traits is interesting because growing cells and tissues require increased protein synthesis and it can be assumed that the genes underlying these QTL are involved in protein synthesis.

Of the 16 QTL for which a pleiotropic effect was detected, none mapped to the chromosomal position of the gene that encoded the protein tested. Therefore, we cannot directly identify the candidate protein or gene as suggested by Consoli et al. [41]. Interpretation of the 16 pleiotropic QTL detected in the current study is clearly more complex, since a variation in genotype probably affects a gene that modifies the metabolic pathway of the protein identified in the pQTL. Moreover, because of the low density of the duck genetic map and its incompletely annotated genome, it is impossible to formulate strong hypotheses on the genes or the gene functions that are highlighted by the different QTL. Nevertheless, the trait-protein associations that result in strong pleiotropic QTL are consistent and are the basis for preliminary explanations regarding the involved metabolic pathways.

Conclusions

Through the identification of polymorphic genomic regions that are related to product quality and liver protein levels in overfed ducks, our aim was to better understand the metabolic mechanisms that are involved in the genetic variation of duck traits of economic value, such as fatty liver and breast (*magret*) quality. By analyzing co-localized phenotypic and proteomic QTL, we identified pleiotropic loci that affect metabolic pathways linked to glycolysis or lipogenesis. However, further investigation is required to confirm the protein biomarkers that were found to impact the genetic variability of phenotypic traits. Thus, the livers of these mule ducks are currently being phenotyped, both via transcriptomics and metabolomics approaches, in order to perform new QTL analyses based on "-omics" data and confirm or invalidate the metabolic pathways described in this paper. To further our understanding of the proteome, the proteomics approach presented here could be combined with mass spectrometry. Finally, once all "omics" QTL analyses are completed, it will be interesting to analyze QTL "hot spot" regions, which potentially harbor strong candidate genes with important regulatory functions in the liver.

Additional files

> **Additional file 1: Table S1.** List of identified protein spots for which QTL were detected. List of 104 protein spots with gene/protein symbol, protein name, spot number, accession number, Mascot score, number of amino acids, molecular weight and calculated isoelectric point.
>
> **Additional file 2: Table S2.** Single-trait QTL detection based on protein quantification. List of 176 pQTL (with successfully identified proteins) with APL chromosome number, protein name, spot number, QTL location (cM), maximum likelihood ratio, P-value, threshold reached, confidence interval, substitution effect and gene position on APL chromosome.
>
> **Additional file 3: Table S3.** Single-trait QTL detection of zootechnical traits. List of 80 QTL with APL chromosome number, protein name, spot number, QTL location (cM), maximum likelihood ratio, P-value, threshold reached, confidence interval, substitution effect and gene position on APL chromosome.

Authors' contributions
All authors were involved in the conception of the study. CME designed the experiment, and CM obtained the funds required to perform the study. YF and NMG performed the proteomic analyses, and YF and CME computed the genetic analyses. Data interpretations were done by LL, CM, AV, CME and YF. All authors read and approved the final manuscript.

Author details
[1] GenPhySE, INRA, INPT, INP-ENVT, Université de Toulouse, 31326 Castanet Tolosan, France. [2] IPREM-EMM, UMR5254, Université de Pau et des Pays de l'Adour, 40004 Mont de Marsan Cedex, France.

Acknowledgements
The authors acknowledge I David for providing the ClipTest software.

Competing interests
The authors declare that they have no competing interests.

Funding
The funding of the proteomic data was provided by the research chair of C. Molette, obtained from the "Institut National Polytechnique de Toulouse" and the "Institut National de la Recherche Agronomique".

References
1. Damerval C, Hébert Y, de Vienne D. Is the polymorphism of protein amounts related to phenotypic variability? A comparison of two-dimensional electrophoresis data with morphological traits in maize. Theor Appl Genet. 1987;74:194–202.
2. Damerval C, Maurice A, Josse JM, de Vienne D. Quantitative trait loci underlying gene product variation: a novel perspective for analyzing regulation of genome expression. Genetics. 1994;137:289–301.
3. Bourgeois M, Jacquin F, Cassecuelle F, Savois V, Belghazi M, Aubert G, et al. A PQL (protein quantity loci) analysis of mature pea seed proteins identifies loci determining seed protein composition. Proteomics. 2011;11:1581–94.
4. Holdt LM, von Delft A, Nicolaou A, Baumann S, Kostrzewa M, Thiery J, et al. Quantitative trait loci mapping of the mouse plasma proteome (pQTL). Genetics. 2013;193:601–8.
5. Kileh-Wais M, Elsen JM, Vignal A, Feves K, Vignoles F, Fernandez X, et al. Detection of QTL controlling metabolism, meat and liver quality traits of the overfed interspecific hybrid mule duck. J Anim Sci. 2013;91:588–604.
6. François Y, Marie-Etancelin C, Vignal A, Viala D, Davail S, Molette C. Mule duck "foie gras" show different metabolic states according to their quality phenotypes by using a proteomic approach. J Agric Food Chem. 2014;62:7140–50.
7. Marie-Etancelin C, Basso B, Davail S, Gontier K, Fernandez X, Vitezica ZG, et al. Genetic parameters of product quality and hepatic metabolism in fattened mule ducks. J Anim Sci. 2011;89:669–79.
8. Théron L, Astruc T, Bouillier-Oudot M, Molette C, Vénien A, Peyrin F, et al. The fusion of lipid droplets is involved in fat loss during cooking of duck "foie gras". Meat Sci. 2011;89:377–83.
9. Fillon V, Vignoles M, Crooijmans RP, Groenen MA, Zoorob R, Vignal A. Fish mapping of 57 BAC clones reveals strong conservation of synteny between galliformes and anseriformes. Anim Genet. 2007;38:303–7.
10. Vignal A, Rue O, Klopp C, Faraut T, Li N, Huang Y, et al. SNP detection for QTL mapping in ducks. In Proceedings of the XXI plant and animal genome meeting, 11–16 Jan 2013. San Diego; 2013.
11. Huang Y, Li Y, Burt DW, Chen H, Zhang Y, Qian W, et al. The duck genome and transcriptome provide insight into an avian influenza virus reservoir species. Nat Genet. 2013;45:776–83.
12. Li H, Durbin R. Fast and accurate short read alignment with Burrows–Wheeler transform. Bioinformatics. 2009;25:1754–60.
13. McKenna A, Hanna M, Banks E, Sivachenko A, Cibulskis K, Kernytsky A, et al. The genome analysis toolkit: a MapReduce framework for analyzing next-generation DNA sequencing data. Genome Res. 2010;20:1297–303.
14. Skinner BM, Robertson LBW, Tempest HG, Langley EJ, Ioannou D, Fowler KE, et al. Comparative genomics in chicken and Pekin duck using FISH mapping and microarray analysis. BMC Genomics. 2009;10:357.
15. Green P, Falls K, Crooks S. Documentation for CRIMAP. St Louis: Washington University; 1990.
16. SAS version 9.1.3. Cary: SAS Institute Inc.; 2002.
17. Elsen JM, Mangin B, Goffinet B, Boichard D, Le Roy P. Alternative models for QTL detection in livestock. I-general introduction. Genet Sel Evol. 1999;31:213.
18. Gilbert H, Le Roy P, Moreno C, Robelin D, Elsen JM. QTLMAP, a software for QTL detection in outbred population. Ann Hum Genet. 2008;72:694.
19. Filangi O, Moreno C, Gilbert H, Legarra A, Le Roy P, Elsen JM. QTLMap, a software for QTL detection in outbred populations. In Proceedings of the 9th world congress on genetics applied to livestock production, 1–8 Aug 2010, Leipzig; 2010.
20. Lander ES, Botstein D. Mapping mendelian factors underlying quantitative traits using RFLP linkage maps. Genetics. 1989;121:185–99.
21. Knott SA, Elsen JM, Haley CS. Methods for multiple marker mapping of quantitative trait loci in half-sib populations. Theor Appl Genet. 1966;93:71–80.
22. Goffinet B, Le RP, Boichard D, Elsen JM, Mangin B. Alternative models for QTL detection in livestock. III. Heteroskedastic model and models corresponding to several distributions of the QTL effect. Genet Sel Evol. 1999;31:341–50.
23. Churchill GA, Doerge RW. Empirical threshold values for quantitative trait mapping. Genetics. 1994;138:963–71.
24. Visscher PM, Thompson R, Haley CS. Confidence intervals in QTL mapping by bootstrapping. Genetics. 1996;143:1013–20.
25. Roldan DL, Dodero AM, Bidinost F, Taddeo HR, Allain D, Poli MA, et al. Merino sheep: a further look at quantitative trait loci for wool production. Animal. 2010;4:1330–40.
26. Gilbert H, Le Roy P. Comparison of three multi-trait methods for QTL detection. Genet Sel Evol. 2003;35:281–304.
27. David I, Elsen JM, Concordet D. CLIP test: a new fast, simple and powerful method to distinguish between linked or pleiotropic quantitative trait loci in linkage disequilibria analysis. Heredity (Edinb). 2013;110:232–8.
28. Bastian M, Heymann S, Jacomy M. Gephi. An open source software for exploring and manipulating networks. In: Proceedings of the third International AAAI conference on weblogs and social media, 17–20 May 2009, San Jose; 2009. https://gephi.org/publications/gephi-bastian-feb09.pdf. Gephi 0.9.1 (Feb 14 2016).
29. Villa-Vialaneix N, Liaubet L, Laurent T, Cherel P, Gamot A, SanCristobal M. The structure of a gene co-expression network reveals biological functions underlying eQTLs. PLoS One. 2013;8:e60045.
30. Civelek M, Lusis AJ. Systems genetics approaches to understand complex traits. Nat Rev Genet. 2014;15:34–48.

31. Liaubet L, Lobjois V, Faraut T, Tircazes A, Benne F, Iannuccelli N, et al. Genetic variability of transcript abundance in pig peri-mortem skeletal muscle: eQTL localized genes involved in stress response, cell death, muscle disorders and metabolism. BMC Genomics. 2011;12:548.

32. Cookson W, Liang L, Abecasis G, Moffatt M, Lathrop M. Mapping complex disease traits with global gene expression. Nat Rev Genet. 2009;10:184–94.

33. Lagarrigue S, Daval S, Bordas A, Douaire M. Hepatic lipogenesis gene expression in two experimental egg-laying lines divergently selected on residual food consumption. Genet Sel Evol. 2000;32:205–16.

34. Szapacs ME, Kim HYH, Porter NA, Lieber DC. Identification of proteins adducted by lipid peroxidation products in plasma and modifications of apolipoprotein A with a novel biotinylated phospholipid probe. J Proteome Res. 2008;7:4237–46.

35. Lagarrigue S, Pitel F, Carré W, Abasht B, Le Roy P, Neau A, et al. Mapping quantitative trait loci affecting fatness and breast muscle weight in meat-type chicken lines divergently selected on abdominal fatness. Genet Sel Evol. 2006;38:85–97.

36. Wang SZ, Hu XX, Wang ZP, Li XC, Wang QG, Wang YX, et al. Quantitative trait loci associated with body weight and abdominal fat traits on chicken chromosomes 3, 5 and 7. Genet Mol Res. 2012;11:956–65.

37. Zhou H, Evock-Clover CM, McMurtry JP, Ashwell CM, Lamont SJ. Genome-wide linkage analysis to identify chromosomal regions affecting phenotypic traits in the chicken. IV. Metabolic traits. Poult Sci. 2007;86:267–76.

38. Berg JM, Tymoczko JL, Stryer L. Glycolysis is an energy-conversion pathway in many organisms. In: Berg JM, Tymoczko JL, Stryer L, editors. Biochemistry. 5th ed. New York: WH Freeman; 2002.

39. Peterfy M. Lipase maturation factor 1: a lipase chaperone involved in lipid metabolism. Biochim Biophys Acta. 2012;1821:790–4.

40. Rahman SA, Nessa A, Hussain K. Molecular mechanisms of congenital hyperinsulinism. J Mol Endocrinol. 2015;54:119–29.

41. Consoli L, Lefèvre A, Zivy M, de Vienne D, Damerval C. QTL analysis of proteome and transcriptome variations for dissecting the genetic architecture of complex traits in maize. Plant Mol Biol. 2002;48:575–81.

10

Derivation of economic values for production traits in aquaculture species

Kasper Janssen[1]*⬭, Paul Berentsen[2], Mathieu Besson[1,3] and Hans Komen[1]

Abstract

Background: In breeding programs for aquaculture species, breeding goal traits are often weighted based on the desired gains but economic gain would be higher if economic values were used instead. The objectives of this study were: (1) to develop a bio-economic model to derive economic values for aquaculture species, (2) to apply the model to determine the economic importance and economic values of traits in a case-study on gilthead seabream, and (3) to validate the model by comparison with a profit equation for a simplified production system.

Methods: A bio-economic model was developed to simulate a grow-out farm for gilthead seabream, and then used to simulate gross margin at the current levels of the traits and after one genetic standard deviation change in each trait with the other traits remaining unchanged. Economic values were derived for the traits included in the breeding goal: thermal growth coefficient (TGC), thermal feed intake coefficient (TFC), mortality rate (M), and standard deviation of harvest weight (σ_{HW}). For a simplified production system, improvement in TGC was assumed to affect harvest weight instead of growing period. Using the bio-economic model and a profit equation, economic values were derived for harvest weight, cumulative feed intake at harvest, and overall survival.

Results: Changes in gross margin showed that the order of economic importance of the traits was: TGC, TFC, M, and σ_{HW}. Economic values in € (kg production)$^{-1}$ (trait unit)$^{-1}$ were: 0.40 for TGC, −0.45 for TFC, −7.7 for M, and −0.0011 to −0.0010 for σ_{HW}. For the simplified production system, similar economic values were obtained with the bio-economic model and the profit equation. The advantage of the profit equation is its simplicity, while that of the bio-economic model is that it can be applied to any aquaculture species, because it can include any limiting factor and/or environmental condition that affects production.

Conclusions: We confirmed the validity of the bio-economic model. TGC is the most important trait to improve, followed by TFC and M, and the effect of σ_{HW} on gross margin is small.

Background

In Europe, over 80% of aquaculture production originates from breeding programs, which in most cases apply family selection with the aim of improving multiple traits simultaneously [1]. Breeding goal traits are often weighted based on desired gains rather than economic values [2], which compromises economic gain [3, 4].

In aquaculture species, economic values are available only for a few species, although their importance has repeatedly been underlined, e.g. [5, 6]. Profit equations have been used to derive economic values for Nile tilapia (*Oreochromis niloticus*) [7], common carp (*Cyprinus carpio*) [8], Australian abalones (*Haliotis rubra* and *H. laevigata*) [9], and crayfish (*Cherax tenuimanus*) [10]. Besson et al. [11, 12] used a bio-economic model to derive economic values for African catfish (*Clarias gariepinus*) that were produced in a land-based aquaculture system in which water is treated and recirculated and for growth rate in European seabass (*Dicentrarchus labrax*) under varying temperature conditions, respectively.

For livestock species with simple and highly controlled production systems, such as pig production, economic values can be derived from a profit equation, e.g. [13]. For

*Correspondence: kasper.janssen@wur.nl
[1] Animal Breeding and Genomics, Wageningen University and Research, Droevendaalsesteeg 1, 6708 PB Wageningen, The Netherlands
Full list of author information is available at the end of the article

production systems with a higher degree of complexity, partly due to seasonal variation, such as in dairy cattle and sheep farming, profit equations may fail to provide an adequate description of the farming system and bio-economic models are required [14–16]. In general, bio-economic models provide a more accurate description of farming systems than profit equations and are, therefore, increasingly used to estimate economic values [2].

Fish farms are complex production systems for two reasons. First, fish are kept outdoors in most farming systems and, thus, are exposed to fluctuating environmental conditions. Seasonal variation in temperature causes variation in growth rate of fish, because of their ectothermic nature. Fish are harvested at a constant weight rather than at a constant age, hence the length of a production cycle depends on the stocking date. Second, production output of a farm is determined by constraints such as oxygen availability [11] and stocking density. Stocking density constrains production output for many important aquaculture species, including Atlantic salmon (*Salmo salar*), European seabass, and gilthead seabream (*Sparus aurata*). Thus, bio-economic models could prove useful to derive economic values for aquaculture species.

The objectives of this study were: (1) to develop such a bio-economic model, (2) to apply the model to determine the economic importance and economic values for various traits in a case-study on gilthead seabream, and (3) to validate the model by comparison with a profit equation for a simplified production system.

Methods
Traits
The breeding goal considered here includes growth rate, feed intake rate, mortality rate, and uniformity in harvest weight. Growth rate affects revenues, feed costs and juvenile costs; feed intake rate affects feed costs; mortality rate affects feed costs and juvenile costs. Feed and juveniles are major costs in production [17], thus including growth and feed intake in the breeding goal is common practice in livestock [18, 19]. Uniformity, i.e. size variation around the mean harvest weight, determines the distribution of fish over price categories at harvest, and thus affects revenues via the average sales price of fish.

Economic values are specific for the unit in which a trait is expressed [20]. Here, growth rate is expressed in units of thermal growth coefficient (TGC) [21]. TGC is a standardized measure of growth in fish that takes stocking weight and temperature variation over the lifespan of a fish into account. TGC is widely used [22], is more accurate than other measures of growth rate [23], and is relatively robust to differences in temperature regimes [24, 25]. Feed intake is assumed to be determined by the same variables as bodyweight and gain in bodyweight,

because energy requirement is largely determined by bodyweight and gain in bodyweight [26]. In this study, feed intake rate is, therefore, expressed in units of thermal feed intake coefficient TFC, a TGC analogue. TFC takes stocking weight and temperature variation over the lifespan of a fish into account. The TFC model is independent of the TGC model, i.e. a modelled change in growth rate will not affect modelled feed intake rate and vice versa, which is a prerequisite to derive economic values. Mortality rate (M) is expressed as % of mortality per day. Uniformity is expressed as the standard deviation of harvest weight (σ_{HW}) in grams.

Bio-economic model
The bio-economic model developed by Besson et al. [12] was adapted to simulate production systems with seasonal variation in temperature and in which density constrains production output, in this case a typical grow-out farm for gilthead seabream in Greece. The model is a deterministic simulation model that is programmed in R version 2.12.2. [27]. The model simulates operation of the farm during an average year. The farm consists of 20 cages of 2800 m^3 each and produces about 550 tons annually. As shown in Fig. 1, the model consists of three hierarchical parts: a fish model, a cage model, and a farm model. Inputs into the fish model are: stocking date, temperature coefficients, TGC, and TFC. Outputs of the fish model for each stocking date are: bodyweight per day per fish, feed consumption per day per fish, and harvest date. Inputs into the cage model are: outputs of the fish model, M, cage volume, and feed prices. Outputs of the cage model for each stocking date are per production cycle of a cage: fish production, number of juveniles stocked, feed consumption, and feed costs. A production cycle is the period between stocking and harvesting a cage. Inputs of the farm model are: outputs of the cage model, number of cages, price of juveniles, price of packing, and sales prices. Outputs of the farm model are total per year: fish production, number of juveniles stocked, feed consumption, feed costs, juvenile costs, packing costs, revenues from fish sales, and gross margin.

The model was used to derive economic values of the traits mentioned above. Economic values give the expected change in profit from a small change in trait level, keeping the level of all other traits constant. Genetic change does not affect fixed costs, hence change in profit due to genetic change equals change in gross margin. When change in trait level equals the additive genetic standard deviation (σ_A) [15], the resulting change in gross margin indicates how important that trait is, because σ_A is indicative of the rate at which breeding values can be improved [28]. To determine the relative importance of the traits and to derive economic values, the model was

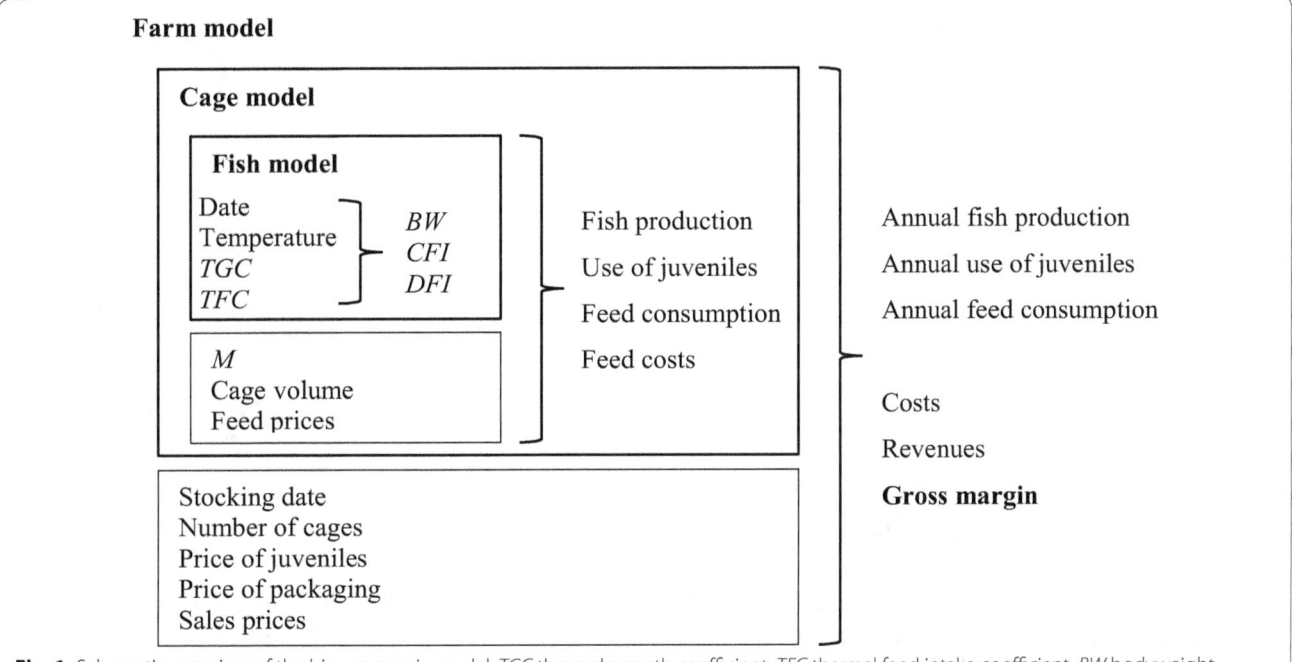

Fig. 1 Schematic overview of the bio-economic model. *TGC* thermal growth coefficient, *TFC* thermal feed intake coefficient, *BW* bodyweight, *CFI* cumulative feed intake, *DFI* daily feed intake, *M* mortality rate

run under two situations: first before genetic change and second, after a change of one σ_A in one trait with the other traits kept constant. For the trait 'uniformity', minimum and maximum values of the possible range of σ_A were used, because the actual value was unknown. Trait levels were changed in the desired direction of the genetic change. Economic values were expressed per kg of fish produced in the situation before genetic change [29] and were calculated as:

Economic value

$$= \left(\frac{gross\ margin_A - gross\ margin_B}{trait\ level_A - trait\ level_B} \right) \Big/ fish\ production_B, \quad (1)$$

where subscripts indicate before (*B*) and after (*A*) genetic change.

Model equations

The "Estimation of model coefficients" section describes the derivation of model coefficients from farm data. These coefficients (see Table 1) are used as the equations' coefficients of the bio-economic model. The three parts of the bio-economic model are described in the following three subsections.

Estimation of model coefficients

Coefficients in the equations to describe temperature, fish growth, feed intake, and number of fish per cage were

derived from recent farm data of the company Andromeda S.A., which is hereafter referred to as 'data'. The data included daily records of temperature, feed provided, and mortality, and regular records of bodyweight from 15 cages of a farm located in Vonitsa, Northern Greece during the period 2013 through 2015.

Seasonal variation in daily water temperature throughout the year followed a sinusoidal pattern. Therefore, the equation to describe daily temperature ($T_{t_{s,a}}$) in °C was [30]:

$$T_{t_{s,a}} = TM - TA \cdot sin\left(2\pi \cdot \left(t_{s,a} - t_A\right)/365\right), \quad (2)$$

where *TM* is the average annual temperature (°C), *TA* is the range of temperatures around *TM* (°C), t_A is the time of the year at which $T_{t_{s,a}}$ equaled *TM*, and $t_{s,a}$ represents the date defined as:

$$t_{s,a} = s + a, \quad (3)$$

where stocking date s ($s = 1, \ldots, n$) equals 1 on January 1 2013 and a ($a = 0, \ldots, n$) is the age of the fish (days). To estimate *TM*, *TA*, and t_A, Eq. 2 was fitted to the data by means of non-linear least-squares regression in R. Table 1 shows the resulting coefficients.

Bodyweight in seabream can be predicted from the stocking weight and the sum of daily effective temperatures. Daily effective temperature is the daily temperature minus 12 °C, where 12 °C represents the minimum temperature for seabream growth [31]. Therefore, the

Table 1 Estimated coefficients used in model equations

Symbol	Meaning	Value	Standard error	Unit
TM	Annual mean temperature	19.57	0.0119	°C
TA	Amplitude of temperature	−4.806	0.0167	°C
t_A	Date at which temperature equals TM	−32.49	0.2057	Day
TGC	Thermal growth coefficient	12.6	0.0847	$g^{2/3}$/(day degrees · 1000)
TFC	Thermal feed intake coefficient	8.25	0.157	$g^{0.544}$/(day degrees · 1000)
p	Weight exponent to predict cumulative feed intake	0.544	0.00282	–
M	Mortality rate	0.0300	0.000164	%/day

equation to describe bodyweight (in g) at $t_{s,a}$ ($BW_{t_{s,a}}$) was [32]:

$$BW_{t_{s,a}} = \left(BW_{t_{s,0}}^{2/3} + \frac{TGC}{1000} \cdot \sum_{i=t_{s,0}}^{(t_{s,a})-1} (T_i - 12) \right)^{3/2}, \quad (4)$$

where $BW_{t_{s,0}}$ is bodyweight at stocking (in g), and $\sum_{i=t_{s,0}}^{(t_{s,a})-1} (T_i - 12)$ represents the sum of effective temperatures (day degrees) over the lifespan of a fish excluding $t_{s,a}$. To estimate TGC, Eq. 4 was fitted to the data by means of non-linear least-squares regression in R. Instead of fixing exponents 2/3 and 3/2, fitting these to the data resulted in values of 0.612 and 1/0.612 but this barely improved accuracy of the model. Values of 2/3 and 3/2 were preferred, because standardization of growth models allows for a better comparison of growth rate across studies. Analogous to $BW_{t_{s,a}}$, the model to describe cumulative feed intake (in g) at $t_{s,a}$ ($CFI_{t_{s,a}}$) was:

$$CFI_{t_{s,a}} = \left(BW_{t_{s,0}}^{p} + \frac{TFC}{1000} \cdot \sum_{i=t_{s,0}}^{t_{s,a}} (T_i - 12) \right)^{1/p} - BW_{t_{s,0}}, \quad (5)$$

where p is a weight exponent, and $\sum_{i=t_{s,0}}^{t_{s,a}} (T_i - 12)$ represents the sum of effective temperatures (day degrees) over the lifespan of a fish, including $t_{s,a}$. The term $BW_{t_{s,0}}$ was subtracted from $\left(BW_{t_{s,0}}^{p} + \frac{TFC}{1000} \cdot \sum_{i=t_{s,0}}^{t_{s,a}} (T_i - 12) \right)^{1/p}$ to force the model through the intercept. To estimate TFC and p, Eq. 5 was fitted to the data by means of non-linear least-squares regression in R. Parameter M (%/day) was assumed to be constant over time, hence the number of fish alive decreased exponentially in time. The model to describe the number of fish at $t_{s,a}$ ($N_{t_{s,a}}$) was:

$$N_{t_{s,a}} = N_{t_{s,0}} \cdot \left(1 - \frac{M}{100\%} \right)^{(t_{s,a})-1}, \quad (6)$$

where $N_{t_{s,0}}$ is the number of fish stocked. To estimate M, Eq. 6 was fitted to the data by means of non-linear least-squares regression in R.

Fish model

Date ($t_{s,a}$) was modelled as in Eq. 3. Temperature ($T_{t_{s,a}}$) was modelled as in Eq. 2. Bodyweight ($BW_{t_{s,a}}$) was modelled as in Eq. 4, where stocking weight ($BW_{t_{s,0}}$) was 4.4 g, equal to the average in the data. Equation 4 was rewritten to calculate the harvest date ($t_{s,h}$) as:

$$\sum_{i=t_{s,0}}^{(t_{s,h})-1} (T_i - 12) = \frac{BW_{t_{s,h}}^{2/3} - BW_{t_{s,0}}^{2/3}}{TGC/1000}, \quad (7)$$

where $BW_{t_{s,h}}$ is the average harvest weight, here set to the desired market weight of 400 g. Solving the right hand side of the equation, yields $\sum_{i=t_{s,0}}^{(t_{s,h})-1} (T_i - 12) = 4084$ day degrees. Cumulative feed intake ($CFI_{t_{s,a}}$) was modelled as in Eq. 5. $CFI_{t_{s,h}}$ was set equal to $CFI_{(t_{s,h})-1}$, because fish are not fed on the day that they are harvested. Daily feed intake ($DFI_{t_{s,a}}$) was modeled as:

$$DFI_{t_{s,a}} = CFI_{(t_{s,a})+1} - CFI_{t_{s,a}}. \quad (8)$$

Cage model

To maximize production, standing stock in a cage reaches the maximum allowable density of 15 kg/m^3 at harvest. For the 2800 m^3 cages, per production cycle fish production is thus 42,000 kg or 100,500 fish. To compensate for mortality, a larger number of fish is stocked than harvested. The number of fish in a cage at $t_{s,a}$ ($N_{t_{s,a}}$) was modeled as:

$$N_{t_{s,a}} = 100,500 \cdot \left(1 - \frac{M}{100\%} \right)^{(t_{s,h}-t_{s,a})}. \quad (9)$$

The number of juveniles stocked per cage ($N_{t_{s,0}}$) was calculated by substituting $t_{s,a}$ for $t_{s,0}$. Daily feed intake per cage (kg) at $t_{s,a}$ ($DFIcage_{t_{s,a}}$) was modeled as:

$$DFIcage_{t_{s,a}} = N_{t_{s,a}} \cdot DFI_{t_{s,a}}/1000. \qquad (10)$$

Total feed consumption per cage (kg) stocked at date $t_{s,0}$ ($TFIcage_{t_{s,0}}$) was calculated as:

$$TFIcage_{t_{s,0}} = \sum_{i=t_{s,0}}^{t_{s,h}} DFIcage_i. \qquad (11)$$

Depending on bodyweight, fish are fed different feed types. Daily feed costs per cage ($DFCcage_{t_{s,a}}$) were calculated as the product of $DFIcage_{t_{s,a}}$ and feed price per size category. Table 2 shows the price of feed types for the fish size categories. Total feed costs per cage (€) stocked at date $t_{s,0}$ ($TFCcage_{t_{s,0}}$) were calculated as:

$$TFCcage_{t_{s,0}} = \sum_{i=t_{s,0}}^{t_{s,h}} DFCcage_i. \qquad (12)$$

Farm model

For the farm model, the cage model was run repeatedly over the whole range of stocking dates, from 1 (January 1th) to 365 days (December 31th) by one-day steps. Per stocking date, age at harvest $(t_{s,h} - t_{s,0})$, $TFIcage_{t_{s,0}}$, $TFCcage_{t_{s,0}}$, and $N_{t_{s,0}}$ were calculated. These results were averaged over all stocking dates to compute the average production cycle of a cage. The period between two successive production cycles is three days [Personal communications Andromeda S.A., 2015]. For the 20 cages that are present on the farm, the number of production cycles per year was calculated as:

$$Production\ cycles\ per\ year = 20 \cdot \frac{365}{average\left(t_{s,h} - t_{s,0}\right) + 3}. \qquad (13)$$

Average results per production cycle were multiplied by the number of production cycles per year to compute outputs at the farm level per year: fish production, number of juveniles stocked, feed consumption, and feed costs. Juvenile costs at the farm level were calculated by multiplying the number of juveniles stocked by the price of juveniles of €0.20 per piece. Packing costs at the farm

level were calculated by multiplying fish production by the price of packing of €0.33 per kg fish. Revenues from fish sales at the farm level were calculated as the product of fish production and average sales price. Average sales price was computed as the proportion of fish of each category in Table 3 multiplied by its corresponding sales price. Three percent of the fish harvested are deformed. The size distribution of the remaining fish was calculated from a normal probability density function with $\mu = 400$ and $\sigma_{HW} = 60$ [Personal communications Andromeda S.A., 2015].

Additive genetic standard deviation of traits

The economic importance of each trait in the breeding goal depends on the change in gross margin, which itself depends on the change in trait level of one σ_A. The genetic coefficient of variation (CVA) can be used to estimate σ_A from the mean trait level (μ) [28]:

$$\sigma_A = \frac{CV_A}{100\%} \cdot \mu. \qquad (14)$$

For TFC, σ_A can be estimated from the genetic variation in $BW_{t_{s,h}}$. For this study, $BW_{t_{s,h}}$ was set equal to 400 g, and $\sum_{i=t_{s,0}}^{(t_{s,h})-1} (T_i - 12)$ was 4084 day degrees (Eq. 7). CVA of bodyweight was estimated to be 10.6% based on data from Navarro et al. [33]. For $BW_{t_{s,h}}$, σ_A was thus 42.4 g. The distribution of $BW_{t_{s,h}}$ was simulated in R as $BW_{t_{s,h},n} = \mu + z_n \cdot \sigma_A$, where $\mu = 400$ and $\sigma_A = 42.4$, and z_n is a standard normal distribution ($z_n \sim N(0,1)$) with $n = 1, \ldots, 10^6$. From this simulation, σ_A of TGC was estimated as (Appendix 1):

$$\sigma_A \text{of } TGC \approx \sqrt{Var(TGC_n)} \approx \sqrt{\left(\frac{1000}{4084}\right)^2 \cdot Var\left(BW_{t_{s,h},n}^{2/3}\right)}$$

$$= \frac{1000}{4084} \sqrt{\frac{1}{10^6 - 1} \cdot \sum_{i=1}^{n} \left(BW_i^{2/3} - 400^{2/3}\right)^2}$$

$$= 0.95 \text{ g}^{2/3}/(\text{day degrees} \cdot 1000). \qquad (15)$$

Table 2 Feed price per fish size category in 2014 [Personal communications Andromeda S.A., 2015]

Fish size (g)	Price (€/kg)
<7	2.21
7–13	1.97
13–30	1.65
30–80	1.26
80–300	1.12
>300	1.17

Table 3 Sales price per fish size category in 2014 [Personal communications Andromeda S.A., 2015]

Category (g)	Price (€/kg)
<100	0
100–200	1.65
200–300	4.15
300–400	4.52
400–600	4.63
>600 g	5.27
Deformed	2.52

For *TFC*, σ_A can be estimated from the genetic variation in both $BW_{t_{s,0}}$ and $CFI_{t_{s,h}}$. For $CFI_{t_{s,h}}$, σ_A can be approximated by (Appendix 2):

$$\sigma_A \text{ of } CFI_{t_{s,h}} \approx \frac{1.75}{r_A} \cdot \sigma_A \text{ of } BW_{t_{s,h}}, \tag{16}$$

where r_A is the genetic correlation between $BW_{t_{s,h}}$ and $CFI_{t_{s,h}}$, which was assumed to be 0.90 [34]. Solving Eq. (16), σ_A of $CFI_{t_{s,h}}$ was equal to 82 g. Based on an average $CFI_{t_{s,h}}$ of 713 g in our study, the *CVA* of $CFI_{t_{s,h}}$ was 12%, which is close to values reported for other species [34, 35]. Genetic variances for $CFI_{t_{s,h}}$ and $BW_{t_{s,0}}$ were simulated to calculate σ_A of *TFC*. In our study, the average $BW_{t_{s,0}}$ was 4.4 g. Based on a *CVA* of 10.6% for bodyweight, σ_A of $BW_{t_{s,0}}$ was equal to 0.45 g. The distribution of $CFI_{t_{s,h}}$ was simulated in R as $CFI_{t_{s,h},n} = \mu + z_n \cdot \sigma_A$, where $\mu = 713$, $\sigma_A = 82$, and z_n is a standard normal distribution ($z_n \sim N(0,1)$) with $n = 1, \ldots, 10^6$. The distribution of $BW_{t_{s,0}}$ was simulated in R as $BW_{t_{s,0},n} = \mu + z_n \cdot \sigma_A$, where $\mu = 4.4$, $\sigma_A = 0.45$ and z_n is a standard normal distribution ($z_n \sim N(0,1)$) with $n = 1, \ldots, 10^6$. A covariance of zero was assumed between $CFI_{t_{s,h}}$ and $BW_{t_{s,0}}$. Based on the simulations, σ_A of *TFC* was estimated as:

$$\sigma_A \text{ of } TFC \approx \sqrt{Var(TFC_n)}$$

$$= \sqrt{Var\left(1000 \cdot \frac{\left(CFI_{t_{s,h},n} + BW_{t_{s,0},n}\right)^P - BW_{t_{s,0},n}^P}{4084}\right)}$$

$$= \frac{1000}{4084} \cdot \sqrt{\frac{1}{10^6 - 1} \cdot \sum_{i=1}^{n} \left(\begin{array}{c}(CFI_i + BW_i)^{0.544} - BW_i^{0.544} \\ -((713 + 4.4)^{0.544} - 4.4^{0.544})\end{array}\right)^2}$$

$$= 0.55 \text{ g}^{0.544}/(\text{degree days} \cdot 1000). \tag{17}$$

For *M*, σ_A can be estimated from the genetic variation in cumulative mortality at harvest ($CM_{t_{s,h}}$). The average $CM_{t_{s,h}}$ was 14.9%. In animal breeding, an underlying liability scale is commonly used to analyze mortality and survival [36]. Heritability of $CM_{t_{s,h}}$ on the liability scale was assumed to be 0.17 [37] and by definition σ_P is equal to 1, hence $\sigma_A = \sqrt{h^2} = \sqrt{0.17}$. Before genetic change, the deviation of the threshold from the mean (x_B) was calculated from the quantile function of a normal distribution in R as $x_B = -qnorm(0.149) = 1.04$. After genetic change by one σ_A, the deviation from the threshold from the mean (x_A) becomes: $x_A = x_B + \sigma_A = 1.04 + \sqrt{0.17} = 1.45$. After genetic change, $CM_{t_{s,h}}$ was calculated from the distribution function of a normal distribution in R as:

$$CM_{t_{s,h}} = (1 - pnorm(x_A)) \cdot 100\%$$
$$= (1 - pnorm(1.45)) \cdot 100\% = 7.34\%. \tag{18}$$

Average age at harvest was equal to 539 days (Table 4). *M* after genetic change was calculated as:

$$M = \left(1 - \left(1 - \frac{CM_{t_{s,h}}}{100}\right)^{\frac{1}{539}}\right) \cdot 100$$

$$\left(1 - \left(1 - \frac{7.34}{100}\right)^{\frac{1}{539}}\right) \cdot 100 = 0.014\%/\text{day}. \tag{19}$$

The difference in *M* before and after genetic change was 0.016, which was treated as the σ_A of *M*.

Genetic improvement of uniformity reduces the environmental variance of bodyweight. For environmental variance of bodyweight, CV_A was calculated as [38]:

$$CV_A = \frac{SD\left(\sigma_E^2\right)}{\sigma_E^2} \cdot 100\%, \tag{20}$$

where $SD\left(\sigma_E^2\right)$ is the genetic standard deviation of environmental variance and σ_E^2 is the mean environmental variance. Environmental variance equals phenotypic variance minus genetic variance [39]. The CV_A of environmental variance of bodyweight is about 20% in rainbow trout [40] and 41.7% in Atlantic salmon (*Salmo salar*) [41]. For seabream, the actual value was unknown, hence a minimum of 20% and maximum of 40% were used to represent both extremes of the possible range of σ_A. In this study, the trait uniformity was expressed on the standard deviation scale instead of the variance scale. On the standard deviation scale, the CV_A is half as large as on the variance scale [42, 43]. For $BW_{t_{s,h}}$, $\overline{\sigma_E} = \sqrt{\sigma_{HW}^2 - \sigma_A^2} = \sqrt{60^2 - 42.4^2} = 42.45$ g. For the minimum CV_A of the environmental standard deviation of bodyweight of 10%, σ_A equals 4.2 g, and for the maximum CV_A of the environmental standard deviation of bodyweight of 20%, σ_A equals 8.5 g.

Validation of the bio-economic model

To validate the bio-economic model, a simplified production system was assumed for which a profit equation can be developed. In this simplified production system, fish were harvested at a constant sum of effective temperatures instead of constant bodyweight. The sum of effective temperatures at harvest was assumed to be unaffected by genetic change. This allowed a profit equation to be set up as a function of the traits: harvest weight ($BW_{t_{s,h}}$), cumulative feed intake at harvest ($CFI_{t_{s,h}}$), and survival at harvest ($S_{t_{s,h}}$). In the bio-economic model, $S_{t_{s,h}} = \frac{N_{t_{s,h}}}{N_{t_{s,0}}} \cdot 100\%$. The bio-economic model was adapted by changing the harvest criterion from a bodyweight of 400 g to a sum of effective temperatures of 4084 day degrees. Thus, an increase in *TGC* resulted in a greater harvest weight instead of a shorter growing period. One σ_A change in *TGC* led to change in $BW_{t_{s,h}}$; one σ_A change in TFC led to change in $CFI_{t_{s,h}}$; one σ_A change in M led to change in $S_{t_{s,h}}$. Economic values were derived from the bio-economic model using Eq. 1 and trait levels of $BW_{t_{s,h}}$, $CFI_{t_{s,h}}$, and $S_{t_{s,h}}$.

In the profit equation, profit at the farm level was described as:

$$Profit = \frac{1000 \cdot Q}{BW_{t_{s,h}}} \cdot \left(BW_{t_{s,h}} \cdot \frac{sales\ price - packing\ costs}{1000} \right.$$
$$\left. - CFI_{t_{s,h}} \cdot \frac{1}{0.5 + S_{t_{s,h}}/200} \cdot \left(\frac{feed\ price}{1000} \right) - \frac{juvenile\ price}{S_{t_{s,h}}/100} \right)$$
$$- fixed\ costs, \tag{21}$$

where Q represents production output of the farm (kg) and was calculated as the product of maximum stocking density, cage volume and number of production cycles per year. Q is not affected by genetic change when the harvest criterion is a sum of effective temperatures of 4084 day degrees. Economic values were calculated as partial derivatives of the profit equation and divided by Q to express them per kg fish production. For $BW_{t_{s,h}}$, the economic value was calculated as:

$$Economic\ value_{BW_{t_{s,h}}} = \frac{\delta Profit}{\delta BW_{t_{s,h}}} \cdot \frac{1}{Q} = \frac{1000}{BW_{t_{s,h}}^2}$$
$$\cdot \left(\frac{CFI_{t_{s,h}} \cdot (feed\ price/1000)}{0.5 + S_{t_{s,h}}/200} + \frac{juvenile\ price}{S_{t_{s,h}}/100} \right). \tag{22}$$

For $CFI_{t_{s,h}}$, the economic value was calculated as:

$$Economic\ value_{CFI_{t_{s,h}}} = \frac{\delta Profit}{\delta CFI_{t_{s,h}}} \cdot \frac{1}{Q}$$
$$= -\frac{feed\ price}{BW_{t_{s,h}} \cdot (0.5 + S_{t_{s,h}}/200)}. \tag{23}$$

For $S_{t_{s,h}}$, the economic value was calculated as:

$$Economic\ value_S = \frac{\delta Profit}{\delta S} \cdot \frac{1}{Q}$$
$$= \frac{CFI_{t_{s,h}} \cdot feed\ price}{BW_{t_{s,h}} \cdot \left(50 + S_{t_{s,h}} + S_{t_{s,h}}^2/200 \right)}$$
$$+ \frac{100,000 \cdot juvenile\ price}{BW_{t_{s,h}} \cdot S_{t_{s,h}}^2}. \tag{24}$$

Results

Production results before genetic change

Tables 4 and 5 show the results of the model for key production variables and costs, respectively. The annual fish production was about 565 tons and gross margin about 759,000€. Average feed costs were €1.18/kg feed and average sales price was €4.49/kg fish.

Table 4 Key production variables of the gilthead seabream farm before genetic change

Item FCR	Value
Number of juveniles stocked (year^{-1})	1,659,945
Feed consumption (kg/year)	1,070,177
Fish production (kg/year)	564,661
Cages stocked (year^{-1})	13.4
Average age at harvest (day)	539
Survival (%)	85.1
Biological FCR[a] (kg feed/kg fish)	1.80
Economic FCR[b] (kg feed/kg fish)	1.92

[a] Biological FCR = feed consumption/(fish production + biomass mortality − biomass juveniles)

[b] Economic FCR = feed consumption/fish production

Production results after genetic change and economic values

The effect of the genetic change on production results is illustrated in Table 6. Changes in gross margin show that the order of economic importance of traits was: TGC, TFC, M, and σ_{HW}. The effect on gross margin of one σ_A change for each trait relative to the effect of a 8.5 g decrease in σ_{HW} was 43-fold for TGC, 28-fold for TFC, and 12-fold for M. Non-linearity was strongest for σ_{HW} (results not presented for TGC, TFC, and M), for which a doubling of change in trait level from −4.2 to −8.5 g led to 7.7% overestimation of the increase in gross margin.

The mechanisms by which changes in trait levels determined changes in gross margin were as follows. An increase in TGC resulted in a lower age at harvest (Eq. 7) and consequently, the number of production cycles per year increased (Eq. 13) and at the farm level, the annual number of juveniles stocked and annual fish production increased. An increase in TGC did not affect daily feed consumption (Eq. 4) and consequently, cumulative feed intake at harvest decreased because the sum of effective temperatures at harvest decreased (Eq. 5) and at the

Table 5 Economic results for the gilthead seabream farm before genetic change

Item	Farm level (€)	Fish level (€/kg)
Feed costs	1,259,917	2.23
Juvenile costs	331,989	0.59
Packing costs	186,338	0.33
Total variable costs	1,778,244	3.15
Total revenues	2,537,166	4.49
Gross margin	758,922	1.34

Table 6 Effect of genetic change on production results relative to the situation without genetic change

Trait	Genetic change (trait unit)	Δ Juveniles stocked (year^{-1})	Δ Feed consumption (kg/year)	Δ Fish production (kg/year)	Δ Gross margin (€)
TGC [a]	+0.95	89,400	−68,409	36,309	213,131
TFC [b]	−0.55	0	−120,300	0	140,891
M [c]	−0.016	−137,294	−34,446	0	69,531
σ_{HW} [d]	−4.2	0	0	0	2636
σ_{HW}	−8.5	0	0	0	4952

[a] Thermal growth coefficient [g$^{2/3}$/(day degrees · 1000)]

[b] Thermal feed intake coefficient [g$^{0.544}$/(day degrees · 1000)]

[c] Mortality rate (%/day)

[d] Standard deviation of harvest weight (g)

farm level, the annual feed consumption decreased. A decrease in TFC decreased total feed consumption per production cycle (Eqs. 5, 11) but the number of juveniles stocked per production cycle and the fish production per production cycle remained unaltered, thus at the farm level, only annual feed consumption decreased. A decrease in M reduced the number of juveniles stocked per production cycle (Eq. 9) and consequently, daily feed intake per cage decreased because the average number of fish per cage per day was smaller (Eq. 10), but fish production per production cycle was unaltered. Thus at the farm level, the annual number of juveniles stocked and annual feed consumption decreased. The effect of σ_{HW} on the average sales price is illustrated in Fig. 2: less variation led to more sales in size category 300 to 400 g (€4.52/kg) at the expense of sales in size category 200 to 300 g (€4.15/kg). Production results were unaltered by a change in σ_{HW}.

Economic values are in Table 7, which shows that the economic value of σ_{HW} was similar for both levels of genetic change.

Table 7 Economic values of traits for gilthead seabream

Trait	Baseline trait level (trait unit)	Genetic change (trait unit)	Economic value [€ (kg production)$^{-1}$ (trait unit)$^{-1}$]
TGC [a]	12.6	+0.95	0.40
TFC [b]	8.25	−0.55	−0.45
M [c]	0.0300	−0.016	−7.7
σ_{HW} [d]	60	−4.2	−0.0011
σ_{HW}	60	−8.5	−0.0010

[a] Thermal growth coefficient [g$^{2/3}$/(day degrees · 1000)]

[b] Thermal feed intake coefficient [g$^{0.544}$/(day degrees · 1000)]

[c] Mortality rate (%/day)

[d] Standard deviation of harvest weight (g)

Comparison of economic values from the bio-economic model and the profit equation

Table 8 shows that, for the simplified production system, the economic values derived from the bio-economic model and the profit equation were similar.

Discussion

Validity of the bio-economic model

For the simplified production system, the profit equation and the bio-economic model return similar economic values, which confirm the validity of the bio-economic model. To further validate the bio-economic model, production results were compared to those of other studies. FCR (Table 4) was within the range of 1.5 to 2 reported by Sola et al. [44] but considerably lower than the 2.3 value reported by EAS-EATiP [45]. Overall survival was 85%, which is within the range reported by EAS-EATiP [45]. A comparison with a cost-breakdown for large-scale production of gilthead seabream and European seabass (*Dicentrarchus labrax*) is in Table 9 [17]. In the FAO data, variable costs are higher, largely because labor, energy, and medicines and veterinary services were not considered to be variable costs in our study. Trends in the increase in productivity per person [46] support the

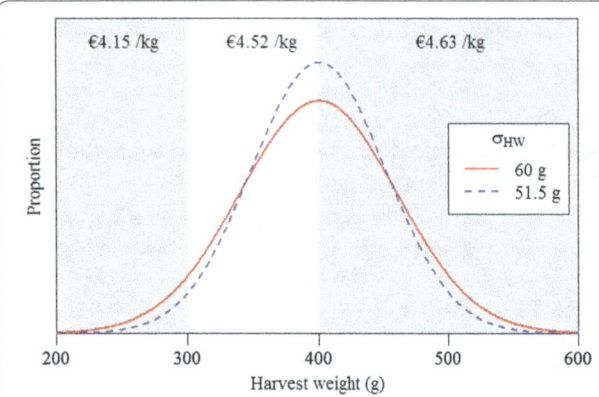

Fig. 2 Distribution of harvest weight over sales price categories at different standard deviations of harvest weight (σ_{HW})

Table 9 Cost-breakdown for gilthead seabream production

Item	Proportion of total costs (%)	
	Our study[a]	Barazi-Yeroulanos [17]
Feed	50	48
Juveniles	13	11
Marketing (incl. packing)	7	18
Labor	–	3
Energy	–	4
Medicines and veterinary services	–	2
Other	–	4
Total variable costs	70	89
Total fixed costs	–	11

[a] Relative to revenues

assumption that labor should be treated more as a fixed than a variable cost. Medicine costs may vary, but veterinary costs are likely to be fixed per farm. Energy costs are to a larger extent determined by farm layout than by realized production and thus can be considered as fixed. Altogether, total variable costs may have been slightly underestimated in our study, but FCR and overall survival matched well to current industry standards.

Breeding goal
In the breeding goal, TGC, TFC, and M are equivalent to respectively $BW_{t_{s,h}}$, $CFI_{t_{s,h}}$, and $S_{t_{s,h}}$, when $BW_{t_{s,0}}$ is much smaller than $BW_{t_{s,h}}$ (Appendixes 1, 2). When the sum of effective temperatures is the harvest criterion, one σ_A change in TGC, TFC, and M led to changes in $BW_{t_{s,h}}$, $CFI_{t_{s,h}}$, and $S_{t_{s,h}}$ that were very similar to the σ_A of these traits (Table 8), which demonstrates their equivalence. If the economic values of TGC, TFC, and M were calculated for the sum of effective temperatures instead of harvest weight as the harvest criterion, they would be slightly lower for TGC [0.34€ (kg production)$^{-1}$ (g$^{0.544}$ /(day degrees · 1000))$^{-1}$] and unaltered for TFC and M. In agreement with Wilton and Goddard [47], economic values were similar for both harvest criteria. Although

both sets of traits are equivalent in the breeding goal, there are pros and cons to each one. $BW_{t_{s,h}}$ is commonly used as a selection criterion and thus its use in the breeding goal is straightforward. However, $BW_{t_{s,h}}$ is a management parameter that is strongly influenced by the growing period and temperature regime. TGC corrects for heterogeneity in stocking weight, growing period, and temperature regime, and, therefore, allows for a better comparison of breeding values across conditions than $BW_{t_{s,h}}$ [11, 24, 25].

FCR could be used as an alternative to TFC in the breeding goal. An advantage of feed intake compared to FCR is that it relates directly to feed costs [48]. An advantage of FCR is that it illustrates the effect of improvement in efficiency on, for example, environmental impacts, as in Besson et al. [49]. Feed intake is often considered more appropriate as a breeding goal trait than FCR [18, 19], with a common argument that traits expressed as ratio's are disadvantageous in animal breeding [19]. Selection for a ratio, e.g. FCR, results in a lower selection response than selection for both components of the ratio, e.g. feed intake and growth [50]. However, in the same way that FCR is a ratio, growth is the ratio of feed intake to FCR, thus a breeding goal that includes both growth and FCR is equivalent to a breeding goal that includes growth and feed intake. The economic value of growth depends on which other trait, feed intake or FCR, is included in the breeding goal [48].

Economic values
Bio-economic models and profit equations are both suitable to derive economic values. An advantage of a profit equation compared to a bio-economic model is its simplicity. However, its applicability is limited to specific situations, because environmental conditions are ignored. For example, the profit equation cannot be used to derive economic values for a range of temperature regimes, as was done in Besson et al. [11] by using the bio-economic model. Such properties may be of particular interest for breeding programs that aim at supplying many farms. In addition, alternative constraints on production output

Table 8 Economic values derived from the bio-economic model and profit equation

Trait	Baseline trait level (trait unit)	Genetic change (trait unit)	Economic value [€ (kg production)$^{-1}$ (trait unit)$^{-1}$]	
			Bio-economic model	Profit equation
$BW_{t_{s,h}}$[a]	400	43.6	0.0074	0.0072
$CFI_{t_{s,h}}$[b]	713	−80.0	−0.0031	−0.0032
$S_{t_{s,h}}$[c]	85.1	7.66	0.016	0.019

[a] Harvest weight (g)

[b] Cumulative feed intake at harvest (g)

[c] Survival at harvest (%)

such as oxygen availability cannot be dealt with by the profit equation but can be incorporated in the bio-economic model, as discussed later. Furthermore, the profit equation is rigid in terms of trait definition, which has led to the false assumption that harvest weight changes following genetic improvement, whereas in the bio-economic model genetic improvement of growth rate leads to a reduction in the growing period.

From a profit function, economic values can be computed from either its partial derivative with respect to trait level, or from an increase or decrease in trait level relative to the current mean. In this study, simulated changes in trait levels correspond to desired directions of genetic change of one genetic standard deviation. However, for a non-linear profit function, Goddard [51] demonstrated that economic values that maximize profit in the next generation may depend on selection responses. Dekkers et al. [52] showed that economic gain is slightly higher when economic values are derived as the partial derivative of a non-linear profit equation at the genetic level of the next generation than at the genetic level of the current generation. This implies two things:

(1) Economic values are closer to optimum when the simulated change in trait level resembles its expected rather than its desired direction.
(2) Economic values are closer to optimum when the simulated change in trait level equals the difference between trait levels in the current and next generation than when it is the partial derivative at current genetic levels.

In our study, expected and desired directions of change in trait levels were identical, except for TFC, which may increase in practice due to its genetic correlation with TGC [34]. A genetic standard deviation generally provides a better proxy for the difference between trait levels in the current and next generation than an infinitesimal change, and hence will result in an economic value that is closer to optimum than the conventional partial derivative at the current trait level.

This is the first time that economic values have been derived for uniformity in aquaculture, here expressed as σ_{HW}. In recent years, there has been increasing interest to improve uniformity [40, 53–55]. Improvement in uniformity affects average sales price and reduces the need for size-grading. However, for seabream production, reducing the need for size-grading would not result in major cost-savings, because seabream is size-graded only once during grow-out. Thus, a potential effect on grading frequency was excluded from the economic value of uniformity. Furthermore, uniformity has been suggested to affect feed intake, growth rate and mortality [56, 57].

Economic consequences of changes in other traits were accounted for in their respective economic values. By exploiting genetic correlations, selection for uniformity may be used to improve the other traits in the breeding goal.

Application to other aquaculture species

In its current form, the bio-economic model can be easily applied for the derivation of economic values for other species produced in systems where stocking density limits production output, such as cages and flow-through tanks. This would require different values for the coefficients of Table 1, maximum stocking density, stocking and harvest weight, and input and output prices. Equations 4 and 5 require some species-specific modifications, such as alternative values for exponents 2/3 and 3/2 in Eq. 4 [58] or a different minimum temperature for growth.

Adaptations to the model are required for species that are reared in production systems for which constraints on production output are different, such as recirculating aquaculture systems and ponds. When the constraint on production output is different from stocking density, the number of fish stocked per production cycle (Eq. 9) is determined by other parameters. For recirculating aquaculture systems, treatment capacity of the biofilter can be a constraint on production output [12]. In this case, daily nitrogen excretion by fish is the parameter that determines the number of fish stocked per production cycle. Daily nitrogen excretion by fish can be predicted from the difference between daily feed consumption and daily gain in bodyweight, as described in Besson et al. [12]. In both cages and ponds, oxygen availability can be a constraint on production output. In this case, daily oxygen consumption per fish is the parameter that determines the number of fish stocked per production cycle. Daily oxygen consumption per fish can be predicted from daily feed consumption and daily gain in bodyweight, as described in Besson et al. [11]. With the above modifications, the same bio-economic model was applied for the derivation of economic values for African catfish produced in recirculating aquaculture systems [12], European seabass produced in cages [11], gilthead seabream produced in cages (this study), turbot produced in tanks (unpublished results), and Nile tilapia produced in ponds (unpublished results).

Conclusions

We developed a bio-economic model to derive economic values for a wide range of aquaculture species. Its validity was confirmed by the comparison to a profit equation for a simplified production system and by comparison of the production results to those of other studies. Application of the bio-economic model to gilthead seabream resulted in economic values for TGC, TFC, M, and σ_{HW}. TGC was the most important trait to improve, followed by TFC and M. The effect of σ_{HW} on gross margin was small.

Authors' contributions
KJ developed the bio-economic model, performed the analysis, and wrote the manuscript. HK and PB contributed to discussions and writing of the manuscript. MB helped in developing the bio-economic model and contributed to discussions. All authors read and approved the final manuscript.

Author details
[1] Animal Breeding and Genomics, Wageningen University and Research, Droevendaalsesteeg 1, 6708 PB Wageningen, The Netherlands. [2] Business Economics Group, Wageningen University and Research, Hollandseweg 1, 6706 KN Wageningen, The Netherlands. [3] Génétique Animale Biologie Intégrative, INRA, AgroParisTech, Université Paris-Saclay, 78350 Jouy-en-Josas, France.

Acknowledgements
We are grateful for the extensive production data provided by Andromeda S.A. and their feedback on model assumptions. We thank Piter Bijma for his help in the computation of genetic standard deviations.

Competing interests
The authors declare that they have no competing interests.

Funding
The research leading to these results has received funding from the European Union's Seventh Framework Programme (KBBE.2013.1.2-10) under grant agreement no. 613611.

Appendices

Appendix 1: Genetic variation in *TGC*

Genetic variation in TGC depends on genetic variation both in $BW_{t_{s,0}}$ and $BW_{t_{s,h}}$:

$$Var(A_{TGC}) = Var\left(1000 \cdot \frac{A_{BW_{t_{s,h}}}^{2/3} - A_{BW_{t_{s,0}}}^{2/3}}{\sum_{i=t_{s,0}}^{(t_{s,h})-1}(T_i - 12)}\right), \quad (25)$$

where A_{TGC} is the genotype for TGC, $A_{BW_{t_{s,h}}}$ is the genotype for harvest weight, and $A_{BW_{t_{s,0}}}$ is the genotype for stocking weight. Equation 25 can be rewritten as:

$$Var(A_{TGC}) = \left(\frac{1000}{\sum_{i=t_{s,0}}^{(t_{s,h})-1}(T_i - 12)}\right)^2 \cdot \left(Var\left(A_{BW_{t_{s,h}}}^{2/3}\right)\right.$$
$$\left. + Var\left(A_{BW_{t_{s,0}}}^{2/3}\right) - 2 \cdot cov\left(A_{BW_{t_{s,h}}}^{2/3}, A_{BW_{t_{s,0}}}^{2/3}\right)\right). \quad (26)$$

Because $BW_{t_{s,0}}$ is much smaller than $BW_{t_{s,h}}$, $Var\left(A_{BW_{t_{s,0}}}^{2/3}\right) - 2 \cdot cov\left(A_{BW_{t_{s,h}}}^{2/3}, A_{BW_{t_{s,0}}}^{2/3}\right)$ is much smaller than $Var\left(A_{BW_{t_{s,h}}}^{2/3}\right)$ [59]. Thus, Eq. 26 can be reduced to Eq. 15.

Appendix 2: Genetic variation in cumulative feed intake at harvest

The regression coefficient of the genotype for $CFI_{t_{s,h}}$ ($A_{CFI_{t_{s,h}}}$) on the difference between $A_{BW_{t_{s,h}}}$ and $A_{BW_{t_{s,0}}}$, can be calculated as:

$$b\left(A_{CFI_{t_{s,h}}}, A_{BW_{t_{s,h}}} - A_{BW_{t_{s,0}}}\right) = r_A \cdot \sqrt{\frac{Var\left(A_{CFI_{t_{s,h}}}\right)}{Var\left(A_{BW_{t_{s,h}}} - A_{BW_{t_{s,0}}}\right)}}, \quad (27)$$

where $b\left(A_{CFI_{t_{s,h}}}, A_{BW_{t_{s,h}}} - A_{BW_{t_{s,0}}}\right)$ is the regression coefficient, and r_A is the genetic correlation coefficient. For the regression of $A_{CFI_{t_{s,h}}}$ on $A_{BW_{t_{s,h}}} - A_{BW_{t_{s,0}}}$, the intercept corresponds to feed consumption to meet maintenance energy requirements ($CFI_{maintenance}$) at zero growth. Assuming a digestible energy content of the diet of 17 kJ/g, $CFI_{maintenance}$ is calculated as [26]:

$$CFI_{maintenance} = \sum_{i=t_{s,0}}^{t_{s,h}} 47.89 \cdot (BW_i/1000)^{0.80}/17 = 20 \text{ g}. \quad (28)$$

For $A_{BW_{t_{s,h}}} - A_{BW_{t_{s,0}}} = 400 - 4.4 = 395.6$ g, $A_{CFI_{t_{s,h}}}$ equals $1.80 \cdot 395.6 = 713$ g, where 1.80 is the biological FCR (Table 4). The regression coefficient can thus be approximated as $(713 - 20)/395.6 = 1.75$ and Eq. 27 can be rewritten as:

$$1.75 = r_A$$
$$\cdot \sqrt{\frac{Var\left(A_{CFI_{t_{s,h}}}\right)}{Var\left(A_{BW_{t_{s,h}}}\right) + Var\left(A_{BW_{t_{s,0}}}\right) - 2 \cdot cov\left(A_{BW_{t_{s,h}}}, A_{BW_{t_{s,0}}}\right)}}. \quad (29)$$

Because $BW_{t_{s,0}}$ is much smaller than $BW_{t_{s,h}}$, $Var\left(A_{BW_{t_{s,0}}}\right) - 2 \cdot cov\left(A_{BW_{t_{s,h}}}, A_{BW_{t_{s,0}}}\right)$ is much smaller than $Var\left(A_{BW_{t_{s,h}}}\right)$ [59]. Thus Eq. 29 can be reduced to Eq. 16.

References
1. Janssen K, Chavanne H, Berentsen P, Komen H. Impact of selective breeding on European aquaculture. Aquaculture. 2016;. doi:10.1016/j.aquaculture.2016.03.012.
2. Nielsen HM, Amer PR, Byrne TJ. Approaches to formulating practical breeding objectives for animal production systems. Acta Agric Scand A Anim. 2014;64:2–12.

3. Shook GE. Major advances in determining appropriate selection goals. J Dairy Sci. 2006;89:1349–61.

4. Gibson JP, Kennedy BW. The use of constrained selection indexes in breeding for economic merit. Theor Appl Genet. 1990;80:801–5.

5. Gjedrem T, Baranski M. Selective breeding in aquaculture: an introduction. Dordrecht: Springer; 2009.

6. Gjedrem T, Thodesen J. Selection. In: Gjedrem T, editor. Selection and breeding programs in aquaculture. Dordrecht: Springer; 2005. p. 89–111.

7. Ponzoni RW, Nguyen NH, Khaw HL. Investment appraisal of genetic improvement programs in Nile tilapia (Oreochromis niloticus). Aquaculture. 2007;269:187–99.

8. Ponzoni RW, Nguyen NH, Khaw HL, Ninh NH. Accounting for genotype by environment interaction in economic appraisal of genetic improvement programs in common carp Cyprinus carpio. Aquaculture. 2008;285:47–55.

9. Zuniga-Jara S, Marin-Riffo MC. A bioeconomic model of a genetic improvement program of abalone. Aquacult Int. 2014;22:1533–62.

10. Henryon M, Purvis IW, Berg P. Definition of a breeding objective for commercial production of the freshwater crayfish, marron (Cherax tenuimanus). Aquaculture. 1999;173:179–95.

11. Besson M, Komen H, Aubin J, De Boer IJM, Poelman M, Quillet E, et al. Economic values of growth and feed efficiency for fish farming in recirculating aquaculture system with density and nitrogen output limitations: a case study with African catfish (Clarias gariepinus). J Anim Sci. 2014;92:5394–405.

12. Besson M, Vandeputte M, van Arendonk JAM, Aubin J, de Boer IJM, Quillet E, et al. Influence of water temperature on the economic value of growth rate in fish farming: the case of sea bass (Dicentrarchus labrax) cage farming in the Mediterranean. Aquaculture. 2016. doi:10.1016/j.aquaculture.2016.04.030.

13. Knap PW. Breeding robust pigs. Austr J Exp Agric. 2005;45:763–73.

14. Hietala P, Wolfova M, Wolf J, Kantanen J, Juga J. Economic values of production and functional traits, including residual feed intake, in Finnish milk production. J Dairy Sci. 2014;97:1092–106.

15. van Middelaar CE, Berentsen PBM, Dijkstra J, van Arendonk JAM, de Boer IJM. Methods to determine the relative value of genetic traits in dairy cows to reduce greenhouse gas emissions along the chain. J Dairy Sci. 2014;97:5191–205.

16. Byrne TJ, Amer PR, Fennessy PF, Cromie AR, Keady TWJ, Hanrahan JP, et al. Breeding objectives for sheep in Ireland: a bio-economic approach. Livest Sci. 2010;132:135–44.

17. Barazi-Yeroulanos L. Synthesis of Mediterranean marine finfish aquaculture—a marketing and promotion strategy. In: Studies and reviews. General Fisheries Commission for the Mediterranean. no. 88. Rome: FAO; 2010. p. 1–198.

18. Emmerson DA. Commercial approaches to genetic selection for growth and feed conversion in domestic poultry. Poult Sci. 1997;76:1121–5.

19. Veerkamp RF, Pryce JE, Spurlock D, Berry D, Coffey M, Løvendahl P, et al. Selection on feed intake or feed efficiency: a position paper from gDMI breeding goal discussions. Interbull Bull. 2013;47:15–22.

20. Wolfová M, Wolf J. Strategies for defining traits when calculating economic values for livestock breeding: a review. Animal. 2013;7:1401–13.

21. Iwama GK, Tautz AF. A simple growth model for Salmonids in hatcheries. Can J Fish Aquat Sci. 1981;38:649–56.

22. Jobling M. The thermal growth coefficient (TGC) model of fish growth: a cautionary note. Aquacult Res. 2003;34:581–4.

23. Cho CY. Feeding systems for rainbow trout and other salmonids with reference to current estimates of energy and protein requirements. Aquaculture. 1992;100:107–23.

24. Sae-Lim P, Kause A, Mulder HA, Martin KE, Barfoot AJ, Parsons JE, et al. Genotype-by-environment interaction of growth traits in rainbow trout (Oncorhynchus mykiss): a continental scale study. J Anim Sci. 2013;91:5572–81.

25. Trong TQ, Mulder HA, van Arendonk JAM, Komen H. Heritability and genotype by environment interaction estimates for harvest weight, Growth rate, And shape of Nile tilapia (Oreochromis niloticus) grown in river cage and VAC in Vietnam. Aquaculture. 2013;384–387:119–27.

26. Lupatsch I, Kissil GW, Sklan D. Comparison of energy and protein efficiency among three fish species gilthead sea bream (Sparus aurata), European sea bass (Dicentrarchus labrax) and white grouper (Epinephelus aeneus): energy expenditure for protein and lipid deposition. Aquaculture. 2003;225:175–89.

27. R Core Team. R: A Language and environment for statistical computing. 2015. http://www.R-project.org/.

28. Houle D. Comparing evolvability and variability of quantitative traits. Genetics. 1992;130:195–204.

29. Groen AF. Economic values in cattle-breeding. 2. Influences of production circumstances in situations with output limitations. Livest Prod Sci. 1989;22:17–30.

30. Cacho OJ. Protein and fat dynamics in fish: a bioenergetic model applied to aquaculture. Ecol Model. 1990;50:33–56.

31. Mayer P, Estruch V, Blasco J, Jover M. Predicting the growth of gilthead sea bream (Sparus aurata L.) farmed in marine cages under real production conditions using temperature- and time-dependent models. Aquacult Res. 2008;39:1046–52.

32. Mayer P, Estruch VD, Jover M. A two-stage growth model for gilthead sea bream (Sparus aurata) based on the thermal growth coefficient. Aquaculture. 2012;358–359:6–13.

33. Navarro A, Zamorano MJ, Hildebrandt S, Ginés R, Aguilera C, Afonso JM. Estimates of heritabilities and genetic correlations for growth and carcass traits in gilthead seabream (Sparus auratus L.), under industrial conditions. Aquaculture. 2009;289:225–30.

34. Quinton CD, Kause A, Koskela J, Ritola O. Breeding salmonids for feed efficiency in current fishmeal and future plant-based diet environments. Genet Sel Evol. 2007;39:431.

35. Kause A, Tobin D, Dobly A, Houlihan D, Martin S, Mantysaari EA, et al. Recording strategies and selection potential of feed intake measured using the X-ray method in rainbow trout. Genet Sel Evol. 2006;38:389–409.

36. Falconer DS, Mackay TFC. Introduction to quantitative genetics. 3rd ed. Harlow: Longman; 1989.

37. Vehvilainen H, Kause A, Quinton C, Koskinen H, Paananen T. Survival of the currently fittest: genetics of rainbow trout survival across time and space. Genetics. 2008;180:507–16.

38. Mulder HA, Bijma P, Hill WG. Prediction of breeding values and selection responses with genetic heterogeneity of environmental variance. Genetics. 2007;175:1895–910.

39. Hazel LN. The genetic basis for constructing selection indexes. Genetics. 1943;28:476–90.

40. Sae-Lim P, Kause A, Janhunen M, Vehvilainen H, Koskinen H, Gjerde B, et al. Genetic (co)variance of rainbow trout (Oncorhynchus mykiss) body weight and its uniformity across production environments. Genet Sel Evol. 2015;47:46.

41. Sonesson AK, Odegard J, Ronnegard L. Genetic heterogeneity of within-family variance of body weight in Atlantic salmon (Salmo salar). Genet Sel Evol. 2013;45:41.

42. Hill WG, Mulder HA. Genetic analysis of environmental variation. Genet Res (Camb). 2010;92:381–95.

43. Sell-Kubiak E, Bijma P, Knol EF, Mulder HA. Comparison of methods to study uniformity of traits: application to birth weight in pigs. J Anim Sci. 2015;93:900–11.

44. Sola L, Moretti A, Crosetti D, Karaiskou N, Magoulas A, Rossi AR, et al. Gilthead seabream—Sparus aurata. In: D Crossetti, S Lapègue, I Olesen, T Svaasand, editors. Genetic effects of domestication, culture and breeding of fish and shellfish, and their impacts on wild populations. Genimpact Final Scientific Report. Viterbo; 2007. p. 47–54.

45. EAS-EATiP. Performance of the sea bass and sea bream sector in the Mediterranean. In Minutes of a Workshop held within Aquaculture Europe: 16 October 2014; San Sebastian; 2014.

46. University of Stirling. Study of the market for aquaculture produced seabass and seabream species; 2004. http://ec.europa.eu/fisheries/documentation/studies/aquaculture_market_230404_en.pdf. Accessed 12 April 2016.

47. Wilton JW, Goddard ME. Selection for carcass and feedlot traits considering alternative slaughter end points and optimized management. J Anim Sci. 1996;74:37–45.

48. Goddard ME. Consensus and debate in the definition of breeding objectives. J Dairy Sci. 1998;81:6–18.

49. Besson M, Aubin J, Komen H, Poelman M, Quillet E, Vandeputte M, et al. Environmental impacts of genetic improvement of growth rate and feed conversion ratio in fish farming under rearing density and nitrogen output limitations. J Clean Prod. 2016;116:100–9.

50. Gunsett FC. Linear index selection to improve traits defined as ratios. J Anim Sci. 1984;59:1185–93.

51. Goddard ME. Selection indexes for non-linear profit-functions. Theor Appl Genet. 1983;64:339–44.

52. Dekkers JCM, Birke PV, Gibson JP. Optimum linear selection indexes for multiple generation objectives with nonlinear profit-functions. Anim Sci. 1995;61:165–75.

53. Mulder HA, Bijma P, Hill WG. Selection for uniformity in livestock by exploiting genetic heterogeneity of residual variance. Genet Sel Evol. 2008;40:37.

54. Khaw HL, Ponzoni RW, Yee HY, Aziz MA, Mulder HA, Marjanovic J, et al. Genetic variance for uniformity of harvest weight in Nile tilapia (Oreochromis niloticus). Aquaculture. 2016;451:113–20.

55. Marjanovic J, Mulder HA, Khaw HL, Bijma P. Genetic parameters for uniformity of harvest weight in the GIFT strain of Nile tilapia estimated using double hierarchical generalized linear models. Genet Sel Evol. 2016;48:41.

56. Jobling M. Simple indices for the assessment of the influences of social environment on growth performance, exemplified by studies on Arctic charr. Aquacult Int. 1995;3:60–5.

57. Gilmour KM, DiBattista JD, Thomas JB. Physiological causes and consequences of social status in salmonid fish. Integr Comp Biol. 2005;45:263–73.

58. Dumas A, France J, Bureau DP. Evidence of three growth stanzas in rainbow trout (Oncorhynchus mykiss) across life stages and adaptation of the thermal-unit growth coefficient. Aquaculture. 2007;267:139–46.

59. Rutten MJM, Komen H, Bovenhuis H. Longitudinal genetic analysis of Nile tilapia (Oreochromis niloticus L.) body weight using a random regression model. Aquaculture. 2005;246:101–13.

11

Inter- and intra-reproducibility of genotypes from sheep technical replicates on Illumina and Affymetrix platforms

Donagh P. Berry[1]*, Aine O'Brien[1], Eamonn Wall[2], Kevin McDermott[2], Shane Randles[2], Paul Flynn[3], Stephen Park[4], Jenny Grose[5], Rebecca Weld[3] and Noirin McHugh[1]

Abstract

Background: Accurate genomic analyses are predicated upon access to accurate genotype input data. The objective of this study was to quantify the reproducibility of genotype data that are generated from the same genotype platform and from different genotyping platforms.

Methods: Genotypes based on 51,121 single nucleotide polymorphisms (SNPs) for 84 animals that were each genotyped on Illumina and Affymetrix platforms and for another 25 animals that were each genotyped twice on the same Illumina platform were compared. Genotypes based on 11,323 SNPs for an additional 21 animals that were genotyped on two different Illumina platforms by two different service providers were also compared. Reproducibility of the results was measured as the correlation between allele counts and as genotype and allele concordance rates.

Results: A mean within-animal correlation of 0.9996 was found between allele counts in the 25 duplicate samples that were genotyped on the same Illumina platform and varied from 0.9963 to 1.0000 per animal. The mean (minimum, maximum) genotype and allele concordance rates per animal between the 25 duplicate samples were equal to 0.9996 (0.9968, 1.0000) and 0.9993 (0.9937, 1.0000), respectively. The concordance rate between the two different Illumina platforms was also near 1. A mean within-animal correlation of 0.9738 was found between genotypes that were generated on the Illumina and Affymetrix platforms and varied from 0.9505 to 0.9812 per animal. The mean (minimum, maximum) within-animal genotype and allele concordance rates between the Illumina and Affymetrix platforms were equal to 0.9711 (0.9418, 0.9798) and 0.9845 (0.9695, 0.9889), respectively. The genotype concordance rate across all genotypes increased from 0.9711 to 0.9949 when the SNPs used were restricted to those with three high-resolution genotype clusters which represented 75.2% of the called genotypes.

Conclusions and implications: Our results suggest that, regardless of the genotype platform or service provider, high genotype concordance rates are achieved especially if they are restricted to high-quality extracted DNA and SNPs that result in high-quality genotypes.

Background

The development of the now commonly termed single nucleotide polymorphism (SNP) chips [1, 2] facilitates the routine generation of genotypes for (hundreds of) thousands of SNPs at a very low cost. There are only a few commercial providers of these SNP chips with most, if not all, studies confined to either Illumina (Illumina Inc, San Diego, CA, USA) or Affymetrix (Affymetrix Inc, San Diego, CA, USA) SNP chips. High concordance rates between genotypes that are generated from both vendors is essential to facilitate switching between platforms; moreover, high reproducibility of genotypes from duplicate biological samples is important for the integrity of downstream statistical analyses.

However, little is known, at least in sheep, on the concordance rate between genotypes that are generated by

*Correspondence: Donagh.berry@teagasc.ie
[1] Animal and Grassland Research and Innovation Centre, Moorepark, Teagasc, Fermoy, Co. Cork, Ireland
Full list of author information is available at the end of the article

both platforms on the same animals. In a comparison based on 134 bovine technical replicates, which were both genotyped on the Illumina BovineSNP50 Beadchip, Berry et al. [3] reported mean genotype and allele concordance rates per individual of 0.9989 and 0.9993, respectively. In a comparison between six human technical replicates, Hong et al. [4] documented a mean (standard deviation) genotype concordance rate between Illumina and Affymetrix platforms of 98.80% (0.34%). The objective of our study was to quantify the genotype concordance rate for 84 sheep samples that were each genotyped with a panel of 51,121 SNPs on both an Illumina and an Affymetrix platform. Reproducibility of genotypes that were obtained twice from the same Illumina platform or from two different Illumina platforms was also quantified.

Methods

DNA was extracted by a single company (Weatherby's, Ireland) from 89 sheep from multiple breeds and used first to generate genotypes based on 51,135 biallelic SNPs using the commercially available Illumina OvineSNP50 Beadchip (http://www.illumina.com/documents/products/datasheets/datasheet_ovinesnp50.pdf); intensity-only SNPs were not considered in the analysis. Genotyping on the Illumina platform was undertaken by a single commercial company (Weatherby's, Ireland). Genotype calling was conducted using GenomeStudio Genotyping Module v1.0 (Illumina Dan Diego). The manifest and cluster file were provided by Illumina.

These 51,135 SNPs were then provided to Affymetrix to generate a custom genotyping chip but four of these SNPs were not included on the Affymetrix chip. In addition, no genotypes for 10 of the remaining 51,131 SNPs were generated on the Illumina platform. Thus, none of these 14 SNPs were included in the subsequent analyses. Genotyping on the Affymetrix platform was undertaken by a separate commercial company (Identigen, Ireland) using the previously extracted DNA by Weatherby's (Ireland) for the Illumina platform. Illumina genotypes were called blind to the genotypes from the Affymetrix platform, and vice versa.

Four and two of the 89 samples that were genotyped on the Affymetrix platform and the Illumina platform, respectively, failed to achieve a 90% call rate (with one of these samples failing to reach the call rate threshold on both platforms). These five samples were not considered further, thus the analysis of the inter-platform reproducibility was based on 51,121 SNPs and 84 individuals.

Separately, 25 animals were genotyped twice on the Illumina OvineSNP50 Beadchip and another 21 samples were genotyped on both the Illumina OvineSNP50 Beadchip and a custom low-density (15,000 SNPs) Illumina

Infinium platform that was developed in collaboration with the International Sheep Genomics Consortium. A total of 11,323 SNPs, which were common to both the Illumina OvineSNP50 Beadchip and the custom Illumina platform, were considered in the subsequent reproducibility analysis. The Illumina OvineSNP50 and low-density genotypes were generated using DNA extracted from separate biological samples, i.e., DNA samples used for the Illumina OvineSNP50 platform were extracted and genotyped by Weatherby's (Ireland) and those used for the Illumina low-density platform were extracted and genotyped by Neogen (GeneSeek, A Neogen Company, Lincoln).

The following statistics were used to compare concordance rates between the duplicate genotypes from the same Illumina platform (n = 25), the genotypes from different Illumina platforms (n = 21), or from the Illumina versus Affymetrix platforms (n = 84): (1) correlation between allele counts; (2) genotype concordance rate defined as average proportion of identical genotypes within SNP or within animal when comparing panels, and (3) allele concordance rate defined as the average proportion of commonly called alleles within SNP or within animal when comparing panels; in this case, a genotype that was called on one platform as heterozygous but homozygous on the other platform was assumed to have one allele in common.

Results

Illumina platforms

The mean within-animal correlation between allele counts for the 25 duplicate samples on the Illumina OvineSNP50 platform was 0.9996 and varied from 0.9963 to 1.0000. The within-animal mean (minimum, maximum) allele and genotype concordance rates between these duplicate samples were 0.9996 (0.9968, 1.0000) and 0.9993 (0.9937, 1.0000), respectively. The minimum GC score per duplicate genotype was lower ($P < 0.001$) for discordant genotypes (0.5027) than for concordant genotypes (0.8821). Restricting the comparison to genotypes with a GC score higher than 0.55 improved the mean allele concordance rate across all genotypes from 0.9997 to 0.9999. Re-clustering the genotypes using only the information from the 84 samples from multiple breeds had a minimal effect on the called genotypes; after re-clustering, no homozygous genotype was called as an opposite homozygous and only 3789 of the 4,263,331 called genotypes (i.e., 0.09%) were called as a different genotype (with only one allele different) relative to the genotype called using the Illumina cluster file.

The mean call rate per individual for the same 21 individuals that were genotyped on the two different Illumina platforms was slightly higher ($P < 0.001$) for the Illumina

OvineSNP50 platform (0.995) than for the low-density Illumina platform (0.992). Across all SNPs, the mean allele and genotype concordance rates were equal to 0.9997 and 0.9993, respectively. Mean (minimum, maximum) allele and genotype concordance rates per individual were equal to 0.9997 (0.9972, 0.99996) and 0.9993 (0.9954, 0.9999), respectively. A mean (minimum, maximum) within-individual correlation of 0.9994 (0.9954, 0.99993) was found between allele counts. No homozygous genotype on one panel was called as the opposite homozygous on the other panel. The mean GC score for discordant genotypes (0.524) was lower ($P < 0.001$) than that for concordant genotypes (0.863) that were called in both panels.

Illumina versus Affymetrix platforms

The mean call rate per individual was lower ($P < 0.001$) for the Affymetrix platform (0.974) than for the Illumina platform (0.994). No strong relationship was obvious between individual animal call rates for each platform. On the Illumina platform, 771 SNPs (i.e., 1.51% of all SNPs) had a call rate lower than 0.90, whereas on the Affymetrix platform 4484 SNPs (i.e., 8.78% of all SNPs) had a call rate lower than 0.90; 152 of these SNPs had a call rate lower than 0.90 on both platforms.

Only a very small proportion (i.e., 0.2%) of the homozygous genotypes on one platform were called as opposite homozygous genotypes on the other platform (Table 1). The mean concordance rate per SNP for different minor allele frequency (MAF) bins is in Fig. 1. Concordance rate was best for SNPs with a MAF between 0 and 0.10 and worst for monomorphic SNPs. Concordance rate decreased as the mean SNP quality score decreased (Fig. 1), which is represented as a lower GC score for Illumina genotypes and a higher confidence score for Affymetrix genotypes. Of the 160 SNPs that had an allele concordance rate between both panels lower than 0.50, 60 (i.e., 37.5%) had a mean GC score lower than 0.55, which is the threshold commonly used in association studies (Fig. 2). The mean GC score was lower ($P < 0.001$) for discordant genotypes (0.8549) than for concordant genotypes (0.8894).

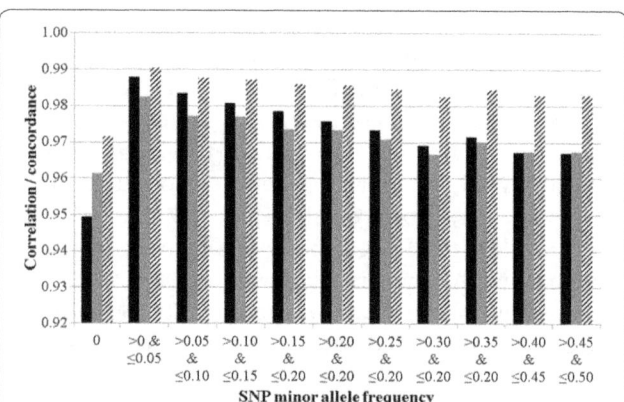

Fig. 1 Mean correlation (*black*), genotype concordance rate (*grey*) and allele concordance rate (*striped*) between Illumina and Affymetrix genotypes by single nucleotide polymorphisms (SNP) minor allele frequency from the Illumina platform

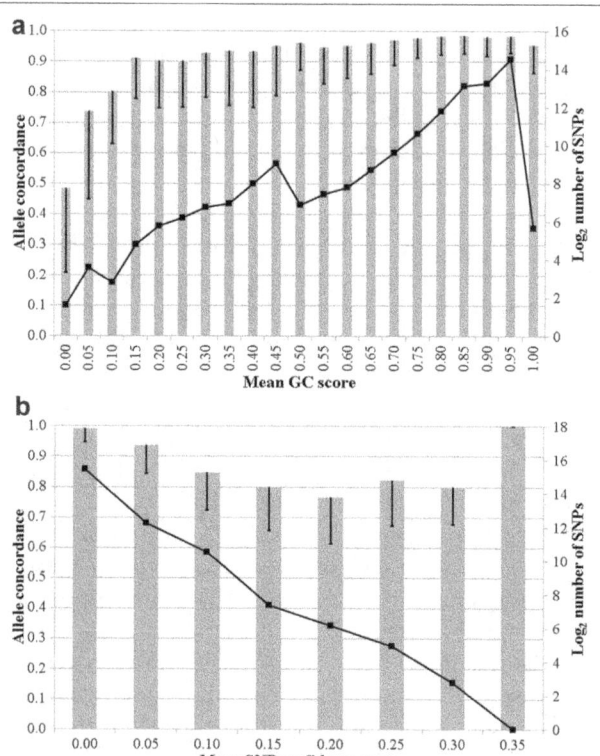

Fig. 2 Mean allele concordance rate per single nucleotide polymorphisms (SNP) stratified by Illumina GC score (**a**) and Affymetrix confidence score (**b**) represented by *grey bars* (one standard deviation represented by *standard error bars*) and number of SNPs per score category (*continuous line*). Please note that a higher Illumina GC score but lower Affymetrix confidence score represents superior quality genotypes

Table 1 Contingency table of the genotypes (0 = AA, 1 = AB, 2 = BB) from Illumina and Affymetrix platforms for all 51,121 SNPs on 84 animals

Illumina	Affymetrix		
	0	1	2
0	97.4	2.24	0.34
1	2.13	95.34	2.53
2	0.33	1.36	98.31

Excluding the SNPs with an allele concordance rate between panels lower than 0.80, the mean genotype (allele) concordance rate per SNP for the remaining

49,859 SNPs was 0.9805 (0.9902). The mean concordance per SNP categorised into the different SNP categories assigned by Affymetrix is in Table 2. Mean call rates were highest for the SNPs that were categorised by Affymetrix as having high resolution clusters.

The mean within-animal correlation between genotypes that were generated on the Illumina and Affymetrix platforms was equal to 0.9738 and varied from 0.9505 to 0.9812. The mean (minimum, maximum) within-animal genotype and allele concordance rates were 0.9711 (0.9418, 0.9798) and 0.9845 (0.9695, 0.9889), respectively.

Discussion

Inaccurate or low reproducibility genotypes have repercussions on genomic predictions [5], genome-wide association studies [4] and other analyses such as parentage verification and assignment as well as estimation of coancestry. The ability to readily switch between providers of genotyping technologies, without impacting the integrity of the data after being collated, can contribute to put greater pressure on vendors to reduce genotyping costs further.

Reproducibility of the Illumina panel

The mean within-animal genotype and allele concordance rates of 0.9993 and 0.9996, respectively between duplicate samples on the Illumina OvineSNP50 platform and also the near unity genotype and allele concordance rates of 0.9993 and 0.9997, respectively between the two Illumina platforms, are excellent and corroborate the respective values of 0.9989 and 0.9993 reported by Berry et al. [3] using duplicate genotypes of 134 cattle that were genotyped on the Illumina BovineSNP50 beadchip. Using six samples from the human HapMap project, Hong et al. [4] reported a mean genotype concordance rate of 0.9940 between duplicate samples on an Illumina platform and of 0.9987 between duplicate samples on an Affymetrix platform; all genotype comparisons undertaken by Hong et al. [4] originated from the same genotyping laboratory.

The range in mean concordance rate per individual genotyped in our study on the same Illumina platform or different Illumina platforms was also minimal, which suggests consistently excellent reproducibility. Although the retrospective nature of the analyses undertaken in the present study did not make it possible to disentangle various effects of the genotyping laboratory, DNA extraction method, or Illumina platform used, the fact that the concordance rate was excellent between genotypes that were generated by two different genotyping laboratories on two different Illumina platforms from DNA extracted by two separate laboratories suggests that all three factors actually have a minimal effect on the generated genotypes. However, only two (experienced) laboratories were compared, which limited the possibility that a laboratory effect impacted genotype. Nonetheless, the high concordance rate between duplicate bovine samples reported by Berry et al. [3], based on genotypes that were generated across multiple laboratories, provides further confidence that there is good genotype concordance across different service providers. Furthermore, most, if not all, of the discrepancies between duplicate genotypes on the platforms used in our study were actually due to a homozygous genotype of one replicate being called as a heterozygous in the other replicate, or vice versa. Moreover, applying stricter quality control on the GC score of the called genotype could improve the reliability of the genotype furthermore; a default threshold GC score of 0.15 is applied in GenomeStudio, thus genotypes with a GC score lower than 0.15 are not called by default. However, our results suggest that a more stringent threshold should be imposed, possibly higher than 0.50 (Fig. 2). This has already been done in some studies in which, only genotypes that had a GC score higher than 0.60 were retained [6].

Reproducibility between panels

The high concordance rate between genotypes that were generated on the two different platforms is consistent with documented reports from human studies that used

Table 2 Number of SNPs (N) and mean correlation, genotype concordance rate, allele concordance rate for each SNP category designated by Affymetrix

Category	N	Correlation	Genotype concordance rate	Allele concordance rate
PolyHighResolution	37,619	0.9931	0.9913	0.9956
NoMinorHom	2135	0.9912	0.9882	0.9933
Monohigh	972	0.9188	0.9336	0.9518
CallRateBelowThres	4288	0.9624	0.9513	0.9752
OffTargetVariant	463	0.8215	0.6951	0.8454
Other	5641	0.8313	0.8024	0.8933

either six duplicate samples (genotype concordance rate of 0.9880; see [4]) or 396 duplicate samples (genotype concordance rate of 0.9989; see [7]) that were genotyped on both Illumina (Infinium array) or Affymetrix platforms. However, Jiang et al. [7] undertook their concordance analysis after quality control of the genotypes, which involved the exclusion of SNPs with a low (i.e., <0.01) MAF and poor (<0.95) call rate, which left only 62.28% of the SNPs on the original Affymetrix platform and 57.04% of SNPs on the original Illumina Infinium platform.

Affymetrix probe sets are classified into six categories (Table 2) by the Affymetrix Axiom software based on quality control metrics; the SNP clustering properties for each of the six categories is graphically illustrated in Liu et al. [8]. A SNP is (1) "PolyHighResolution" if three good resolution clusters (i.e., homozygous wild, heterozygous, homozygous individuals) are formed; (2) "NoMinorHom" if only two clusters are formed with no genotype for one homozygous individual; (3) "MonoHighResolution" if the called genotypes are all monomorphic; (4) "Off-target variants", if three clusters are formed, but with one additional off-target cluster due to sequence dissimilarity between the probes and the target genome regions; (5) "CallRateBelowThreshold" if the call rate of the SNP is below the call rate threshold but the cluster properties are above the threshold, and (6) "Other" if more than one of the cluster properties are below the threshold. Thus, the fact that the concordance rate was higher for SNPs that are defined as "PolyHighResolution" is not unexpected but this category of SNPs represented only 73.5% of all SNPs. However, genotyping a larger number of animals may increase the likelihood of identifying more genotypic variability and could therefore contribute to the clustering property of SNPs classified in our study as "NoMinorHom" being changed to "PolyHighResolution"; "NoMinorHom" SNPs represented 4.2% of the data. Therefore, restricting SNPs to those classified as high-quality is likely to improve the reliability of the genotypes. Furthermore, most studies impose a restriction on the MAF of SNPs prior to inclusion in analyses; concordance rate of monomorphic SNPs was poorer than that of all other SNPs (Fig. 1). Restricting the SNPs to only the segregating "PolyHighResolution" SNPs increased the mean genotype concordance rate across all SNPs from 0.9712 to 0.9949.

In conclusion, our findings indicate that genotype data obtained from the panels investigated here can be readily combined with little expected loss in the integrity of subsequent analyses especially if quality control measures are imposed. However it was not feasible in this retrospective analysis to actually determine the truly correct genotype, thus we cannot make any inference as to which platform was most accurate. It should also be noted that our results are based on high-quality DNA samples using standard DNA extraction methods; thus, we cannot draw conclusions on the absence of discrepancies if lower quality DNA samples (e.g., from embryo biopsies or from high-throughput DNA extraction methods) are used.

Authors' contributions

DPB conceived the study, analysed the data, and drafted the manuscript. AOB facilitated the genotyping of the animals and collation of the genotype data, EW, KM and SR collected the biological samples, PF, SP and JG undertook the genotyping and aided in the interpretation of the results as well as additional requested analyses. NMH oversaw the entire project. All authors discussed the results, made suggestions and corrections. All authors read and approved the final manuscript.

Author details

[1] Animal and Grassland Research and Innovation Centre, Moorepark, Teagasc, Fermoy, Co. Cork, Ireland. [2] Sheep Ireland, Highfield House, Shinagh, Bandon, Co. Cork, Ireland. [3] Weatherbys Ltd, Naas, Ireland. [4] Identigen Ltd, Dublin, Ireland. [5] GeneSeek, A Neogen Company, Lincoln, NE, USA.

Acknowledgements

Financial support from the Irish Department of Agriculture, Stimulus Research Fund project OVIGEN is gratefully acknowledged. The contribution from the International Sheep Genomics Consortium in the development of the low-density custom genotyping platform is also acknowledged. Gratitude is also extended to Affymetrix and, in particular, Alessandro Davassi in (blindly) converting the Affymetrix genotype calls to Illumina format.

Competing interests

The authors declare that they have no competing interests.

References

1. Matukumalli LK, Lawley CT, Schnabel RD, Taylor JF, Allan MF, Heaton MP, et al. Development and characterization of a high density SNP genotyping assay for cattle. PLoS One. 2009;4:e5350.
2. Boichard D, Chung H, Dassonneville R, David X, Eggen A, Fritz S, et al. Design of a bovine low-density SNP array optimized for imputation. PLoS One. 2012;7:e34130.
3. Berry DP, McParland S, Kearney JF, Sargolzaei M, Mullen MP. Imputation of ungenotyped parental genotypes in dairy and beef cattle from progeny genotypes. Animal. 2014;8:895–903.
4. Hong H, Xu L, Liu J, Jones WD, Su Z, Ning B, et al. Technical reproducibility of genotyping SNP arrays used in genome-wide association studies. PLoS One. 2012;7:e44483.
5. Berry DP, Kearney JF. Imputation of genotypes from low-to high-density genotyping platforms and implications for genomic selection. Animal. 2011;5:1162–9.
6. Pryce JE, Johnston J, Hayes BJ, Sahana G, Weigel KA II, McParland S, Spurlock D, Krattenmacher N, Spelman RJ, Wall E, Calus MP. Imputation of genotypes from low density (50,000 markers) to high density (700,000 markers) of cows from research herds in Europe, North America, and Australasia using 2 reference populations. J Dairy Sci. 2014;97:1799–811.
7. Jiang L, Willner D, Danoy P, Xu H, Brown MA. Comparison of the performance of two commercial genome-wide association study genotyping platforms in Han Chinese samples. G3 (Bethesda). 2013;3:23–9.
8. Liu S, Sun L, Li Y, Sun F, Jiang Y, Zhang Y, et al. Development of the catfish 250 K SNP array for genome-wide association studies. BMC Res Notes. 2014;7:135.

12

Genomic prediction from observed and imputed high-density ovine genotypes

Nasir Moghaddar[1,2]*, Andrew A. Swan[1,3] and Julius H. J. van der Werf[1,2]

Abstract

Background: Genomic prediction using high-density (HD) marker genotypes is expected to lead to higher prediction accuracy, particularly for more heterogeneous multi-breed and crossbred populations such as those in sheep and beef cattle, due to providing stronger linkage disequilibrium between single nucleotide polymorphisms and quantitative trait loci controlling a trait. The objective of this study was to evaluate a possible improvement in genomic prediction accuracy of production traits in Australian sheep breeds based on HD genotypes (600k, both observed and imputed) compared to prediction based on 50k marker genotypes. In particular, we compared improvement in prediction accuracy of animals that are more distantly related to the reference population and across sheep breeds.

Methods: Genomic best linear unbiased prediction (GBLUP) and a Bayesian approach (BayesR) were used as prediction methods using whole or subsets of a large multi-breed/crossbred sheep reference set. Empirical prediction accuracy was evaluated for purebred Merino, Border Leicester, Poll Dorset and White Suffolk sire breeds according to the Pearson correlation coefficient between genomic estimated breeding values and breeding values estimated based on a progeny test in a separate dataset.

Results: Results showed a small absolute improvement (0.0 to 8.0% and on average 2.2% across all traits) in prediction accuracy of purebred animals from HD genotypes when prediction was based on the whole dataset. Greater improvement in prediction accuracy (1.0 to 12.0% and on average 5.2%) was observed for animals that were genetically lowly related to the reference set while it ranged from 0.0 to 5.0% for across-breed prediction. On average, no significant advantage was observed with BayesR compared to GBLUP.

Background

The development of high-throughput genotyping based on single nucleotide polymorphisms (SNPs) in livestock species has made the implementation of genomic evaluation more practical. In genomic prediction, the breeding values of selection candidates are evaluated according to their genotypes and a prediction equation derived from a reference population with both phenotypes and genotypes [1]. The accuracy of genomic prediction relies on several factors including linkage disequilibrium (LD) between genome-wide SNPs and quantitative trait loci (QTL) that are responsible for the phenotypic variation of traits of interest [1]. High-density (HD) SNP genotypes can result

in stronger LD between SNPs and QTL which can improve the accuracy of genomic prediction in livestock, e.g. [2–5].

Results of simulation studies in livestock show various degrees of improvement in genomic prediction when using HD genotypes compared to genotypes from moderate-density SNP panels such as 50k. For example, based on simulation studies, Meuwissen and Goddard [6] reported a large gain (>40%) in prediction accuracy from HD genotypes, while VanRaden et al. [7] and Harris and Johnson [8] found zero to only small gains in prediction accuracy. Such differences can be attributed to the assumption made about the distribution of QTL effects in the simulated models. Meuwissen and Goddard [6] and Clark et al. [9] showed that both the number and distribution of QTL effects that control a polygenic trait have a significant impact on the advantage of using HD genotypes in genomic prediction, with only small benefits for the "infinitesimal" model for which most of the

*Correspondence: n.moghaddar@une.edu.au
[2] School of Environmental and Rural Science, University of New England, Armidale, NSW 2351, Australia
Full list of author information is available at the end of the article

variation of a trait is due to a large number of QTL each with a relatively small effect.

Analyses of real data are available from dairy cattle and show zero to relatively small increases in prediction accuracy from HD genotypes. Solberg et al. [10] reported between 0.0 and 9.0% improvement in prediction accuracy across seven production and functional traits in Norwegian Red bulls. VanRaden et al. [7] found up to 6.5% (on average 0.4%) extra accuracy across 28 production traits using HD genotypes in Holstein dairy cattle.

Initially, the first factor that was suggested to affect the accuracy of genomic prediction was the LD between genome-wide SNPs [1, 2]. However, it was later shown that genomic prediction accuracy depends both on co-segregation of SNP alleles in related individuals and information from SNP alleles being in LD with QTL alleles e.g. [11]. Prediction accuracy based on LD is more persistent over distant relationships and the expectation is that higher density SNP arrays are better at capturing effects of QTL that are in LD with SNPs. Therefore, the advantage of using HD genotypes is expected to be greater for animals that are less genetically related to the reference set, and this could apply to both within-breed and across-breed genomic prediction. Thus, denser SNP genotypes may have a favorable effect on the accuracy of genomic prediction in multi-breed and crossbred populations, which are common in the sheep and beef cattle industries. Harris et al. [12] and Erbe et al. [13] showed that there was very limited improvement from using HD genotypes in across-breed prediction in Holstein and Jersey dairy cattle, but differences may be larger in sheep where breeds are genetically more related to each other and have a larger effective population size.

The objective of this study was to compare the accuracy of genomic prediction for weight, ultra-sound scanned fat and muscle traits, and wool quality and quantity traits in Australian sheep breeds based on both observed and imputed HD genotypes (600k Illumina Ovine SNP) to accuracies based on moderate-density SNP genotypes (Illumina ovine SNP50k). Using a reference set comprised of purebred, crossbred or mixed crossbred and purebred animals, prediction accuracies were compared for purebred industry sires for which very accurate estimated breeding values based on a progeny test were available. Furthermore, we contrasted accuracy of genomic prediction within a breed between animals with low and high genetic relatedness to the reference set as well as prediction within and across breeds.

Methods
Reference set, phenotypes and validation population
The genomic prediction reference set consisted of about 20,000 animals that were recorded for a large number

of production traits measured in the "Sheep Cooperative Research Centre Information Nucleus Flock" (INF) and "Sheep Genomics Flock" (SGF). The INF consisted of eight flocks that are located across different regions of Australia and are linked to each other because artificial insemination with common sires was used between 2007 and 2011 [14]. The SGF was a single research flock located in southern New South Wales, Australia, for which data were collected between 2005 and 2006 [15]. All animals in the reference set were from multiple breeds or cross-breds with the sires comprising approximately 40% animals from Terminal breeds [Poll Dorset (PD) and White Suffolk (WS)], 20% from a Maternal breed [Border Leicester (BL)] and 40% from Merino and the dams comprising 80% Merino and 20% BL × Merino crossbreds. The dominant purebred animals were Merinos which included three sheep strains that have different wool qualities, i.e. strong wool, fine wool and ultra-fine wool types. The traits analyzed were live body weights from birth to adult age, ultra-sound scanned muscle and fat depth measured at post-weaning age and wool quantity and quality measured at yearling and adult age. The data used in this study was collected according to the guidelines of the "University of New England Animal Ethics committee" reference number AEC 09/115. The number of records and basic statistics per trait are summarized in Table 1.

A validation population was used to find the empirical accuracy of genomic prediction. The validation population was a group of industry purebred sires with accurate estimated breeding values (EBV) (accuracy ranging from 0.70 to 0.99 and on average 0.92), which were calculated based on progeny records. The phenotypes of INF and SGF animals (genomic prediction reference set) were not used in the calculation of EBV of the validation sires.

Genotypes
The reference and validation populations were genotyped using a 50k SNP panel (Illumina Inc., San Diego, CA, USA). This 50k SNP panel provided 48,559 SNP genotypes after applying quality control based on the following criteria: individual SNP genotypes were removed if their call rates were lower than 90%, or if the GenCal (GC) scores were <0.6, if the heterozygosity rate for a given SNP deviated more than 3 SD from the population mean, if the SNP minor allele frequency was lower than 0.01, and for SNPs located on chromosomes X and Y or SNPs that deviated from Hardy–Weinberg equilibrium ($P < 1 \times 10^{-15}$). Furthermore, an individual sample was removed if the correlation of its genotypes (coded 0, 1 or 2 per locus) with those of another sample was equal or greater than 0.98.

Most of the sires and 1735 progeny from the four main breeds including Merino, BL, PD and WS were

Table 1 Summary statistics of weight, ultra sound scanned and wool traits using a multi-breed reference set

Trait	Size	Mean	SD	Range
B-WT	10,524	4.82	1.06	1.6–8.2
W-WT	12,415	27.20	7.24	7.8–43.5
PW-WT	10,881	41.52	8.79	17–75.8
Y-WT	6846	44.10	10.11	20.5–84.0
H-WT	4701	51.91	11.31	22.2–97.6
A-WT	4272	59.70	13.45	27.2–107.5
P-EMD	10,568	27.75	5.15	9.0–45.0
P-CF	9924	2.86	1.21	0.5–8.1
Y-EMD	3845	23.31	5.00	10.0–43.0
Y-CF	3841	3.12	1.31	0.6–8.5
Y-GFW	4662	3.64	1.04	1.2–7.8
Y-CFW	4423	2.46	0.65	0.93–4.76
Y-FD	3969	19.93	5.39	12.8–41.5
Y-FDCV	3554	19.26	2.86	11.7–30.8
Y-SS	3554	33.80	9.82	13.0–88.0
Y-SL	3554	80.93	13.06	38–136
A-GFW	4541	5.75	1.97	1.50–13.60
A-CFW	4540	4.19	1.39	1.13–9.91
A-FD	3001	18.17	1.84	13.80–24.60
A-FDCV	2436	18.07	2.56	11.80–27.70
A-SS	2414	36.61	10.31	3.00–68.00
A-SL	2413	98.57	18.34	41.00–149.00

B-WT birth weight, *W-WT* weaning weight, *PW-WT* post-weaning weight, *Y-WT* yearling weight, *H-WT* hogget weight, *A-WT* adult weight, *P-EMD* post-weaning eye muscle depth, *P-CF* post-weaning fat, *Y-EMD* yearling eye muscle depth, *Y-CF* yearling fat, *Y-GFW* yearling greasy fleece weight, *Y-CFW* yearling clean fleece weight, *Y-FD* yearling fibre diameter, *Y-FDCV* yearling fibre diameter coefficient of variation, *Y-SS* yearling staple strength, *Y-SL* yearling staple length, *A-GFW* adult greasy fleece weight, *A-CFW* adult clean fleece weight, *A-FD* adult fibre diameter, *A-FDCV* adult fibre diameter coefficient of variation, *A-SS* adult staple strength, *A-SL* adult staple length, *SD* standard deviation

genotyped using the HD (Illumina Inc., San Diego, CA, USA) ovine SNP panel. This SNP panel provided 510,174 SNPs after applying the same quality controls as above. Using all HD genotyped animals as imputation reference set, the un-typed genotypes of the rest of the population were imputed to HD genotypes using the software program FImpute [16]. The accuracy of imputation, which was tested within subsets of animals with observed HD genotypes, was high (on average 0.98).

Statistical methods

For the analysis based on pedigree relationships, the following mixed model was fitted using ASReml 3.0 [17]:

$$\mathbf{y} = \mathbf{Xb} + \mathbf{Z_1a} + \mathbf{Ww} + \mathbf{Z_1Qq} + \mathbf{Z_2s} + \mathbf{e},$$

where $\mathbf{y}$ is a vector of phenotypes, $\mathbf{b}$ is a vector of fixed effects, $\mathbf{a}$ is a vector of random additive polygenic effects, $\mathbf{w}$ is a vector of random maternal effects, $\mathbf{q}$ is a vector of random breed effects, $\mathbf{s}$ is a vector with random sire

by flock interaction effects and $\mathbf{e}$ is a vector of random residual effects. $\mathbf{X}$, $\mathbf{Z_1}$ and $\mathbf{W}$ and $\mathbf{Z_2}$ are incidence matrices relating fixed effect, additive genetic, maternal effects and sire by flock interaction effects to phenotypes. $\mathbf{Q}$ is a matrix with breed proportions for each animal derived from pedigree data. Up to 28 breed effects, including those of the three Merino strains, were estimated via the $\mathbf{Q}$ matrix, however the major breeds were Merino, BL, PD and WS. All random effects are identically and independently distributed except for a which is distributed as: $a \sim N\left(0, \mathbf{A}\sigma_a^2\right)$, where $\mathbf{A}$ is a numerator relationship and σ_a^2 is the additive genetic variance. The fixed effects in the model were birth type, rearing type, gender, age at measurement, weight at measurement and contemporary group which was defined as a cohort of site × birth year × management group. The model used for the estimation of variance components and prediction of genomic breeding values (GBV) was the same except that $\mathbf{A}$ was replaced by $\mathbf{G}$, where $\mathbf{G}$ is a genomic relationship matrix calculated based on 50k or HD SNP genotypes using VanRaden's [18] equation as below:

$$\mathbf{G} = \mathbf{MM'}/2\sum \left(p_j\right)\left(1 - p_j\right),$$

where $\mathbf{M}$ is a matrix of the size n × m (i.e. number of individual by number of SNPs) with coefficients equal to $\left(2 - 2p_j\right)$, $\left(1 - 2p_j\right)$ and $\left(-2p_j\right)$ for genotype $\left(A_1A_1\right)$, $\left(A_1A_2\right)$ and $\left(A_2A_2\right)$ of the jth SNP genotype respectively, p_j is the frequency of allele A_1 for the jth SNP genotype. σ_g^2 is the additive genetic variance estimated from SNPs. Variance components were estimated according to the restricted maximum likelihood (REML) method using either pedigree information or genomic information from 50k or HD genotypes. Genomic EBV (GEBV) were also calculated based on a Bayesian method (BayesR [13]) in which BESSiE [19] was used for prediction of GBV based on the following model:

$$\mathbf{y} = \mathbf{Xb} + \mathbf{M_1m} + \mathbf{Ww} + \mathbf{Z_1Qq} + \mathbf{Z_2s} + \mathbf{e},$$

where $\mathbf{m}$ refers to the random effects of SNPs, $\mathbf{M_1}$ is an incidence matrix relating SNP effects to phenotypes and the other terms are the same as described above. A mixture of four normal distributions for SNP effects with variances $\sigma_1^2 = 0$, $\sigma_2^2 = 0.0001\sigma_g^2$, $\sigma_3^2 = 0.001\sigma_g^2$, and $\sigma_4^2 = 0.01\sigma_g^2$ was considered in BayesR where σ_g^2 is the assumed total genetic variance. The starting values for σ_g^2 were taken from GREML analysis and the prior distribution of the proportion of SNPs in each distribution was the Dirichlet distribution. A total of 50,000 iterations (with 10,000 burn-in) were run for analysis.

The accuracy of GBV was assessed in a separate population of purebred industry rams including Merino, Maternal and Terminal sires (validation set), as the

Pearson correlation coefficient between GBV and an accurate EBV estimated from progeny test. Correlations were estimated for each breed separately, while an effect due to the Merino strain was fitted to avoid GBV accuracy to be biased upward for merinos by evaluating accuracy across strains. The size of the validation set for different traits was 341 to 389 sires for Merino, 79 to 88 for BL, 161 to 188 for PD and 189 to 204 for WS. We also contrasted the accuracy of GBV for animals with high or low genomic relationships with the reference set. Animals with high genomic relatedness were those for which the average value of their 30 highest genomic relationships to the reference population was at least 0.20. Animals with low genetic relatedness were those for which the genomic relationship with any of the individuals in the reference set was not higher than 0.10.

Results

Variance components

Table 2 shows the genetic and residual variance components of the studied traits as well as the estimated heritability based on the genetic covariance matrix among animals that was estimated from pedigree or marker genotypes (50k or HD). Additive genetic variances and heritability estimates based on 50k SNP genotypes tended to be lower than those based on pedigree data (heritability was on average 4.9% lower across different traits). Other variance components including the maternal effect and the sire by site (genotype by environment) interaction effects varied little between different models and are not reported in Table 2. In most cases, estimated residual variances were slightly larger from a model based on 50k genotypes compared with those based on pedigree relationships.

Variance components estimated by using HD genotypes resulted in larger additive genetic variance, smaller residual variance and hence higher heritability across all studied traits, when compared to 50k genotypes. However, the increase in additive variance and heritability was small (up to 4% of the absolute value for heritability). Variance components and heritability estimates were similar between models that used HD genotypes and pedigree. Less than 1% differences were found between heritability estimates based on HD genotypes and pedigree when averaged across all weight, carcass scan and wool traits.

Table 2 Additive (V_A) and residual (V_R) variance components and heritability estimate based on pedigree (PBLUP) and 50k (GBLUP-50k) or HD SNP genotypes (GBLUP-HD)

Trait	PBLUP			GBLUP-50k			GBLUP-HD		
	V_A	V_R	h^2	V_A	V_R	h^2	V_A	V_R	h^{2a}
B-WT	0.24	0.26	0.31	0.21	0.27	0.28	0.25	0.24	0.33
W-WT	4.62	6.62	0.36	4.13	8.36	0.27	4.77	7.95	0.31
PW-WT	8.36	15.59	0.28	7.82	15.85	0.27	9.10	15.14	0.31
H-WT	19.63	14.22	0.51	17.69	17.65	0.41	20.78	16.19	0.47
Y-WT	14.54	12.55	0.44	12.12	14.48	0.33	13.69	12.22	0.40
A-WT	27.22	26.84	0.42	26.53	28.13	0.41	30.0	26.41	0.46
P-EMD	1.32	3.73	0.26	1.41	3.68	0.26	1.56	3.57	0.28
P-CF	0.09	0.32	0.13	0.09	0.32	0.16	0.09	0.32	0.18
Y-EMD	1.56	3.49	0.31	1.97	3.15	0.39	2.04	2.89	0.41
Y-CF	0.16	0.54	0.20	0.18	0.40	0.23	0.21	0.37	0.28
Y-GFW	0.12	0.10	0.49	0.09	0.12	0.35	0.09	0.11	0.39
Y-CFW	0.06	0.06	0.45	0.07	0.08	0.42	0.07	0.07	0.46
Y-FD	1.41	0.40	0.76	1.21	0.34	0.75	1.36	0.29	0.8
Y-FDCV	3.34	2.35	0.54	2.82	2.73	0.45	3.15	2.59	0.49
Y-SL	70.7	33.28	0.67	58.51	44.98	0.56	62.02	42.09	0.59
Y-SS	29.09	50.78	0.33	19.28	55.4	0.22	22.05	54.51	0.26
A-GFW	0.34	0.26	0.55	0.32	0.33	0.47	0.34	0.3	0.51
A-CFW	0.22	0.14	0.57	0.20	0.17	0.52	0.21	0.16	0.54
A-FD	1.60	0.04	0.88	1.34	0.30	0.73	1.80	0.17	0.85
A-FDCV	2.70	2.35	0.54	2.78	2.73	0.45	2.94	2.59	0.49
A-SL	56.53	49.41	0.51	55.86	51.16	0.49	56.52	53.12	0.50
A-SS	29.62	68.34	0.28	27.68	73.79	0.26	32.19	70.53	0.30

[a] Standard error of heritability was between 0.02 and 0.09; for trait abbreviations see Table 1

Genomic prediction

Genomic prediction for weight and scanned carcass traits using a multi-breed/crossbred reference set

Tables 3, 4 and 5 show the accuracy of genomic prediction for weight and scanned carcass traits for Merino, BL, PD and WS sires, based on GBLUP (both for 50k and HD SNP genotypes) and BayesR and using the complete multi-breed reference set. Compared to 50k SNP genotypes, the HD SNP genotypes provided higher prediction accuracy but the extra accuracy was on average small. The maximum improvement in prediction accuracy as absolute value was 7.7% and was on average equal to 1.6, 1.2, 4.3 and 3.1% for Merino, BL, PD and WS sires, respectively. Terminal breeds showed a higher increase in prediction accuracy (3.7%) compared to Merino and Maternal breeds (1.4%), which suggests a tendency for greater improvement in accuracy from HD genotypes for breeds with a lower overall accuracy.

When using HD genotypes, the accuracy of genomic prediction was very similar between GBLUP and BayesR across all traits, with an average absolute value of the difference in genomic prediction accuracy between GBLUP-HD and BayesR of −0.008, −0.006 and 0.03 for Merino, Maternal and Terminal breeds, respectively.

Genomic prediction for wool traits in Merino based on a Merino reference set

Table 6 shows the accuracy of genomic prediction of breeding value for wool traits in Merino sires based on GBLUP—with 50k and HD SNP density, and BayesR using HD SNP density with only Merinos in the reference

set. The extra accuracy resulting from HD genotypes ranged from 0.0 to 8.0% with an average of 5.0%. No considerable difference in accuracy was observed between GBLUP and BayesR.

Genomic prediction within and across breeds from purebred or crossbred reference sets

Table 7 shows the accuracy of genomic prediction within and across breeds for three weight traits and two

Table 4 Accuracy of genomic prediction of weight and scanned traits for Merino, Border Leicester (BL), Poll Dorset (PD) and White Suffolk (WS) sires based on the multi-breed reference set and GBLUP based on HD genotypes

Trait	Size	GBLUP-HD			
		Merino	BL	PD	WS
B-WT	10,524	0.43 (0.04)[a]	0.41 (0.10)	0.12 (0.07)	0.17 (0.07)
W-WT	12,415	0.38 (0.04)	0.29 (0.11)	0.13 (0.07)	0.33 (0.06)
PW-WT	10,881	0.64 (0.04)	0.37 (0.10)	0.15 (0.07)	0.20 (0.07)
H-WT	6846	0.67 (0.04)	0.21 (0.11)	0.04 (0.07)	0.23 (0.07)
Y-WT	4701	0.63 (0.04)	0.33 (0.10)	0.25 (0.07)	0.20 (0.07)
A-WT	4272	0.68 (0.04)	0.42 (0.10)	0.06 (0.07)	0.21 (0.07)
P-EMD	10,568	0.31 (0.05)	0.19 (0.11)	0.50 (0.06)	0.40 (0.06)
P-CF	9924	0.33 (0.05)	0.31 (0.10)	0.37 (0.07)	0.29 (0.07)
Y-EMD	3845	0.43 (0.04)	0.21 (0.11)	0.14 (0.07)	0.39 (0.06)
Y-CF	3841	0.42 (0.04)	0.22 (0.11)	0.24 (0.07)	0.15 (0.07)

[a] Standard error (SE) calculated according to: $\left(\frac{1-r^2}{n-2}\right)^{0.5}$ where r is the correlation coefficient and n is the number of paired observations; for trait abbreviations see Table 1

Table 3 Accuracy of genomic prediction of weight and scanned traits for Merino, Border Leicester (BL), Poll Dorset (PD) and White Suffolk (WS) sires based on the multi-breed reference set and GBLUP based on 50k genotypes

Trait	Size	GBLUP-50k			
		Merino	BL	PD	WS
B-WT	10,524	0.42 (0.04)[a]	0.37 (0.10)	0.10 (0.07)	0.14 (0.07)
W-WT	12,415	0.38 (0.04)	0.30 (0.10)	0.05 (0.07)	0.25 (0.07)
PW-WT	10,881	0.63 (0.04)	0.37 (0.10)	0.10 (0.07)	0.15 (0.07)
H-WT	6846	0.65 (0.04)	0.21 (0.10)	0.02 (0.07)	0.20 (0.07)
Y-WT	4701	0.61 (0.04)	0.33 (0.10)	0.20 (0.07)	0.19 (0.07)
A-WT	4272	0.66 (0.04)	0.43 (0.10)	0.00 (0.07)	0.16 (0.07)
P-EMD	10,568	0.30 (0.04)	0.23 (0.11)	0.45 (0.06)	0.35 (0.06)
P-CF	9924	0.33 (0.05)	0.31 (0.10)	0.32 (0.07)	0.27 (0.07)
Y-EMD	3845	0.39 (0.04)	0.14 (0.11)	0.14 (0.07)	0.39 (0.06)
Y-CF	3841	0.40 (0.04)	0.18 (0.11)	0.24 (0.07)	0.15 (0.07)

[a] Standard error (SE) calculated according to $\left(\frac{1-r^2}{n-2}\right)^{0.5}$ where r is the correlation coefficient and n is the number of paired observations; for trait abbreviations see Table 1

Table 5 Accuracy of genomic prediction of weight and scanned traits for Merino, Border Leicester (BL), Poll Dorset (PD) and White Suffolk (WS) sires based on the multi-breed reference set and BayesR based on HD genotypes

Trait	Size	BayesR			
		Merino	BL	PD	WS
B-WT	10,524	0.43 (0.04)[a]	0.40 (0.10)	0.11 (0.07)	0.17 (0.07)
W-WT	12,415	0.38 (0.04)	0.28 (0.11)	0.13 (0.07)	0.34 (0.07)
PW-WT	10,881	0.64 (0.04)	0.35 (0.10)	0.21 (0.07)	0.22 (0.07)
H-WT	6846	0.65 (0.04)	0.22 (0.11)	0.06 (0.07)	0.23 (0.07)
Y-WT	4701	0.66 (0.04)	0.27 (0.11)	0.27 (0.07)	0.29 (0.07)
A-WT	4272	0.68 (0.04)	0.42 (0.10)	0.11 (0.07)	0.21 (0.07)
P-EMD	10,568	0.31 (0.04)	0.21 (0.11)	0.49 (0.06)	0.40 (0.06)
P-CF	9924	0.32 (0.04)	0.30 (0.10)	0.40 (0.07)	0.27 (0.07)
Y-EMD	3845	0.43 (0.04)	0.18 (0.11)	0.15 (0.07)	0.40 (0.06)
Y-CF	3841	0.42 (0.04)	0.20 (0.11)	0.24 (0.07)	0.15 (0.07)

[a] Standard error (SE) calculated according to: $\left(\frac{1-r^2}{n-2}\right)^{0.5}$ where r is the correlation coefficient and n is the number of paired observations; for trait abbreviations see Table 1

Table 6 Accuracy of genomic prediction of wool traits in Merino sheep based on GBLUP (50k/HD) and BayesR

Trait	Size	GBLUP-50k	GBLUP-HD	BayesR
Y-GFW	4662	0.68 (0.03)[a]	0.69 (0.03)	0.67 (0.03)
Y-CFW	4423	0.62 (0.03)	0.63 (0.03)	0.63 (0.03)
Y-FD	3969	0.69 (0.03)	0.75 (0.03)	0.72 (0.03)
Y-FDCV	3554	0.46 (0.04)	0.47 (0.04)	0.47 (0.04)
Y-SL	3554	0.56 (0.03)	0.62 (0.03)	0.63 (0.03)
Y-SS	3554	0.33 (0.04)	0.41 (0.04)	0.43 (0.04)
A-GFW	4541	0.65 (0.03)	0.69 (0.03)	0.69 (0.03)
A-CFW	4540	0.59 (0.03)	0.63 (0.03)	0.62 (0.03)
A-FD	3001	0.61 (0.03)	0.67 (0.03)	0.74 (0.03)
A-FDCV	2436	0.32 (0.04)	0.36 (0.04)	0.36 (0.04)
A-SL	2414	0.59 (0.04)	0.67 (0.04)	0.66 (0.04)
A-SS	2413	0.40 (0.04)	0.46 (0.04)	0.45 (0.04)

[a] Standard Error (SE) calculated according to: $\left(\frac{1-r^2}{n-2}\right)^{0.5}$ where r is the correlation coefficient and n is the number of paired observations; for trait abbreviations see Table 1

scanned carcass traits. Using HD genotypes and a pure-bred Merino reference set resulted in a small increase in GBV accuracy (0.0 to 2.5%) for Merino sires, which was similar to the increase in genomic prediction accuracy in Tables 3, 4 and 5. A larger increase (0.3 to 9.6%) was observed for Merino sires based on prediction from crossbred Merinos. However, it should be noted that the magnitude of the prediction accuracy for Merino sires from crossbred Merinos is still much lower than the prediction from purebred Merinos.

The data in Table 7 can be used to infer the accuracy of genomic prediction across breeds. The increase in genomic prediction accuracy for BL, PD or WS sires from a purebred Merino reference set, which is genetically distant to the target breeds, was low and showed a small non-significant improvement in prediction accuracy when moving from 50k to HD prediction. However, genomic prediction of PD and WS sires based on a combined crossbred reference set (PD × M + WS × M)

Table 7 Accuracy of genomic prediction within and across breeds from purebred or crossbred reference set

Trait	Reference set	Size	GBV accuracy (50k)				GBV accuracy (HD)			
			Merino	BL	PD	WS	Merino	BL	PD	WS
B-WT	Mer	3159	0.42 (0.04)[a]	−0.14 (0.11)	−0.16 (0.07)	−0.015 (0.07)	0.43 (0.04)	0.08 (0.11)	−0.09 (0.07)	0.09 (0.07)
	BL × Mer	1187	0.37 (0.04)	0.25 (0.11)	0.06 (0.07)	0.073 (0.07)	0.38 (0.04)	0.28 (0.11)	0.06 (0.07)	0.11 (0.07)
	PD × Mer (A)	1616	0.35 (0.04)	−0.09 (0.11)	0.25 (0.07)	0.056 (0.07)	0.38 (0.04)	0.01 (0.11)	0.25 (0.07)	0.06 (0.07)
	WS × Mer (B)	1015	0.33 (0.04)	−0.04 (0.11)	0.04 (0.07)	0.152 (0.07)	0.34 (0.04)	0.01 (0.11)	0.04 (0.07)	0.20 (0.07)
	(A) + (B)	2631	0.39 (0.04)	−0.02 (0.11)	0.25 (0.07)	0.163 (0.07)	0.40 (0.04)	−0.01 (0.11)	0.26 (0.07)	0.18 (0.07)
W-WT	Mer	4586	0.36 (0.04)	−0.09 (0.11)	−0.01 (0.07)	0.001 (0.07)	0.37 (0.04)	0.10 (0.11)	0.02 (0.07)	0.01 (0.07)
	BL × Mer	1495	0.31 (0.04)	0.33 (0.10)	−0.10 (0.07)	−0.047 (0.07)	0.34 (0.04)	0.33 (0.11)	−0.09 (0.07)	0.06 (0.07)
	PD × Mer (A)	936	0.24 (0.05)	0.10 (0.11)	0.10 (0.07)	0.045 (0.07)	0.34 (0.04)	0.10 (0.11)	0.13 (0.07)	0.14 (0.07)
	WS × Mer (B)	876	0.23 (0.05)	0.03 (0.11)	−0.08 (0.07)	0.218 (0.07)	0.32 (0.04)	0.04 (0.11)	0.00 (0.07)	0.33 (0.07)
	(A) + (B)	1812	0.32 (0.04)	0.02 (0.11)	0.19 (0.07)	0.117 (0.07)	0.41 (0.04)	0.02 (0.11)	0.27 (0.07)	0.19 (0.07)
PW-WT	Mer	3935	0.50 (0.04)	−0.01 (0.11)	−0.03 (0.07)	0.076 (0.07)	0.52 (0.04)	−0.01 (0.11)	0.01 (0.07)	0.10 (0.07)
	BL × Mer	1824	0.40 (0.04)	0.36 (0.10)	−0.02 (0.07)	−0.026 (0.07)	0.41 (0.04)	0.37 (0.11)	0.09 (0.07)	0.13 (0.07)
	PD × Mer (A)	1849	0.39 (0.04)	0.01 (0.11)	0.28 (0.07)	0.021 (0.07)	0.46 (0.04)	0.00 (0.11)	0.31 (0.07)	0.07 (0.07)
	WS × Mer (B)	1224	0.33 (0.04)	0.00 (0.11)	0.02 (0.07)	0.230 (0.07)	0.35 (0.04)	0.06 (0.11)	0.08 (0.07)	0.28 (0.07)
	(A) + (B)	3073	0.47 (0.04)	−0.01 (0.11)	0.27 (0.07)	0.251 (0.07)	0.54 (0.04)	−0.01 (0.11)	0.31 (0.07)	0.28 (0.07)
P-EMD	Mer	3449	0.337 (0.04)	−0.059 (0.11)	0.084 (0.07)	0.074 (0.07)	0.337 (0.04)	−0.062 (0.11)	0.084 (0.07)	0.101 (0.07)
	BL × Mer	1602	0.241 (0.04)	0.217 (0.11)	0.124 (0.07)	0.028 (0.07)	0.244 (0.04)	0.232 (0.11)	0.144 (0.07)	0.102 (0.07)
	PD × Mer (A)	1809	0.270 (0.04)	0.004 (0.11)	0.150 (0.07)	0.037 (0.07)	0.284 (0.04)	0.002 (0.11)	0.174 (0.07)	0.042 (0.07)
	WS × Mer (B)	1249	0.190 (0.04)	0.000 (0.11)	0.044 (0.07)	0.134 (0.07)	0.201 (0.04)	0.000 (0.11)	0.046 (0.07)	0.141 (0.07)
	(A) + (B)	2544	0.250 (0.04)	0.001 (0.11)	0.160 (0.07)	0.152 (0.07)	0.254 (0.04)	0.002 (0.11)	0.181 (0.07)	0.157 (0.07)
PW-CF	Mer	2685	0.314 (0.04)	0.076 (0.11)	0.073 (0.07)	−0.099 (0.07)	0.318 (0.04)	0.091 (0.11)	0.024 (0.07)	−0.005 (0.07)
	BL × Mer	1186	0.136 (0.05)	0.240 (0.11)	0.044 (0.07)	0.044 (0.07)	0.139 (0.04)	0.253 (0.11)	0.064 (0.07)	0.065 (0.07)
	PD × Mer (A)	1295	0.134 (0.05)	0.121 (0.11)	0.296 (0.07)	0.069 (0.07)	0.138 (0.04)	0.126 (0.11)	0.322 (0.07)	0.080 (0.07)
	WS × Mer (B)	1250	0.130 (0.05)	0.000 (0.11)	0.001 (0.07)	0.074 (0.07)	0.133 (0.04)	0.000 (0.11)	0.003 (0.07)	0.116 (0.07)
	(A) + (B)	2540	0.170 (0.05)	0.021 (0.11)	0.286 (0.07)	0.076 (0.07)	0.184 (0.04)	0.024 (0.11)	0.296 (0.07)	0.121 (0.07)

BL Border Leicester, *PD* Poll Dorset, *WS* White Suffolk

[a] Standard error (SE) calculated according to: $\left(\frac{1-r^2}{n-2}\right)^{0.5}$ where r is the correlation coefficient and n is the number of paired observations; for trait abbreviations see Table 1

showed a greater improvement in prediction accuracy (up to 8.0%). It should be noted that this accuracy was still low, even when using HD genotypes.

Genomic prediction for animals highly or lowly related to the reference set

Figures 1 and 2 compare the accuracy of genomic prediction for two groups of Merino sires used as validation animals, one with a high and one with a low genomic relationship to the purebred Merino reference set. For highly related animals, the gain in accuracy from using HD genotypes was very low (on average 0.8%) but it was significantly higher for lowly related animals (up to 12% and on average 5.2%).

Regression of EBV on GBV

Table 8 shows the regression coefficient of the accurate (>0.90) breeding values that were based on progeny data on the estimated genomic breeding values. Regression coefficients estimates were between 0.74 and 0.94 and were on average higher for GBLUP or BayesR methods based on HD SNPs compared to GBLUP based on

moderate density SNPs. No significant difference in regression coefficient was observed between GBLUP and BayesR prediction methods based on HD SNPs.

Discussion

This study investigates the possible improvement in accuracy of genomic prediction of breeding values for weight, scanned carcass and wool quantity and quality traits in Australian sheep when using high-density SNP genotypes. First, we compared the variance components that were estimated based on relationships derived from 50k and HD genotypes to those based on pedigree relationships. Estimated additive genetic variances based on HD genotypes were larger than those based on the 50k SNP panel, which suggests that the HD panel captures more genetic variation; this is likely due to higher LD between SNPs and QTL. Estimated genetic variances based on the HD panel were similar while the estimates based on the 50k panel were lower than those based on pedigree data. However, the **A** and **G** matrices are not necessarily on the same scale (e.g. the **G** matrix is derived as a genomic relationship) so these estimates cannot be directly compared. Haile-Mariam et al. [20] also reported that the additive genetic variances and heritabilities estimated from Bovine50k genotypes were lower than those based on pedigree BLUP for 29 production traits in Australian dairy cattle. Legarra [25] argued that the relationship matrices used to estimate genetic variances should be comparable, i.e. the same average relationship and the same average inbreeding. In any case, the difference between 50k and HD panels is the most relevant comparison and this is not affected by scaling.

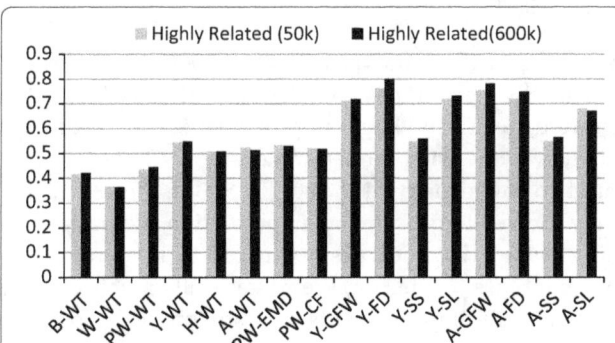

Fig. 1 Accuracy of genomic prediction for animals that are genetically highly related to the reference set based on GBLUP using 50k or HD marker genotypes

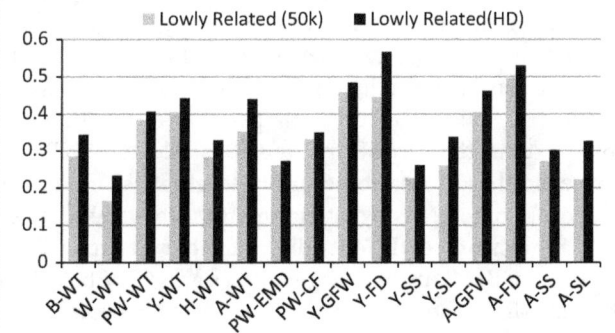

Fig. 2 Accuracy of genomic prediction for animals that are genetically lowly related to the reference set based on GBLUP using 50k or HD marker genotypes

Table 8 Regression coefficient of genomic breeding values from accurate (>90%) pedigree breeding values for wool traits based on GBLUP 50k and HD and BayesR

Trait	GBLUP-50k	GBLUP-HD	BayesR
Y-GFW	0.85	0.83	0.83
Y-CFW	0.82	0.88	0.87
Y-FD	0.81	0.86	0.86
Y-FDCV	0.74	0.77	0.76
Y-SL	0.81	0.88	0.88
Y-SS	0.75	0.77	0.78
A-GFW	0.86	0.94	0.93
A-CFW	0.82	0.85	0.85
A-FD	0.79	0.80	0.80
A-FDCV	0.83	0.83	0.84
A-SL	0.85	0.87	0.86
A-SS	0.78	0.79	0.80

For trait abbreviations see Table 1

HD SNP panels provided higher prediction accuracies but the increase had only practical significance for individuals that were not closely related to the reference population. The average improvement in prediction accuracy was small, ~2.2% which is likely due to the effect of closer relationships providing information that is not much improved by higher marker density. SNPs can capture co-segregation of alleles (family relationships) as well as the LD between SNPs and QTL [5, 11, 21, 22]. Co-segregation is based on linkage between SNPs and QTL which exists over much larger chromosomal regions, therefore not requiring a very high SNP density for adequate prediction. Van der Werf et al. [22] pointed out that prediction from closer relatives is similar to prediction in populations with a lower effective size in which fewer effective chromosome segments are segregating. This observation leads to the same conclusion, i.e. that higher SNP density will have a limited effect on the prediction accuracy when the relationship between reference and target set is stronger.

Previous reports based on real data in dairy cattle also showed a very limited improvement in prediction accuracy when using HD genotypes [7, 8], which confirm results from some simulation studies [12, 23]. However, Meuwissen and Goddard [6] showed a larger gain in prediction accuracy, using a simulation model that included more QTL with large effects, e.g. all the genetic variation of a polygenic trait was due to three to 30 QTL segregating on one chromosome. Meuwissen and Goddard [6] and Clark et al. [9] showed that the use of denser SNP panels was more beneficial if traits are controlled by fewer QTL with larger effects. Our results show limited extra accuracy from HD genotypes, which could indicate that the distribution of QTL effects is closer to the infinitesimal model assumption.

Genomic prediction in a multi-breed reference set could potentially benefit from across-breed prediction when using HD genotypes, as has been suggested in various studies [24, 26, 27]. However, we observed only a small (from 0 to a slightly positive value) increase in accuracy when using information from other breeds. Across-breed prediction could be lower due to differences in both QTL and SNP allele frequencies, incomplete LD between SNPs and QTL across breeds and different allele substitution effects at QTL in different breeds, e.g. due to epistatic interactions [28]. Using higher density SNPs would address only the incomplete LD aspect but not the other two factors. In this study, a slightly greater improvement in GBV accuracy from using HD genotypes was observed for purebred Merinos (5%) based on a Merino reference set compared to a larger multi-breed reference set. Very limited prediction accuracy from HD genotypes was found for PD and WS breeds based

on the Merino sheep reference set, which is likely due to the large genetic distance between Merino and PD or WS as terminal breeds. These results are in line with those of other across-breed prediction studies, e.g. [12, 27] who reported small to no across-breed prediction accuracy from a combined Holstein and Jersey dairy cattle reference set. Interestingly, our results showed a notable (on average 5%) improvement in genomic prediction of PD or WS sheep based on a combined crossbred PD or WS reference set. This suggests that HD SNP panels could be useful to improve LD between SNPs and QTL within diverse breeds or between closely-related breeds, in which case it is also more likely that QTL effects are similar. However, predictions across more distant breeds will not benefit from HD genotypes due to lower levels of LD and possibly larger differences in QTL effects.

Some studies have shown that using moderate-density SNP panels (~50k) provide a more marked improvement in genomic prediction accuracy over low-density SNP panels in different livestock species. Moghaddar et al. [29] compared prediction based on panels of 5k, 10k, 20k and 50k SNPs and showed on average a 11 to 13% gain in prediction accuracy for different production traits in Merino sheep. In dairy cattle, Moser et al. [30] reported on average 10% extra accuracy by switching from very low-density SNP genotypes (3000 to 5000) to moderate-density SNP genotypes (50k). Other studies have also reported relatively large improvements in prediction accuracy from using moderate-density SNP panels compared to low-density SNP sets [3, 5, 31]. However, this study showed improvements in prediction accuracy from using ovine HD genotypes compared to moderate-density genotypes (ovine 50k) seems generally much smaller, but significant improvements were still observed for individuals distantly related to the reference population. This is consistent with the theory about genomic prediction accuracy [32].

The regression coefficient of EBV on GBV was on average higher (less biased) based on HD SNPs than on 50k SNPs. This could be related to the larger additive genetic variances that were estimated when using HD genotypes and are more similar to the estimates of additive genetic variance based on pedigree data. Bias could also occur if selected SNPs were used for genomic prediction. To some extent, the BayesR method uses selected SNPs, in the sense that it uses some priors to emphasize a larger effect for some SNPs by giving them more weight. However, regression coefficients did not differ between GBV based on GBLUP using HD genotypes and GBV based on the BayesR method, which suggests that this explanation is less likely.

Regression coefficients of EBV on GBV were generally lower than 1.00 (0.74 to 0.94). This may be due to the **G**-matrix not being expressed at the same scale as the numeric relationship matrix (**A**) used in the genetic evaluation that produces the EBV, or because of differences in the method for accounting for genetic groups in the reference and validation populations. The **A**-matrix is based on pedigree relationships whereas GBV are calculated with a **G**-matrix that uses relationships across various subpopulations within the population. Since this study was mainly aimed at evaluating genomic prediction accuracy, we did not attempt to rescale the **G**-matrix, since accuracy is calculated as a correlation which is independent of scale. Furthermore, the averages of diagonal and off-diagonal elements of **A** and **G** were similar (1.01 and 0.00 for **A**, 1.00 and 0.00 for **G** based on 50k SNP density and 1.03 and 0.00 for **G** based on HD density) as was suggested by Legarra [25] as a requirement to obtain unbiased estimation of breeding values.

Conclusions

Our results show that the use of high-density (600k) SNP genotypes for the genomic prediction of weight and wool production traits in a multi-breed sheep population resulted in a small improvement in accuracy compared to a moderate SNP density (50k). Improvement in accuracy was greater for individuals that were distantly related to the reference set. Prediction accuracy based on a reference set from other breeds was low and showed limited improvement with HD genotypes. Results of GBLUP and BayesR were not significantly different.

Authors' contributions
NM performed the statistical analysis and drafted the manuscript. AAS participated in the design of the study, data analysis and commented on discussions. JHJV designed and coordinated the study and supervised the statistical analysis and writing of the manuscript. All authors read and approved the final manuscript.

Author details
[1] Cooperative Research Centre for Sheep Industry Innovation, Armidale, NSW 2351, Australia. [2] School of Environmental and Rural Science, University of New England, Armidale, NSW 2351, Australia. [3] Animal Genetics and Breeding Unit (AGBU), University of New England, Armidale, NSW 2351, Australia.

Acknowledgements
The authors wish to gratefully acknowledge the contribution of research staff involved with the "Information Nucleus Program", D. Brown for helpful consultation and providing industry sires' breeding values, C. Gondro and K. Gore for performing quality control on genotypes, B. Sunduimijid and H. Daetwyler for HD imputation, B. Hayes for helpful consultation.

Competing interests
The authors declare that they have no competing interests.

References
1. Meuwissen THE, Hayes BJ, Goddard ME. Prediction of total genetic value using genome-wide dense marker maps. Genetics. 2001;157:1819–29.
2. Goddard ME, Hayes BJ. Genomic selection. J Anim Breed Genet. 2007;124:323–30.
3. Solberg TR, Sorenson AK, Woolliams JA, Meuwissen TH. Genomic selection using different marker types and densities. J Anim Sci. 2008;86:2447–54.
4. Meuwissen TH. Accuracy of breeding values of 'unrelated' individuals predicted by dense SNP genotyping. Genet Sel Evol. 2009;41:35.
5. Habier D, Fernando RL, Dekkers JC. Genomic selection using low-density marker panels. Genetics. 2009;182:343–53.
6. Meuwissen TH, Goddard ME. Accurate prediction of genetic values for complex traits by whole-genome resequencing. Genetics. 2011;185:623–31.
7. VanRaden PM, Null DJ, Sargolzaei M, Wiggans GR, Tooker ME, Vole BJ, et al. Genomic imputation and evaluation using high-density Holstein genotypes. J Dairy Sci. 2013;96:668–78.
8. Harris BL, Johnson DL. The impact of high density SNP chips on genomic evaluation in dairy cattle. Interbull Bull. 2010;42:40–3.
9. Clark SA, Hickey JM, van der Werf JHJ. Different models of genetic variation and their effect on genomic evaluation. Genet Sel Evol. 2011;43:18.
10. Solberg TR, Heringstad B, Svendsen M, Grove H, Meuwissen TH. Genomic predictions for production and functional traits in Norwegian Red from BLUP analyses of imputed 54K and 777K SNP data. Interbull Bull. 2011;44:240–3.
11. Habier D, Fernando RL, Dekkers JC. The impact of genetic relationships on genome-assisted breeding values. Genetics. 2007;177:2389–97.
12. Harris BL, Creagh FE, Winkelman AM, Johnson DL. Experiences with the Illumina high density bovine beadchip. Interbull Bull. 2011;44:3–7.
13. Erbe M, Hayes BJ, Matukumalli LK, Goswami S, Bowman PJ, Reich CM, et al. Improving accuracy of genomic predictions within and between dairy cattle breeds with imputed high-density single nucleotide polymorphism panels. J Dairy Sci. 2012;95:4114–29.
14. Van der Werf JHJ, Kinghorn BP, Banks RG. Design and role of an information nucleus in sheep breeding programs. Anim Prod Sci. 2010;50:998–1003.
15. White JD, Allingham PG, Gorman CM, Emery DL, Hynd P, Owens J, et al. Design and phenotyping procedures for recording wool, skin, parasite resistance, growth, carcass yield and quality traits of the Sheep GENOMICS mapping flock. Anim Prod Sci. 2012;52:157–71.
16. Sargolzaei M, Chesnais JP, Schenkel FS. A new approach for efficient genotype imputation using information from relatives. BMC Genomics. 2014;15:478.
17. Gilmour AR, Gogel BG, Cullis BR, Thompson R. ASReml user guide R release 3.0. Hemel Hempstead: VSN International Lt; 2009.
18. VanRaden PM. Efficient methods to compute genomic predictions. J Dairy Sci. 2008;91:4414–23.
19. Boerner V. Tier BESSiE a program for multivariate linear model BLUP and bayesian analysis of large scale genomic data. Proc Assoc Advmt Breed Genet. 2015;21:390–2.
20. Haile-Mariam M, Nieuwhof GJ, Beard KT, Konstatinov KV, Hayes BJ. Comparison of heritabilities of dairy traits in Australian Holstein-Friesian cattle from genomic and pedigree data and implications for genomic evaluations. J Anim Breed Genet. 2013;130:20–31.
21. Wientjes YCJ, Veerkamp RF, Calus MPL. The effect of linkage disequilibrium and family relationships on the reliability of genomic prediction. Genetics. 2013;193:621–31.
22. Van der Werf JHJ, Clark SA, Lee SH. Predicting genomic selection accuracy from heterogeneous sources. Proc Assoc Advmt Breed Genet. 2015;21:161–4.
23. VanRaden PM, O'Connell JR, Wiggans GR, Weigel KA. Genomic evaluations with many more genotypes. Genet Sel Evol. 2011;43:10.
24. de Roos APW, Hayes BJ, Goddard ME. Reliability of genomic breeding values across multiple populations. Genetics. 2009;183:1545–53.
25. Legarra A. Comparing estimates of genetic variance across different relationship models. Theor Popul Biol. 2016;107:26–30.
26. Ibanez-Escriche N, Fernando RL, Toosi A, Dekkers JCM. Genomic selection of purebreds for crossbred performance. Genet Sel Evol. 2009;41:12.
27. Pryce JE, Gredler B, Bolormaa S, Bowman PJ, Egger-Danner C, Fuerst C, et al. Short communication: genomic selection using a multi- breed, across-country reference population. J Dairy Sci. 2011;4:2625–30.

28. Moghaddar N, Swan AA, van der Werf JHJ. Genomic prediction of weight and wool traits in a multi-breed sheep population. Anim Prod Sci. 2013;54:544–9.

29. Moghaddar N, Van der Werf JHJ. Genomic prediction in Merino sheep for varying reference population size and marker density. In: Proceeding of the 33rd international society for animal genetics. Cairns; 2012.

30. Moser G, Khatkar MS, Hayes BJ, Raadsma HW. Accuracy of direct genomic values in Holstein bulls and cows using subsets of SNP markers. Genet Sel Evol. 2010;42:37.

31. Weigel KA, de los Campos G, Gonzalez-Recio O, Naya H, Wu XL, Rosa GJM, et al. Predictive ability of direct genomic values for lifetime net merit of Holstein sires using selected subsets of single nucleotide polymorphism markers. J Dairy Sci. 2009;92:5248–57.

32. Goddard ME. Genomic selection: prediction of accuracy and maximisation of long term response. Genetica. 2009;136:245–57.

13

Estimation of genetic connectedness diagnostics based on prediction errors without the prediction error variance–covariance matrix

John B. Holmes[1]*, Ken G. Dodds[2] and Michael A. Lee[1]

Abstract

Background: An important issue in genetic evaluation is the comparability of random effects (breeding values), particularly between pairs of animals in different contemporary groups. This is usually referred to as genetic connectedness. While various measures of connectedness have been proposed in the literature, there is general agreement that the most appropriate measure is some function of the prediction error variance–covariance matrix. However, obtaining the prediction error variance–covariance matrix is computationally demanding for large-scale genetic evaluations. Many alternative statistics have been proposed that avoid the computational cost of obtaining the prediction error variance–covariance matrix, such as counts of genetic links between contemporary groups, gene flow matrices, and functions of the variance–covariance matrix of estimated contemporary group fixed effects.

Results: In this paper, we show that a correction to the variance–covariance matrix of estimated contemporary group fixed effects will produce the exact prediction error variance–covariance matrix averaged by contemporary group for univariate models in the presence of single or multiple fixed effects and one random effect. We demonstrate the correction for a series of models and show that approximations to the prediction error matrix based solely on the variance–covariance matrix of estimated contemporary group fixed effects are inappropriate in certain circumstances.

Conclusions: Our method allows for the calculation of a connectedness measure based on the prediction error variance–covariance matrix by calculating only the variance–covariance matrix of estimated fixed effects. Since the number of fixed effects in genetic evaluation is usually orders of magnitudes smaller than the number of random effect levels, the computational requirements for our method should be reduced.

Background

A goal of genetic evaluation is to predict genetic merit, while optimising accuracy and minimising bias. Ideally, a breeder of seed stock should be able to compare all individuals in an evaluation irrespective of contemporary group. This is problematic when there is little or no genetic connectedness between groups, unless there is a belief that the model assumptions, specifically assumptions concerning genetic relationships between animals, completely describe the population in question, which is not the case in general. Estimation and reporting of genetic connectedness are important as there are, taking the example of the New Zealand sheep industry, hundreds of flocks evaluated over disparate environments and within each, there are many more contemporary groups. There is sharing of genetic material (rams) between groups and individual seedstock breeders and a centrally co-ordinated progeny test to increase genetic connectedness [1], but many flocks or groups of flocks likely lack genetic connectedness to allow comparison,

*Correspondence: jholmes@maths.otago.ac.nz
[1] Department of Mathematics and Statistics, University of Otago, Cumberland St., Dunedin 9016, New Zealand
Full list of author information is available at the end of the article

therefore, in New Zealand, genetic connectedness is reported to seed stock (rams) breeders [2].

In the work of Foulley et al. [3, 4] and Laloë et al. [5, 6], genetic connectedness is regarded as a measure of predictability, where predictability is the random effect extension of estimability [7]. More recently, this was the approach to connectedness taken by Kerr et al. [8]. An estimable function [9, 10] is defined in the context of a fixed effect model. In particular, a function is said to be estimable if vectors $\mathbf{a}$ and $\mathbf{k}$ exist such that $E(\mathbf{a}'y) = \mathbf{k}'\boldsymbol{\beta}$. For random effects, all linear combinations can be predicted, regardless of their distribution [3], even if they are not estimable when treated as fixed effects. To get around this, connectedness was defined as the loss of information due to a lack of orthogonality [4] measured by using the Kullback–Leibler divergence. It was shown in Laloë [5] that for a linear mixed model, the expected information is a function of the ratio of the posterior and prior variance for $\mathbf{u}$, alternatively known as the prediction error variance–covariance matrix (PEV) and the relationship matrix, respectively. They also showed that the expected information could be re-arranged to give a co-efficient of determination (CD) statistic [5, 6]. To reduce the computational cost of this measure, simulation and the repeated use of iterative solvers were proposed [11].

Alternative measures of connectedness have been designed either to ease interpretability or minimise computational cost [12–14]. Usually these measures attempt to measure the level of genetic linkage between contemporary groups. They often also allow for the possibility that the model is incorrectly specified, such as omitting genetic groups. They include methods based on PEV, the variance–covariance matrix of estimated fixed effects $Var(\hat{\boldsymbol{\beta}})$, the covariance structure fitted for the random effects (the relationship matrix), or a combination of these. Those based on PEV include the ratio in determinants between full and reduced models [4], differences in PEV of contrasts [12] and correlations of random effect contrasts [15]. Methods based on the variance–covariance matrix of estimated fixed effects include variance of differences between estimated fixed effects (VED) [12], and correlations between estimated fixed effects referred to as connectedness rating (CR) [16]. The fixed effect usually considered is contemporary group (such as flock by year or herd by year). Methods based on the relationship matrix include genetic drift variance [17] and direct genetic links [18, 19].

The focus here is on measures of connectedness that are functions of the PEV or the variance covariance matrix of estimated fixed effects, the links between them and the changes observed as the fitted effect structure is changed. The inclusion of genotype data was also considered to assess the impact changes in the relationship

matrix have on the relationship between PEV and the variance–covariance matrix of estimated fixed effects and on the connectedness measure being considered.

The first of the measures that we investigated was the PEV of contemporary group differences ($PEVD_{ij}$) [12]. This is calculated from $\mathbf{Z}$, the incidence matrix indicating which animals have records, $\mathbf{x}_{ij}$, a vector of contrasts comparing two groups i and j and $Var(\hat{\mathbf{u}} - \mathbf{u})$, the prediction error variance–covariance matrix of random effects.

$$PEVD_{ij} = \mathbf{x}'_{ij}\mathbf{Z}\,Var(\hat{\mathbf{u}} - \mathbf{u})\mathbf{Z}'\mathbf{x}_{ij}.$$

If the groups i and j being compared are contemporary groups such that $\mathbf{x}'_{ij}\mathbf{u}$ is the difference in the mean random effect between group i and j, PEVD can be simplified to a function of the prediction error variance–covariance matrix of random effects averaged by contemporary group.

$$PEVD_{ij} = \overline{Var(\hat{\mathbf{u}} - \mathbf{u})}_{ii} + \overline{Var(\hat{\mathbf{u}} - \mathbf{u})}_{jj} - 2\overline{Var(\hat{\mathbf{u}} - \mathbf{u})}_{ij}.$$

The coefficient of determination ($CD(\mathbf{x}_{ij})$) [5, 6] is also calculated from $\mathbf{Z}$, $\mathbf{x}_{ij}$ and $Var(\hat{\mathbf{u}} - \mathbf{u})$ but it also includes $Var(\mathbf{u})$.

$$CD(\mathbf{x}_{ij}) = \frac{\mathbf{x}'_{ij}\mathbf{Z}\,Var(\hat{\mathbf{u}})\mathbf{Z}'x_{ij}}{\mathbf{x}'_{ij}\mathbf{Z}\,Var(\mathbf{u})\mathbf{Z}'x_{ij}}$$
$$= \frac{\mathbf{x}'_{ij}\mathbf{Z}(Var(\mathbf{u}) - Var(\hat{\mathbf{u}} - \mathbf{u}))\mathbf{Z}'x_{ij}}{\mathbf{x}'_{ij}\mathbf{Z}\,Var(\mathbf{u})\mathbf{Z}'x_{ij}}.$$

Flock correlation (r) [15] is calculated from the elements of the prediction error variance–covariance matrix of random effects averaged by contemporary group.

$$r_{ij} = \frac{\overline{Var(\hat{\mathbf{u}} - \mathbf{u})}_{ij}}{\sqrt{\overline{Var(\hat{\mathbf{u}} - \mathbf{u})}_{ii}\,\overline{Var(\hat{\mathbf{u}} - \mathbf{u})}_{jj}}}.$$

For the variance of differences in management unit effects (VED), Kennedy and Trus [12] used the variances and covariances of estimated contemporary group fixed effects, where $\hat{\boldsymbol{\beta}}_i$ is the estimated effect for contemporary group i and $\hat{\boldsymbol{\beta}}_j$ is the estimated effect for contemporary group j.

$$VED_{ij} = Var(\hat{\boldsymbol{\beta}})_{ii} + Var(\hat{\boldsymbol{\beta}})_{jj} - 2Var(\hat{\boldsymbol{\beta}})_{ij}.$$

The basis for using VED is that $Var(\hat{\boldsymbol{\beta}})$ is an approximation of $\overline{Var(\hat{\mathbf{u}} - \mathbf{u})}$ [12] . In this scenario, VED should estimate the PEV of contemporary group differences, PEVD. As a connectedness rating (CR), [16] used the variances and covariances of estimated contemporary group fixed effects, where $\hat{\boldsymbol{\beta}}_i$ is the estimated effect for contemporary group i and $\hat{\boldsymbol{\beta}}_j$ is the estimated effect for contemporary group j.

$$CR_{ij} = \frac{Var(\hat{\beta})_{ij}}{\sqrt{Var(\hat{\beta})_{ii}Var(\hat{\beta})_{jj}}}.$$

Using the same argument as for VED, CR approximates the flock correlation. The aim of this paper is to give an exact measure of $\overline{Var(\hat{u} - u)}$ using functions of the variance-covariance matrix of the estimated fixed effects. We also demonstrate that, under certain circumstances, the approximations provide poor estimates of $\overline{Var(\hat{u} - u)}$ and hence are poor predictors of genetic connectedness.

For the remainder of this paper, $Var(\hat{u} - u)$ will be referred to as PEV and $\overline{Var(\hat{u} - u)}$ as PEVMean.

Materials and methods
Data
The data available, collected by New Zealand seed stock (ram) breeders and previously used in Holmes et al. [20], consisted of 40,837 animals with live-weight recorded at eight months of age. These animals were born between 2011 and 2013. Together with ancestors, 84,802 animals with pedigree information were obtained from the database of the New Zealand genetic evaluation system for sheep, Sheep Improvement Limited (SIL) [2]. A total of 269 animals were genotyped using the 50K Illumina SNP chip and of these, 21 had live-weight records. A total of 31,615 animals without genotype information were descendants of a genotyped animal. As these data were previously collected by commercial seed stock breeders, special animal ethics authorisation was not required.

Methods
Models
For modelling purposes, we considered the following variables as fixed effects. The contemporary group variable was flock-sex-contemporary group combination, as is standard for growth traits in SIL. There were 202 flock-sex-contemporary groups in the dataset. The combination of birth and rearing rank (four levels) and age of dam (three levels) were treated as categorical variables. Date of birth was treated as a continuous covariate and defined as the difference (in days) between the animals date of birth and the average date of birth in its flock and year combination. Weaning weight was fitted as a continuous covariate. Three models were fitted. Model 1 fitted flock-sex-contemporary group combination as the only fixed effect. Model 2 fitted flock-sex-contemporary group combination, date of birth, and birth rearing rank as fixed effects. Model 3 fitted all available fixed effects. The animal genetic effect was fitted into all models as a random effect. Two variations on the variance-covariance matrix of the random animal effect were considered. These were $\mathbf{A}$ and $\mathbf{H}$. Matrix $\mathbf{A}$ used only the pedigree information

available to construct the variance-covariance matrix. The method of Meuwissen and Luo [21] was used to construct the inverse of $\mathbf{A}$ required for the mixed-model equations. Matrix $\mathbf{H}$ used genotype and pedigree information to construct the variance-covariance matrix. The genomic component of the variance-covariance matrix $\mathbf{G}$ was constructed using the first method of VanRaden [22] and the inverse of $\mathbf{H}$ was constructed using the method outlined in Aguilar et.al. [23]. The variance components were estimated for Model 3 using $\mathbf{A}$ to model the covariance structure of the animal effect in ASReml [24]. Estimates of variance components were $\sigma_g^2 = 1.81$ and $\sigma_e^2 = 7.43$ resulting in a heritability of 0.20. Standard errors for the variance components were 0.13 and 0.11 respectively. The variance components were then fixed at these values for all other models, regardless of whether the variance-covariance matrix of the random effect was $\mathbf{A}$ or $\mathbf{H}$.

Functions of the fixed effects considered
Three functions of the variance-covariance matrix of estimated fixed effects were compared to the directly calculated PEVMean. Function 1 is the approximation $Var(\hat{\beta}_1)$, where $\hat{\beta}_1$ is the vector of contemporary group fixed effects. The elements of this function were used to calculate CR [16] and VED [12]. Function 2 is the function of the variance-covariance matrix of estimated fixed effects that gives PEVMean for a model with only one fixed effect fitted.

$$PEVMean = Var(\hat{\beta}) - \sigma_e^2(\mathbf{X}'\mathbf{X})^{-1}.$$

Function 3 is the function of the variance-covariance matrix of estimated fixed effects that gives PEVMean for a model with multiple fixed effects fitted.

$$\begin{aligned}PEVMean = {} & (\mathbf{X}_1'\mathbf{X}_1)^{-1}\mathbf{X}_1'\mathbf{X}_2 Var(\hat{\beta}_2)\mathbf{X}_2'\mathbf{X}_1(\mathbf{X}_1'\mathbf{X}_1)^{-1} \\ & + (\mathbf{X}_1'\mathbf{X}_1)^{-1}\mathbf{X}_1'\mathbf{X}_2 Var(\hat{\beta}_2, \hat{\beta}_1) \\ & + Var(\hat{\beta}_1, \hat{\beta}_2)\mathbf{X}_2'\mathbf{X}_1(\mathbf{X}_1'\mathbf{X}_1)^{-1} \\ & + Var(\hat{\beta}_1) - \sigma_e^2(\mathbf{X}_1'\mathbf{X}_1)^{-1}.\end{aligned}$$

The derivations and notations for function 2 and function 3 are in the "Appendix".

Correction factors used in function 2 and function 3
Both function 2 and function 3 are matrix additions to function 1, $Var(\hat{\beta}_1)$. Therefore, the extra calculations required can be regarded as correction factors to obtain PEVMean. In function 2, we subtracted $\sigma_e^2(\mathbf{X}_1'\mathbf{X}_1)^{-1}$ from function 1, where $(\mathbf{X}_1'\mathbf{X}_1)^{-1}$ is a diagonal matrix with entries ii equal to $\frac{1}{n_i}$, where n_i is the number of observations in contemporary group i. Therefore, $\sigma_e^2(\mathbf{X}_1'\mathbf{X}_1)^{-1}$ is the correction factor for the number of

records. Due to the inverse relationship with contemporary group size, this correction is more pronounced for small contemporary groups. Function 3 is the addition of $(\mathbf{X}_1'\mathbf{X}_1)^{-1}\mathbf{X}_1'\mathbf{X}_2 Var(\hat{\boldsymbol{\beta}}_2)\mathbf{X}_2'\mathbf{X}_1(\mathbf{X}_1'\mathbf{X}_1)^{-1} + (\mathbf{X}_1'\mathbf{X}_1)^{-1}\mathbf{X}_1'\mathbf{X}_2 Var(\hat{\boldsymbol{\beta}}_2,\hat{\boldsymbol{\beta}}_1) + Var(\hat{\boldsymbol{\beta}}_1,\hat{\boldsymbol{\beta}}_2)\mathbf{X}_2'\mathbf{X}_1(\mathbf{X}_1'\mathbf{X}_1)^{-1}$ to function 2. This addition is therefore the correction to account for the inclusion of other fixed effects in the model.

Calculation of connectedness measures and their comparison

The fixed effect variance covariance matrix $Var(\hat{\boldsymbol{\beta}})$ and PEV were extracted from the inverse of the mixed model equations. PEVMean was calculated from PEV. From this, the PEV of contemporary group differences (PEVD) and flock correlation were calculated. From $Var(\hat{\boldsymbol{\beta}}_1)$, VED and CR were calculated. All calculations used R [25].

The three functions described earlier were compared using correlations between the elements of PEVMean and the corresponding elements of the function in question. Diagonal elements were considered separately from off-diagonal elements.

As mentioned in the "Background" section, CR is the analogue to the flock correlation and VED is the analogue to PEVD under the assumption that $Var(\hat{\boldsymbol{\beta}}_1)$ approximates PEVMean. Therefore, correlations between the flock correlation and CR and between VED and PEVD were calculated to assess whether variance of differences or correlation functions of $Var(\hat{\boldsymbol{\beta}}_1)$ gave a more accurate approximation to the corresponding functions of PEVMean than the individual elements of $Var(\hat{\boldsymbol{\beta}}_1)$ did for the individual elements of PEVMean. Both Pearson and Spearman correlations were considered for all examples to assess whether a linear relationship or just the relative rank was maintained.

Results

Model 1: Flock-sex-contemporary group interaction is the only fixed effect fitted

Correlations between the elements of PEVMean and the elements of function 1 and function 2 are in Table 1. For function 1, correlations were high for diagonal elements (Pearson: 0.994 for **A**, 0.994 for **H**. Spearman: 0.932 for **A**, 0.928 for **H**), regardless of whether **A** or **H** was used as the variance–covariance matrix of the animal random effect. The off-diagonal elements of PEVMean and $Var(\hat{\boldsymbol{\beta}}_1)$ were exactly equivalent. As expected from the derivations earlier, function 2 produced an exact one to one correspondence with PEVMean.

A high correlation between the elements of PEVMean and the elements of function 1 and function 2 was observed because the correction to function 1 that is required to obtain PEVMean, when only one fixed effect is fitted, is the correction for the number of records. As

Table 1 Pearson and Spearman correlations of PEVMean with functions 1, 2 and 3 for three models and two relationship matrices (A and H)

Model		Function		
		1	2	3
1 **A**	Diagonals Pearson	0.994	1	NA
	Diagonals Spearman	0.932	1	NA
	Off-diagonal Pearson	1	1	NA
	Off-diagonal Spearman	1	1	NA
1 **H**	Diagonals Pearson	0.994	1	NA
	Diagonals Spearman	0.928	1	NA
	Off-diagonal Pearson	1	1	NA
	Off-diagonal Spearman	1	1	NA
2 **A**	Diagonals Pearson	0.994	1.000*	1
	Diagonals Spearman	0.932	0.999	1
	Off-diagonal Pearson	0.995	0.995	1
	Off-diagonal Spearman	0.625	0.625	1
2 **H**	Diagonals Pearson	0.994	1.000*	1
	Diagonals Spearman	0.928	1.000*	1
	Off-diagonal Pearson	0.996	0.996	1
	Off-diagonal Spearman	0.710	0.710	1
3 **A**	Diagonals Pearson	0.994	1.000*	1
	Diagonals Spearman	0.935	0.980	1
	Off-diagonal Pearson	0.481	0.481	1
	Off-diagonal Spearman	0.423	0.423	1
3 **H**	Diagonals Pearson	0.994	1.000*	1
	Diagonals Spearman	0.931	0.985	1
	Off-diagonal Pearson	0.534	0.534	1
	Off-diagonal Spearman	0.491	0.491	1

Measure 3 is not applicable for Model 1. Correlations marked with a* round to 1 as opposed to being exactly 1

mentioned earlier, the correction factor for the number of records was a diagonal matrix and the off-diagonal elements of $Var(\hat{\boldsymbol{\beta}})$ were unchanged when converting to PEVMean. The diagonal elements of PEVMean will be less than $Var(\hat{\boldsymbol{\beta}})$ (Fig. 1), in particular for contemporary groups with few records. This also means that CR consistently gave lower values than the flock correlation.

The basis for using VED was that $Var(\hat{\boldsymbol{\beta}})$ approximated PEVMean. By the same logic, CR should also approximate the flock correlation. Correlations of CR with the flock correlation and of VED with PEVD are in Table 2. Pearson correlations of CR with the flock correlation were lower than the correlation between the elements of function 1 and PEVMean, which are in Table 1. Spearman correlations of CR with the flock correlation were higher. Correlations between VED and PEVD were high, but Pearson correlations were higher than Spearman correlations. This was as expected based on the high correlations for both the diagonals and off-diagonals. However,

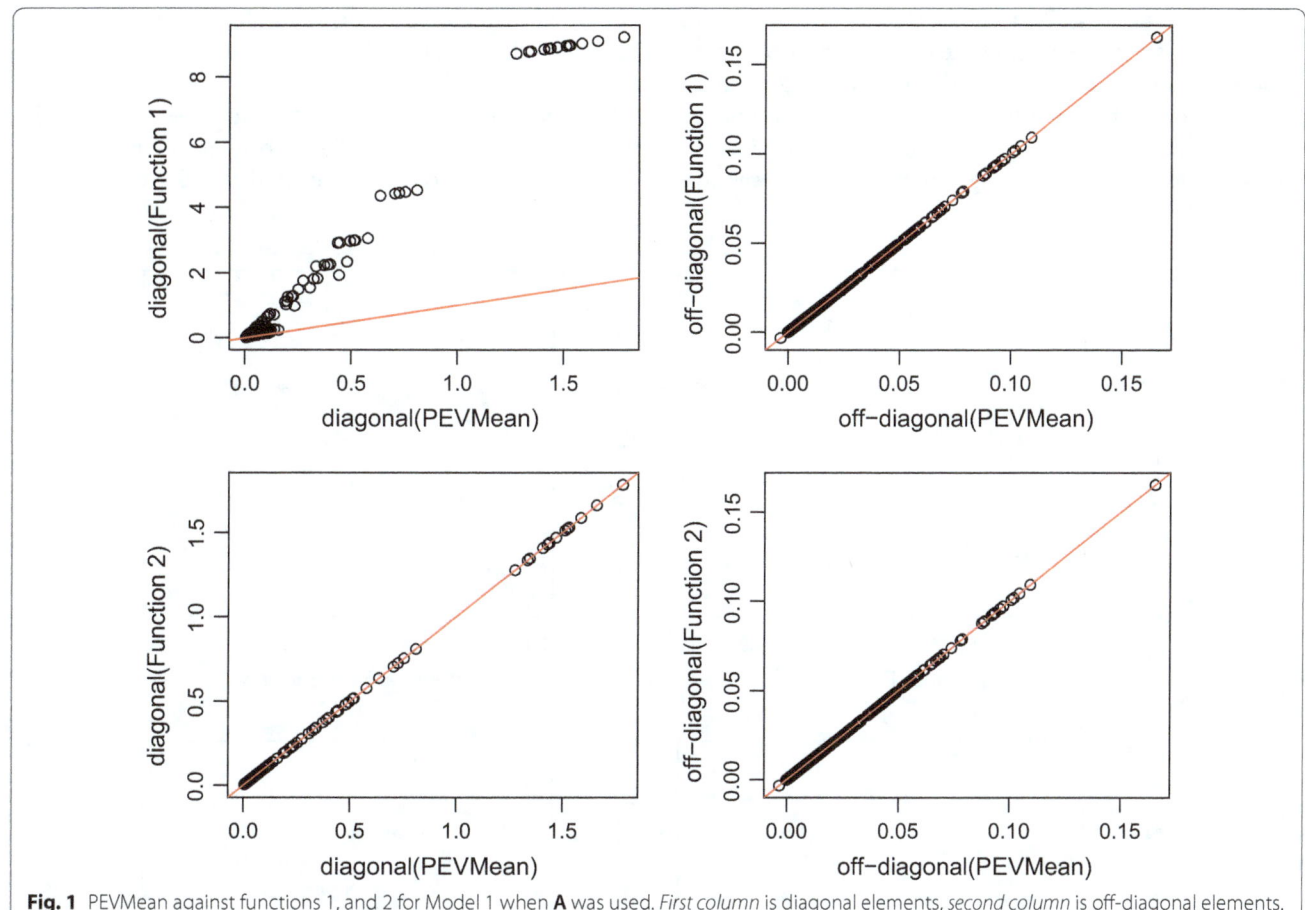

Fig. 1 PEVMean against functions 1, and 2 for Model 1 when **A** was used. *First column* is diagonal elements, *second column* is off-diagonal elements. The *red line* is equality

Table 2 Pearson and Spearman correlations of the flock correlation with CR and PEVD with VED for three models and two relationship matrices (A and H)

Model	Correlation type	Flock correlation against CR	PEVD against VED
1 **A**	Pearson	0.943	0.994
	Spearman	0.999	0.942
1 **H**	Pearson	0.945	0.994
	Spearman	0.999	0.938
2 **A**	Pearson	0.914	0.994
	Spearman	0.534	0.942
2 **H**	Pearson	0.927	0.994
	Spearman	0.636	0.938
3 **A**	Pearson	0.430	0.994
	Spearman	0.258	0.939
3 **H**	Pearson	0.481	0.994
	Spearman	0.345	0.934

the values of VED were in a higher range than PEVD due to the inflation of diagonal elements of $Var(\hat{\beta})$ compared to PEVMean. The inflation of VED compared to PEVD,

due to not applying the correction factor for the number of records, was most pronounced for small contemporary groups.

Model 2: Contemporary group, date of birth and birth rearing rank fitted

Correlations between the elements of PEVMean and the elements of function 1, function 2 and function 3 are in Table 1. Correlations between the elements of PEVMean and function 1 were high for diagonal elements but lower for off-diagonal elements. Due to the inclusion of non-contemporary group fixed effects, elements of function 2 did not give an exact correspondence to the elements of PEVMean. In function 2, correlations with the diagonal elements of PEVMean increased compared to function 1, while the off-diagonal elements were unchanged because the correction factor for the number of records applied to diagonals only. As expected from the derivations obtained above, function 3 produced an exact one to one correspondence with PEVMean.

The diagonal elements of function 2 gave almost a one to one correspondence with the diagonal elements of

PEVMean regardless of whether **A** (Fig. 2) or **H** was used. This indicates that the magnitude of the correction factor to account for the other fixed effects was negligible relative to the magnitude of function 2. The correction factor lowered the off-diagonal elements of $Var(\hat{\boldsymbol{\beta}}_1)$ uniformly. For both diagonal and off-diagonal elements, the relative

impact of including the correction for other fixed effects in the model was therefore higher for elements with a lower absolute value.

Inclusion of other fixed effects lowered the correlation between CR and the flock correlation and between VED and PEVD compared to model 1. CR usually gave

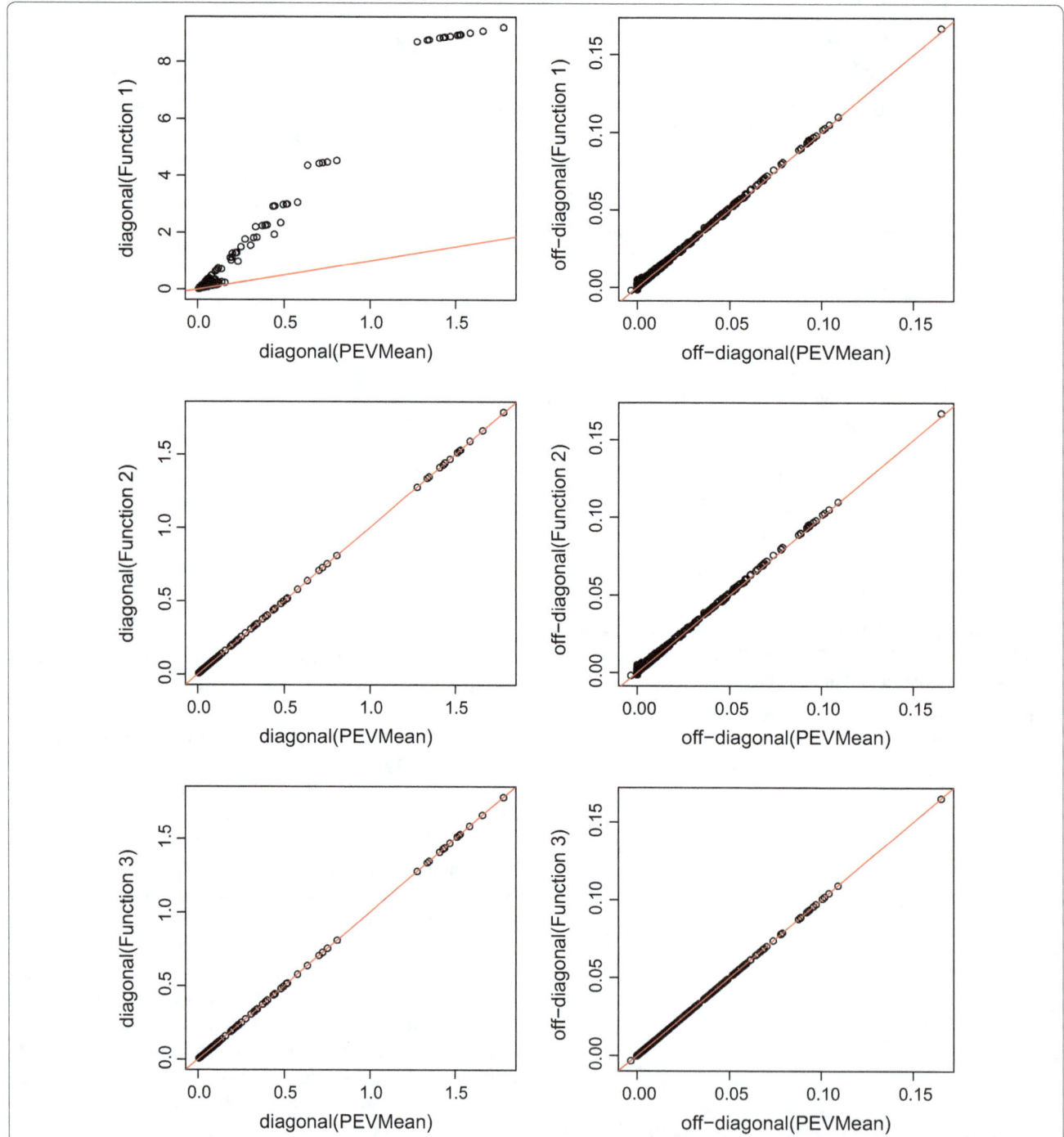

Fig. 2 PEVMean against functions 1, 2, and 3 for Model 2 when **A** was used. *First column* is diagonal elements, *second column* is off-diagonal elements. The *red line* is equality

lower values than the flock correlation. Exceptions were due to both the diagonal and off-diagonal elements of $Var(\hat{\beta}_1)$ that overestimated the corresponding element of PEVMean. Correlations between VED and PEVD were high; with Pearson correlations higher than Spearman correlations. As in Model 1, VED had a higher range than PEVD.

Model 3: Contemporary group, age of dam, date of birth, birth rearing rank and flock × sex interaction fitted

Correlations between the elements of PEVMean and function 1 were high for diagonal elements but lower for off-diagonal elements. Inclusion of additional fixed effects means that, as in Model 2, elements of function 2 did not give an exact correspondence to the elements of PEVMean. Correlations of the diagonal elements of function 2 with the diagonal elements of PEVMean increased compared to function 1, while the off-diagonal elements were unchanged because the correction factor for the number of records applies to diagonals only. As expected from the derivations obtained above, function 3 produced an exact one to one correspondence with PEVMean.

The correction factor to account for the other fixed effects in the model was typically about 35 times larger than in Model 2. As a result, diagonal elements of function 2 were increased compared to diagonal elements of PEVMean (Fig. 3). For the off-diagonal elements, the correction factor accounting for other fixed effects in the model was uniform when the off-diagonal element of PEVMean moved away from zero. There was more variation in the correction factor when the off-diagonal element of PEVMean was near zero. Inflation seen in off-diagonal elements of function 1 compared to off-diagonal elements of PEVMean was due primarily to not correcting for other fixed effects rather than not correcting for the number of records. CR generally gave larger estimates than the flock correlation and over-estimation was most pronounced when off-diagonal elements of PEVMean and hence the flock correlation were near zero.

Inclusion of weaning weight and age of dam in the model decreased the correlations of CR with the flock correlation compared to Models 1 and 2 (Table 2). In particular, flock correlations that approach 0 in this model may have a high CR. The reasons for this will be elaborated in the "Discussion" section. The largest difference between CR and the flock correlation was between contemporary groups 98 and 107 when **A** was used (flock correlation = 0.022, CR = 0.818), and between contemporary groups 147 and 152 when **H** was used (flock correlation = 0.056, CR = 0.803). The correlation between VED and PEVD remained high in Model 3.

Impact of using H compared to A to model the variance–covariance of the animal random effect

The use of **H** instead of **A** did not significantly change the Pearson correlation of PEVMean with the approximations functions 1 and 2, except for the off-diagonals in Model 3 (Table 1). Similarly, it did not result in large differences in the Pearson correlations between CR and the flock correlation or between VED and PEVD, except between CR and the flock correlation in Model 3 (Table 2). The use of **H** increased the Spearman correlations for off-diagonal elements of PEVMean with functions 1 and 2 (Table 1) and of CR with the flock correlation (Table 2) for Models 2 and 3.

Additional file 1: Figure S1 shows the impact of using **H** as opposed to **A**, which was to increase PEVMean, particularly when the value of PEVMean using **A** was near zero. This was particularly obvious for the off-diagonals. The result was an increase in the flock correlation and CR compared to the equivalent model in which **A** was fitted.

Patterns in the correction factor accounting for the inclusion of other fixed effects in the model

The relationship between the correction factor and the PEVMean for the two models (Models 2 and 3), for which the correction factor was relevant is in Fig. 4. The correction factor was similar for both the diagonal and off-diagonal elements. There was no relationship between the value of the correction factor and the value of PEVMean, except for an increase in variability in the correction factor when the element of PEVMean was near zero. The correction factor was approximately 35 times larger in Model 3 than in Model 2, as indicated by traces of the correction factor. The low degree of variation in the correction factor for other fixed effects suggested that the dataset that we used was approximately balanced across contemporary groups.

Patterns in connectedness rating (CR) and variance of estimated differences of management units (VED)
Connectedness rating

The flock correlation was compared to CR (Fig. 5). As mentioned, CR underestimated the flock correlation in Model 1 for all pairs of contemporary groups and for most pairs in Model 2. Conversely, CR overestimated the flock correlation for most pairs in Model 3. In Model 2 and especially in Model 3, there was a collection of contemporary group pairs for which the flock correlation was near zero (completely disconnected), while the corresponding CR estimate was much higher than zero. This was due to the correction factor for the other fitted fixed effects, which was similar for both the diagonal and off-diagonal elements, and had the largest impact on very small covariances and hence correlations. The divergence

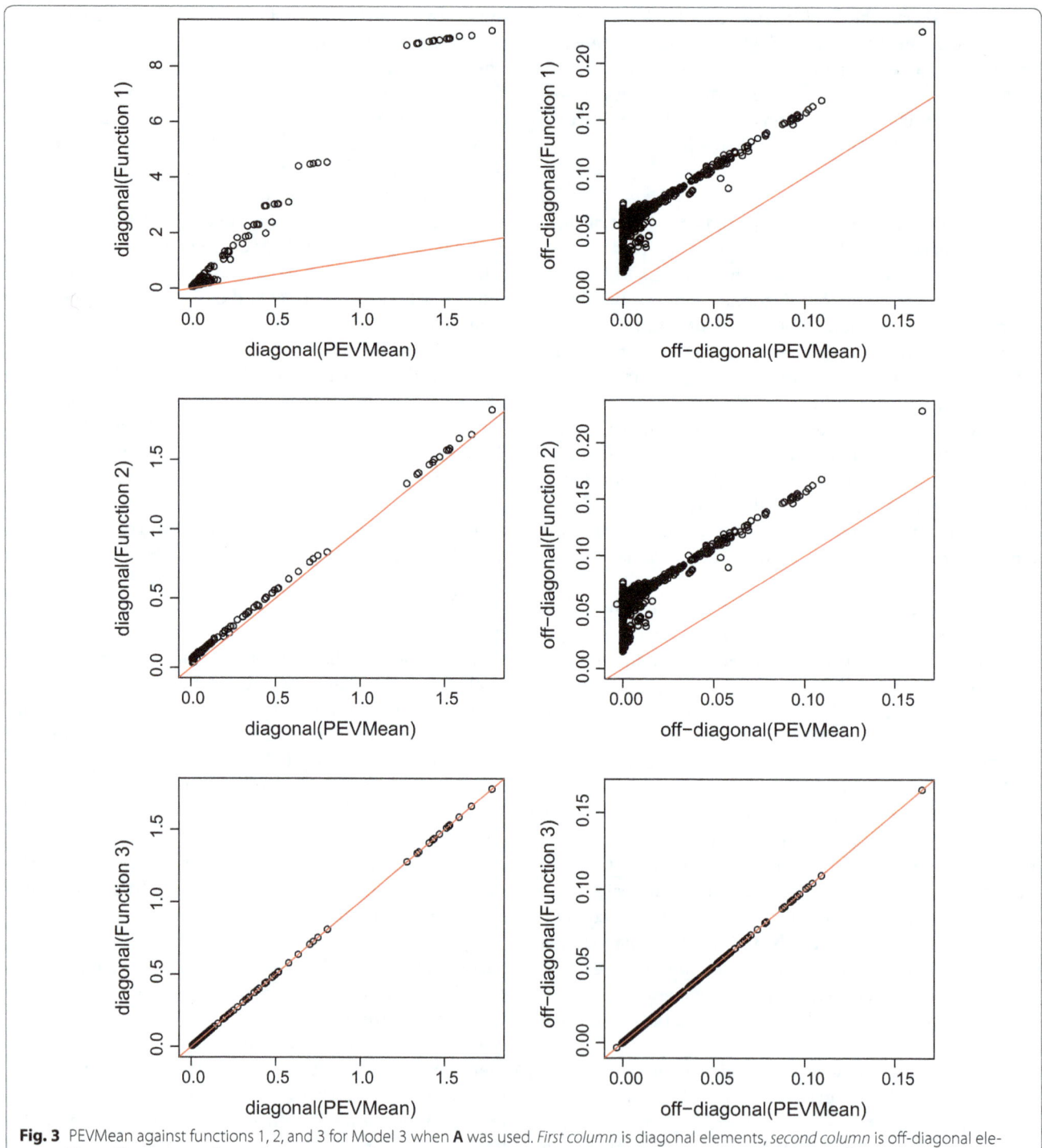

Fig. 3 PEVMean against functions 1, 2, and 3 for Model 3 when **A** was used. *First column* is diagonal elements, *second column* is off-diagonal elements. The *red line* is the 45 degree *line*

between CR and the flock correlation when the flock correlation was near zero was also a function of contemporary group size. Since the variances were inversely dependent on the number of records in the contemporary group, the most pronounced differences between CR and flock correlation occurred between contemporary groups that were not linked and had a large number of records. Additional file 2: Figure S2 shows the relationship between the harmonic mean $\frac{2}{\frac{1}{n_1}+\frac{1}{n_2}}$ and CR when

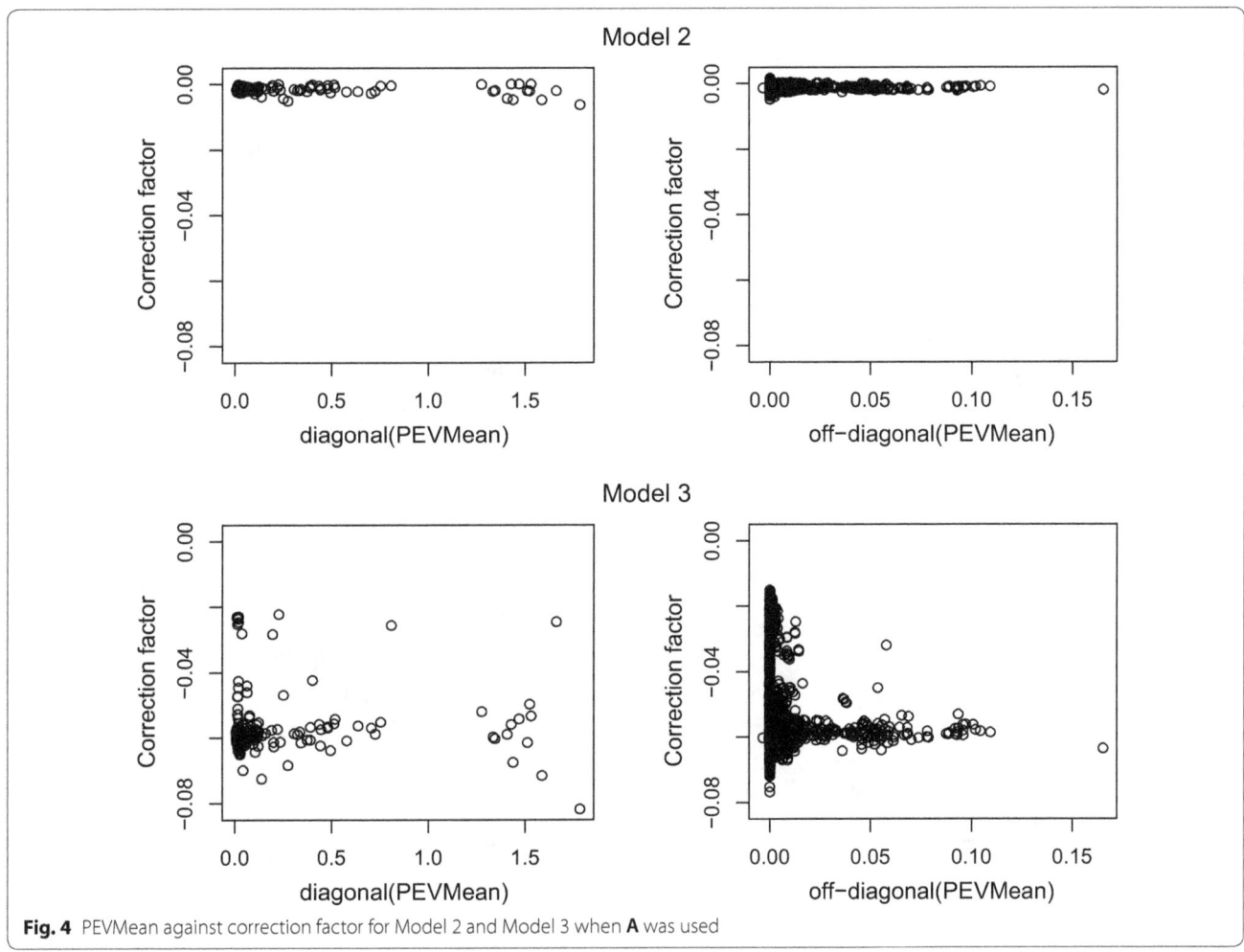

Fig. 4 PEVMean against correction factor for Model 2 and Model 3 when **A** was used

the corresponding flock correlation is low. For Model 2 and especially Model 3, higher harmonic means were associated with higher CR.

Variance of estimated differences of management units (VED)

Unlike CR compared to the flock correlation, VED showed a stronger relationship with PEVD (Fig. 5). However, for all three models, there were certain pairs of contemporary groups that had similar VED, but substantially different PEVD. This variation increased PEVD and was probably due to VED not correcting for the number of records in each contemporary group because VED, PEVD and the correction factor for the number of records were all inversely dependent on the number of records in the contemporary groups in question. Table 3 shows that VED corrected for the number of records was equivalent to PEVD in Model 1, as expected, while the corrected VED showed a near one to one relationship with PEVD for both Models 2 and 3. An almost exact one to one

relationship between corrected VED and PEVD for Models 2 and 3 was due to the correction factor for the other fixed effects being fairly uniform and thus cancelling out in the calculation of variances of differences, which both VED and PEVD are examples of.

Discussion
Sensitivity to the presence of other fixed effects in the model fitted

In the example used by Kennedy and Trus [12], a correlation of 0.995 was found between $Var(\hat{\beta}_1)$ and the mean PEV. However, they only considered a model where contemporary group was the only fixed effect. For the three models that we fitted, the correlation between the variance–covariance matrix of estimated contemporary group fixed effects and the prediction error variance–covariance matrix of contemporary group averages was sensitive to the inclusion of other fixed effects in the model. This sensitivity depended on the correction factor for the other fixed effects included in the model.

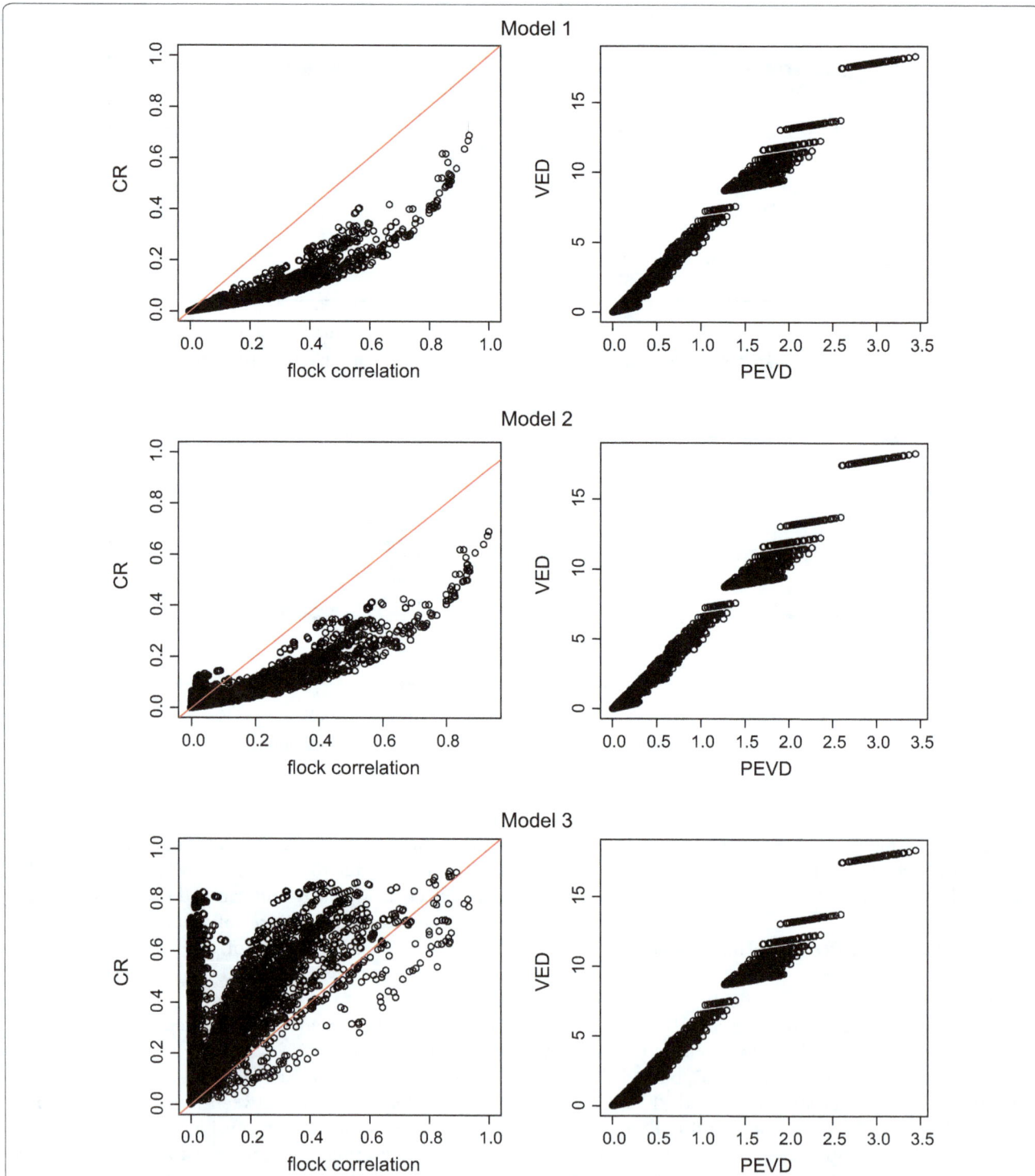

Fig. 5 Flock correlation against CR and PEVD against VED when **A** was used. The *first column* is Flock correlation against CR. The *second column* is PEVD against VED. The *red line* in *first column* is equality

Table 3 Simple linear regression between VED corrected for the number of records and PEVD for three models and two relationship matrices (A and H)

Model	Intercept	Slope	r^2
1, **A**	0	1	1
1, **H**	0	1	1
2, **A**	0.000*	1.001	1.000*
2, **H**	0.000*	1.001	1.000*
3, **A**	0.004	1.002	1.000*
3, **H**	0.004	1.002	1.000*

Numbers with a * only round to and are not exactly 0 or 1

Situations where it is unnecessary to use the correction factor for other fixed effects included in the model

If we assume that the incidence matrices for the contemporary group effect X_1 and the other fixed effects X_2 are orthogonal, then $X_1'X_2 = 0$. In this scenario, the correction factor for the other fixed effects included in the model becomes zero and the calculation of PEVMean from the variance–covariance matrix of estimated fixed effects can be done as if the contemporary group is the only fixed effect. An individual element ij of matrix $X_1'X_2$ represents the number of observations of effect j in contemporary group level i if the other effect is a factor and is the sum of the covariate values for effect j in the contemporary level i if effect j is continuous. In practice, $X_1'X_2 = 0$ would be limited to the situation where the other fixed effects considered in the model are continuous, centred on zero and balanced across all levels of the contemporary group effect, i.e. the mean of the other variables is zero for all contemporary group levels.

Situations where parts of the correction factor for the other fixed effects in the model can be ignored

If all the columns of the other fixed effects present in the model lie in the null-space of $X_1' Var(\mathbf{y})^{-1}$, where X_1 is the incidence matrix of contemporary group effects and $Var(\mathbf{y}) = \mathbf{Z} Var(\mathbf{u}) \mathbf{Z}' + \sigma_e^2 \mathbf{I}$ is the variance–covariance matrix of the observations, then $Var(\hat{\boldsymbol{\beta}}_2, \hat{\boldsymbol{\beta}}_1) = 0$ and the correction factor for the other fitted fixed effects reduces to $(X_1'X_1)^{-1}X_1'X_2 Var(\hat{\boldsymbol{\beta}}_2)X_2'X_1(X_1'X_1)^{-1}$. The variance–covariance matrix of estimated contemporary group effects $Var(\hat{\boldsymbol{\beta}}_1)$ is unchanged when moving from the reduced model, (only contemporary group is fitted) compared to a full model where other fixed effects are fitted. To measure how close the model considered could come to such a state, the covariance ratio [26] was considered. The covariance ratio is the ratio of determinants for $Var(\hat{\boldsymbol{\beta}})$ between a full and reduced model. Therefore, it is similar to the γ statistic proposed by Foulley et al.

[3]. In our particular case, we considered the covariance ratio of contemporary group effects between a full and reduced model. If the correction factor reduced to $(X_1'X_1)^{-1}X_1'X_2 Var(\hat{\boldsymbol{\beta}}_2)X_2'X_1(X_1'X_1)^{-1}$, the covariance ratio was equal to 1. A covariance ratio that diverged from 1 indicates that estimates of $Var(\hat{\boldsymbol{\beta}})_1$ are influenced by the addition of more fixed effects. The covariance ratios of the three models fitted are in Table 4. The covariance ratio for Model 1 compared to Model 2 (0.406 when **A** was used and 0.452 when **H** was used) is close to one, while for Model 1 compared to Model 3, it was not (0.005 when **A** was used, 0.006 when **H** was used).

Correction factor for other fixed effects in the model when those effects are balanced across contemporary groups.

When all other effects in the model are balanced across contemporary group, defined as having equal means (if continuous) or occurring for the same proportion of observations (if factors) for all contemporary groups, then the elements in each row of the incidence matrix $(X_1'X_1)^{-1}X_1'X_2$ are the same. Therefore, $(X_1'X_1)^{-1}X_1'X_2 = \mathbf{1r}'$, where $\mathbf{1}$ and $\mathbf{r}$ are column vectors of length p_1 and p_2, respectively, and p_1, p_2 are the number of contemporary group and non-contemporary group effect levels in the model. As a consequence, $(X_1'X_1)^{-1}X_1'X_2 Var(\hat{\boldsymbol{\beta}}_2)X_2'X_1(X_1'X_1)^{-1} = \mathbf{1r}' Var(\hat{\boldsymbol{\beta}}_2)\mathbf{r1}' = \mathbf{r}' Var(\hat{\boldsymbol{\beta}}_2)\mathbf{r11}' = c\mathbf{11}'$, where c is the constant $\mathbf{r}' Var(\hat{\boldsymbol{\beta}}_2)\mathbf{r}$ and $\mathbf{11}'$ a $p_1 \times p_1$ matrix of ones. In this situation, the relationship between VED and PEVD simplifies to the result below when contemporary group is the only fixed effect fitted.

Table 4 Covariance ratio for the variance–covariance matrix of estimated contemporary group fixed effects for three models and two relationship matrices (A and H)

	$Var(\hat{\boldsymbol{\beta}})$		
	Model 1	**Model 2**	**Model 3**
A			
$Var(\hat{\boldsymbol{\beta}})^{-1}$			
Model 1	1	2.462	210.041
Model 2	0.406	1	85.239
Model 3	0.005	0.001	1
H			
$Var(\hat{\boldsymbol{\beta}})^{-1}$			
Model 1	1	2.213	166.744
Model 2	0.452	1	75.354
Model 3	0.006	0.013	1

Covariance ratio is defined as $det(Var(\hat{\boldsymbol{\beta}})_A Var(\hat{\boldsymbol{\beta}})_B^{-1})$ where A and B represent nested models. The model indicated in the column heading is A, the model in the row heading is B

$$
\begin{aligned}
PEVD_{ij} =\, & Var(\hat{\boldsymbol{\beta}}_1)_{ii} + Var(\hat{\boldsymbol{\beta}}_1)_{jj} - 2Var(\hat{\boldsymbol{\beta}}_1)_{ij} \\
& + c(\mathbf{11}')_{ii} + (\mathbf{1r}'Var(\hat{\boldsymbol{\beta}}_2, \hat{\boldsymbol{\beta}}_1))_{ii} \\
& + c(\mathbf{11}')_{jj} + (\mathbf{1r}'Var(\hat{\boldsymbol{\beta}}_2, \hat{\boldsymbol{\beta}}_1))_{jj} \\
& - 2c(\mathbf{11}')_{ij} - 2(\mathbf{1r}'Var(\hat{\boldsymbol{\beta}}_2, \hat{\boldsymbol{\beta}}_1))_{ij} \\
& + \left(Var\left(\hat{\boldsymbol{\beta}}_1, \hat{\boldsymbol{\beta}}_2\right)\mathbf{r1}'\right)_{ii} + (Var(\hat{\boldsymbol{\beta}}_1, \hat{\boldsymbol{\beta}}_2)\mathbf{r1}')_{jj} \\
& - 2(Var(\hat{\boldsymbol{\beta}}_1, \hat{\boldsymbol{\beta}}_2)\mathbf{r1}')_{ij} - \sigma_e^2(\mathbf{X}_1'\mathbf{X}_1)_{ii}^{-1} - \sigma_e^2(\mathbf{X}_1'\mathbf{X}_1)_{jj}^{-1} \\
=\, & Var(\hat{\boldsymbol{\beta}}_1)_{ii} + Var(\hat{\boldsymbol{\beta}}_1)_{jj} - 2Var(\hat{\boldsymbol{\beta}}_1)_{ij} \\
& + Var(\mathbf{r}'\hat{\boldsymbol{\beta}}_2, \hat{\boldsymbol{\beta}}_1)_i + Var(\mathbf{r}'\hat{\boldsymbol{\beta}}_2, \hat{\boldsymbol{\beta}}_1)_j \\
& - 2Var(\mathbf{r}'\hat{\boldsymbol{\beta}}_2, \hat{\boldsymbol{\beta}}_1)_j + Var(\mathbf{r}'\hat{\boldsymbol{\beta}}_2, \hat{\boldsymbol{\beta}}_1)_i \\
& + Var(\mathbf{r}'\hat{\boldsymbol{\beta}}_2, \hat{\boldsymbol{\beta}}_1)_j - 2Var(\mathbf{r}'\hat{\boldsymbol{\beta}}_2, \hat{\boldsymbol{\beta}}_1)_i \\
& - \sigma_e^2(\mathbf{X}_1'\mathbf{X}_1)_{ii}^{-1} - \sigma_e^2(\mathbf{X}_1'\mathbf{X}_1)_{jj}^{-1} \\
=\, & Var(\hat{\boldsymbol{\beta}}_1)_{ii} + Var(\hat{\boldsymbol{\beta}}_1)_{jj} - 2Var(\hat{\boldsymbol{\beta}}_1)_{ij} \\
& - \sigma_e^2(\mathbf{X}_1'\mathbf{X}_1)_{ii}^{-1} - \sigma_e^2(\mathbf{X}_1'\mathbf{X}_1)_{jj}^{-1} \\
=\, & VED_{ij} - \sigma_e^2(\mathbf{X}_1'\mathbf{X}_1)_{ii}^{-1} - \sigma_e^2(\mathbf{X}_1'\mathbf{X}_1)_{jj}^{-1}
\end{aligned}
$$

Sensitivity to the mean of continuous covariates fitted in the model

To obtain the relationship between PEVMean and the variance–covariance matrix of estimated contemporary group fixed effects, the intercept must be absorbed into the contemporary group effects. The variance of the intercept depends on the mean of the variables included in the model [9]. By absorbing the intercept into the contemporary groups, $Var(\hat{\boldsymbol{\beta}}_1)$ becomes dependent on the means of the other variables included in the model. Since PEVMean itself is invariant to rescaling of continuous fixed effects, the impact of the correction factor for the other fixed effects in the model is itself influenced by the means of the other effects. This can be illustrated by fitting a fourth model. Model 4 is equivalent to Model 3 except that the weaning weight covariate is standardised to have a mean of 0 and standard deviation of 1. The zero mean for weaning weight minimises the influence of the weaning weight covariate on $Var(\hat{\boldsymbol{\beta}}_1)$. While the PEVMean was unchanged when moving from Model 3 to Model 4, Additional file 3: Figure S3 shows that the correction factor for the other fixed effects in the model was reduced. It also reduced but did not eliminate the overestimation of flock correlation when using CR, particularly when the flock correlation was near zero.

Link to postulated mixed model r^2 and correction factor for the inclusion of other fixed effects

To measure the impact of including fixed effects other than contemporary group into the model, we considered the coefficient of determination (r^2). Unlike the general linear model, linear mixed models do not have a commonly agreed r^2 statistic. We considered two methods to measure r_m^2 for the fixed effect component of the model. The first was marginal r^2 [27]. This was calculated as:

$$
r_m^2 = \frac{Var(\hat{y})}{Var(\hat{y}) + \sigma_e^2 + \sigma_g^2},
$$

where $\hat{y}$ were the predicted values for the observation without the random effects. The second method was r_β^2 [28]. This is calculated as a function of the Wald F statistic, $\hat{\boldsymbol{\beta}}'\mathbf{V}(\hat{\boldsymbol{\beta}})^{-1}\hat{\boldsymbol{\beta}}$ with $n - p$ as ν, where n was the number of observations, and p was the number of fixed effects to be estimated.

$$
r_\beta^2 = \frac{(q - 1)F(\hat{\boldsymbol{\beta}}, Var(\mathbf{Y}))}{\nu + (q - 1)F(\hat{\boldsymbol{\beta}}, Var(\mathbf{Y}))}.
$$

While we did find the r^2 statistics useful for indicating improvement in model fit, we did not find any relationship with the correction factor. Therefore, r^2 statistics like those considered should not be used as a diagnostic of the impact that the inclusion of additional fixed effects in the model had on the correction factor.

A diagnostic to assess the need to include the correction factor

The value of the correction factor for calculating PEVMean from $Var(\hat{\boldsymbol{\beta}})$ can be assessed as the trace of the matrix of the correction factor for other fixed effects included in the model. Specifically, the trace was considered as a diagnostic to determine whether it is appropriate to just use $Var(\hat{\boldsymbol{\beta}}_1) - (\mathbf{X}'\mathbf{X})^{-1}\sigma_e^2$ as an approximation to PEVMean. The trace of the correction factor can be written as $2Tr(Var(\hat{\boldsymbol{\beta}}_2, \hat{\boldsymbol{\beta}}_1)(\mathbf{X}_1'\mathbf{X}_1)^{-1}\mathbf{X}_1' + Tr(Var(\hat{\boldsymbol{\beta}}_2)\mathbf{X}_2'\mathbf{X}_1(\mathbf{X}_1'\mathbf{X}_1)^{-1}(\mathbf{X}_1'\mathbf{X}_1)^{-1}\mathbf{X}_1'\mathbf{X}_2)$. This formulation was less computationally demanding when the number of contemporary group fixed effect levels was greater than the number of other fixed effect levels. Traces that were further from zero indicated that the correction factor had a greater impact in the calculation of PEVMean. Table 5 provides the traces of the correction factor for the inclusion of other fixed effects in the model. For Model 3 the trace is approximately 35 times greater than for Model 2, which suggests that ignoring the other fixed effects in Model 3 results in a poor approximation of PEVMean.

Table 5 Trace of the correction factor for the inclusion of additional fixed effects

Model	A	H
2	−0.3310	−0.3298
3	−11.4795	−11.5005

Utility of the method

Solving blocks of the mixed model equations

The exact PEVMean given by function 3 requires the calculation of the variance–covariance matrix for all estimated fixed effects in the model. This can be done directly by calculating $(\mathbf{X}'Var(\mathbf{y})^{-1}\mathbf{X})^{-1}$, where $Var(\mathbf{y}) = \mathbf{Z}Var(\mathbf{u})\mathbf{Z}' + \sigma_e^2\mathbf{I}$. This is computationally demanding since the direct inversion of $Var(\mathbf{y})$ requires $n^2(n+1)/2$ operations, where n is the number of observations. An alternative method is to find the block of the mixed model equation inverse corresponding to the fixed effects. Mathur et al. [16] wrote a program that calculated these blocks for CR. Many software programs have in-built functions that can be used to solve equations of the form $\mathbf{AX} = \mathbf{B}$, where $\mathbf{A}$ and $\mathbf{B}$ are known matrices. Examples include the `solve()` function in R [25]. Using this method to find $Var(\hat{\boldsymbol{\beta}})$, $\mathbf{A}$ would be the mixed model equation matrix and $\mathbf{B}$ would be the first p columns of the identity matrix, where p is the number of fixed effects to be estimated in the model. The elements of PEVMean can then be calculated from $Var(\hat{\boldsymbol{\beta}})$. However this method would also calculate $Var(\hat{\boldsymbol{\beta}}, \hat{\mathbf{u}} - \mathbf{u})$ in addition to $Var(\hat{\boldsymbol{\beta}})$.

Calculating PEVMean from $Var(\hat{\boldsymbol{\beta}})$

After $Var(\hat{\boldsymbol{\beta}})$ is obtained, the number of operations required to obtain the components that go into function 3 is as follows. To avoid re-calculation of the same matrix, we assume that these steps are done in the order outlined in Table 6. Since $\mathbf{X}'\mathbf{X}$ is required to form the mixed model equations, $\mathbf{X}_1'\mathbf{X}_2$ is assumed to have no cost. In the number of operations, p_1 represents the number of contemporary group fixed effects and p_2 represents the number of other fixed effects estimated.

In the models we considered $p_1 >> p_2$. This means that the number of operations required to obtain $PEVMean$ after $Var(\hat{\boldsymbol{\beta}})$ was obtained is of order p_1^2.

Conclusions

For single-trait models in which only one random effect is fitted, a function of the variance-covariance matrix of all fixed effects fitted can be used to calculate the prediction error variance-covariance matrix averaged by contemporary group. Depending on the other fixed effects included, the use of just the elements of the variance–covariance matrix of the estimated contemporary group fixed effects can give suboptimal estimates of connectedness. This is particularly the case when correlation-based measures are used, such as CR. These inaccuracies can be reduced by centring any continuous variables included in the model to have a mean of zero. When difference-based measures such as PEVD are used, the need to consider the other fitted fixed effects is eliminated when those effects are balanced across the contemporary groups effect levels. Nevertheless, there was always a notable improvement in the approximation of PEVMean by subtracting $\sigma_e^2(\mathbf{X}_1'\mathbf{X}_1)^{-1}$ from $Var(\hat{\boldsymbol{\beta}}_1)$.

The proposed formula for calculating PEVMean from $Var(\hat{\boldsymbol{\beta}})$ can be also used to calculate the flock correlation, the prediction error variance of differences, and the PEV component of the coefficient of determination for contrasts between contemporary groups by calculating only the block of the inverse of the mixed model equations corresponding to the fixed effects, rather than the full prediction-error variance–covariance matrix of random effects. By being able to calculate PEVMean exactly from functions of $Var(\hat{\boldsymbol{\beta}})$, a more accurate assessment of connectedness can be obtained in livestock genetic evaluation compared to traditional fixed effect based measures such as connectedness rating and VED, without the computational cost of PEV based measures. A future goal of research is to give tractable solutions to calculate this for industry evaluations which may include millions of animals. In addition, tens of thousands of these animals will typically have genotype data and in the future this number will increase and

Table 6 Operations required to calculate the correction factor

Step	Component	Number of operations
1	$(\mathbf{X}_1'\mathbf{X}_1)^{-1}$	p_1
2	$\mathbf{X}_1'\mathbf{X}_2 Var(\hat{\boldsymbol{\beta}}_2)\mathbf{X}_2'\mathbf{X}_1$	$p_1 p_2^2 + p_1^2 p_2$
3	Multiplying $(\mathbf{X}_1'\mathbf{X}_1)^{-1}$ on both sides of step 2	$2p_1^2$
4	$\mathbf{X}_1'\mathbf{X}_2 Var(\hat{\boldsymbol{\beta}}_2, \hat{\boldsymbol{\beta}}_1)$	$p_1^2 p_2$
5	Multiplying $(\mathbf{X}_1'\mathbf{X}_1)^{-1}$ on the left side of step 4	p_1^2
6	Addition to obtain correction factor for other fixed effects	$2p_1^2$
7	Addition of step 6 to $Var(\hat{\boldsymbol{\beta}}_1)$	p_1^2
8	Completing $PEVMean$	p_1
	Total calculations	$2p_1 + 6p_1^2 + p_1 p_2(2p_1 + p_2)$

hence will require a re-evaluation of the connectedness measures used in the New Zealand sheep industry. Better measures of genetic connectedness between groups will allow seed stock breeders to make better decisions on the appropriateness of comparing animals in evaluations, which will, in an industry such as the New Zealand sheep industry, lead to increased genetic gain.

Appendix

Derivation of the *PEVMean* as a function of the variance–covariance matrix of estimated fixed effects only

The equation of a linear mixed model has the following matrix form:

$$\mathbf{y} = \mathbf{X}\boldsymbol{\beta} + \mathbf{Z}\mathbf{u} + \mathbf{e}, Var(\mathbf{u}) = \mathbf{G}, Var(\mathbf{e}) = \mathbf{R}.$$

Solutions for $\boldsymbol{\beta}, \mathbf{u}$ can be found by solving the mixed model equations derived by Henderson [29]:

$$\mathbf{X}'\mathbf{R}^{-1}\mathbf{X}\hat{\boldsymbol{\beta}} + \mathbf{X}'\mathbf{R}^{-1}\mathbf{Z}\hat{\mathbf{u}} = \mathbf{X}'\mathbf{R}^{-1}\mathbf{y} \quad (1)$$

$$\mathbf{Z}'\mathbf{R}^{-1}\mathbf{X}\hat{\boldsymbol{\beta}} + (\mathbf{Z}'\mathbf{R}^{-1}\mathbf{Z} + \mathbf{G}^{-1})\hat{\mathbf{u}} = \mathbf{Z}'\mathbf{R}^{-1}\mathbf{y}. \quad (2)$$

The exact relationship between *PEV* and the variance of estimated fixed effects $Var(\hat{\boldsymbol{\beta}})$ was found by taking the variance on both sides of Eq. (1) and applying the results for the variances from mixed model equations [10].

Formula for function 2

If contemporary group is the only fixed effect included, $\mathbf{X}'\mathbf{X}$ is a diagonal matrix with the entry $(\mathbf{X}'\mathbf{X})_{ii}$ corresponding to the number of observations in contemporary group i. The entries of $\mathbf{X}'\mathbf{Z}$ are an incidence matrix indicating which contemporary group a particular animal belongs to. In this setting, the matrix $(\mathbf{X}'\mathbf{X})^{-1}\mathbf{X}'\mathbf{Z}$ is the linear transformation from $\mathbf{u}$ to $\bar{\mathbf{u}}$, where $\bar{\mathbf{u}}$ is the vector of breeding values averaged by contemporary group. This simplifies Eq. 4 as follows.

$$(\mathbf{X}'\mathbf{X})^{-1} Var(\mathbf{X}'\mathbf{Z}(\hat{\mathbf{u}} - \mathbf{u}))(\mathbf{X}'\mathbf{X})^{-1} = (\mathbf{X}'\mathbf{X})^{-1}(Var(\mathbf{X}'\mathbf{X}\hat{\boldsymbol{\beta}})$$
$$- \sigma_e^2 \mathbf{X}'\mathbf{X})(\mathbf{X}'\mathbf{X})^{-1}$$
$$Var((\mathbf{X}'\mathbf{X})^{-1}\mathbf{X}'\mathbf{Z}(\hat{\mathbf{u}} - \mathbf{u})) = Var(\hat{\boldsymbol{\beta}}) - \sigma_e^2(\mathbf{X}'\mathbf{X})^{-1}$$
$$Var(\overline{\hat{\mathbf{u}} - \mathbf{u}}) = Var(\hat{\boldsymbol{\beta}}) - \sigma_e^2(\mathbf{X}'\mathbf{X})^{-1}$$

Thus, in this scenario $PEVMean = Var(\hat{\boldsymbol{\beta}}) - \sigma_e^2(\mathbf{X}'\mathbf{X})^{-1}$ as shown above.

Formula for function 3

If contemporary group is not the only fixed effect included, the incidence matrix, $\mathbf{X}$, is split into two parts. $\mathbf{X}_1$ is the incidence matrix for contemporary groups and $\mathbf{X}_2$ is the incidence matrix for other contemporary

$$Var(\mathbf{X}'\mathbf{R}^{-1}\mathbf{X}\hat{\boldsymbol{\beta}} + \mathbf{X}'\mathbf{R}^{-1}\mathbf{Z}\hat{\mathbf{u}}) = Var(\mathbf{X}'\mathbf{R}^{-1}\mathbf{y})$$
$$Var(\mathbf{X}'\mathbf{R}^{-1}\mathbf{X}\hat{\boldsymbol{\beta}}) + Var(\mathbf{X}'\mathbf{R}^{-1}\mathbf{Z}\hat{\mathbf{u}}) = Var(\mathbf{X}'\mathbf{R}^{-1}\mathbf{y})$$
$$\mathbf{X}'\mathbf{R}^{-1}(\mathbf{X} Var(\hat{\boldsymbol{\beta}})\mathbf{X}' + \mathbf{Z} Var(\hat{\mathbf{u}})\mathbf{Z}')\mathbf{R}^{-1}\mathbf{X} = \mathbf{X}'\mathbf{R}^{-1}(Var(\mathbf{Z}\mathbf{u}) + Var(\mathbf{e}))\mathbf{R}^{-1}\mathbf{X}$$
$$\mathbf{X}'\mathbf{R}^{-1}(\mathbf{X} Var(\hat{\boldsymbol{\beta}})\mathbf{X}' + \mathbf{Z} Var(\hat{\mathbf{u}})\mathbf{Z}')\mathbf{R}^{-1}\mathbf{X} = \mathbf{X}'\mathbf{R}^{-1}(\mathbf{Z} Var(\mathbf{u})\mathbf{Z}' + \mathbf{R})\mathbf{R}^{-1}\mathbf{X} \quad (3)$$
$$\mathbf{X}'\mathbf{R}^{-1}(\mathbf{X} Var(\hat{\boldsymbol{\beta}})\mathbf{X}' - \mathbf{R})\mathbf{R}^{-1}\mathbf{X} = \mathbf{X}'\mathbf{R}^{-1}(\mathbf{Z} Var(\mathbf{u})\mathbf{Z}' - \mathbf{Z} Var(\hat{\mathbf{u}})\mathbf{Z}')\mathbf{R}^{-1}\mathbf{X}$$
$$\mathbf{X}'\mathbf{R}^{-1}(\mathbf{X} Var(\hat{\boldsymbol{\beta}})\mathbf{X}' - \mathbf{R})\mathbf{R}^{-1}\mathbf{X} = \mathbf{X}'\mathbf{R}^{-1}\mathbf{Z}(Var(\mathbf{u}) - Var(\hat{\mathbf{u}}))\mathbf{Z}'\mathbf{R}^{-1}\mathbf{X}$$
$$\mathbf{X}'\mathbf{R}^{-1}\mathbf{X} Var(\hat{\boldsymbol{\beta}})\mathbf{X}'\mathbf{R}^{-1}\mathbf{X} - \mathbf{X}'\mathbf{R}^{-1}\mathbf{X} = \mathbf{X}'\mathbf{R}^{-1}\mathbf{Z} Var(\hat{\mathbf{u}} - \mathbf{u})\mathbf{Z}'\mathbf{R}^{-1}\mathbf{X}$$

To simplify the result, we assumed that $\mathbf{R} = \sigma_e^2\mathbf{I}$ where $\mathbf{I}$ is the identity matrix. This simplified the result in Eq. (3) to:

$$\mathbf{X}'\mathbf{X} Var(\hat{\boldsymbol{\beta}})\mathbf{X}'\mathbf{X} - \sigma_e^2\mathbf{X}'\mathbf{X} = \mathbf{X}'\mathbf{Z} Var(\hat{\mathbf{u}} - \mathbf{u})\mathbf{Z}'\mathbf{X}$$
$$Var(\mathbf{X}'\mathbf{X}\hat{\boldsymbol{\beta}}) - \sigma_e^2\mathbf{X}'\mathbf{X} = Var(\mathbf{X}'\mathbf{Z}(\hat{\mathbf{u}} - \mathbf{u})). \quad (4)$$

For the derivations of function 2 and function 3, it was assumed that the intercept was absorbed into the contemporary group fixed effect.

groups. In this setting, the matrix $(\mathbf{X}_1'\mathbf{X}_1)^{-1}\mathbf{X}_1'\mathbf{Z}$ is the linear transformation from u to $\bar{u}$ with respect to contemporary groups. To derive function 3, Eq. 4 was re-written partitioning $\mathbf{X}$ as described and similarly partitioning $\hat{\boldsymbol{\beta}}$ into $\hat{\boldsymbol{\beta}}_1, \hat{\boldsymbol{\beta}}_2$, which are the vectors of estimated contemporary group and non-contemporary group fixed effects respectively.

$$
\begin{pmatrix} \mathbf{X}_1'\mathbf{Z} \\ \mathbf{X}_2'\mathbf{Z} \end{pmatrix} Var(\hat{\mathbf{u}} - \mathbf{u}) \begin{pmatrix} \mathbf{Z}'\mathbf{X}_1 & \mathbf{Z}'\mathbf{X}_2 \end{pmatrix}
$$

$$
= \begin{pmatrix} \mathbf{X}_1'\mathbf{X}_1 & \mathbf{X}_1'\mathbf{X}_2 \\ \mathbf{X}_2'\mathbf{X}_1 & \mathbf{X}_2'\mathbf{X}_2 \end{pmatrix} \begin{pmatrix} Var(\hat{\boldsymbol{\beta}}_1) & Var(\hat{\boldsymbol{\beta}}_1, \hat{\boldsymbol{\beta}}_2) \\ Var(\hat{\boldsymbol{\beta}}_2, \hat{\boldsymbol{\beta}}_1) & Var(\hat{\boldsymbol{\beta}}_2) \end{pmatrix}
$$

$$
\times \begin{pmatrix} \mathbf{X}_1'\mathbf{X}_1 & \mathbf{X}_1'\mathbf{X}_2 \\ \mathbf{X}_2'\mathbf{X}_1 & \mathbf{X}_2'\mathbf{X}_2 \end{pmatrix} - \sigma_e^2 \begin{pmatrix} \mathbf{X}_1'\mathbf{X}_1 & \mathbf{X}_1'\mathbf{X}_2 \\ \mathbf{X}_2'\mathbf{X}_1 & \mathbf{X}_2'\mathbf{X}_2 \end{pmatrix}. \tag{5}
$$

To complete the derivation, the top left block of Equation 5 which corresponds to $Var(\mathbf{X}_1'\mathbf{Z}(\hat{\mathbf{u}} - \mathbf{u}))$ was re-arranged.

Author details

[1] Department of Mathematics and Statistics, University of Otago, Cumberland St., Dunedin 9016, New Zealand. [2] AgResearch, Invermay Research Centre, Puddle Alley, Dunedin 9053, New Zealand.

Acknowledgements

The authors wish to acknowledge NZ Seed stock farmers and Sheep Improvement Limited for providing access to datasets and Beef and Lamb NZ Genetics for providing funding and support for this work. We would also like to thank Benoit Auvray, Sheryl Anne Newman and anonymous reviewers for their comments and suggestions.

Competing interests

The authors declare that they have no competing interests.

$$
Var(\mathbf{X}_1'\mathbf{Z}(\hat{\mathbf{u}} - \mathbf{u})) = \mathbf{X}_1'\mathbf{X}_1 Var(\hat{\boldsymbol{\beta}}_1)\mathbf{X}_1'\mathbf{X}_1 + \mathbf{X}_1'\mathbf{X}_2 Var(\hat{\boldsymbol{\beta}}_2)\mathbf{X}_2'\mathbf{X}_1
$$
$$
+ \mathbf{X}_1'\mathbf{X}_2 Var(\hat{\boldsymbol{\beta}}_2, \hat{\boldsymbol{\beta}}_1)\mathbf{X}_1'\mathbf{X}_1 + \mathbf{X}_1'\mathbf{X}_1 Var(\hat{\boldsymbol{\beta}}_1, \hat{\boldsymbol{\beta}}_2)\mathbf{X}_2'\mathbf{X}_1 - \sigma_e^2 \mathbf{X}_1'\mathbf{X}_1
$$
$$
Var((\mathbf{X}_1'\mathbf{X}_1)^{-1}\mathbf{X}_1'\mathbf{Z}(\hat{\mathbf{u}} - \mathbf{u})) = (\mathbf{X}_1'\mathbf{X}_1)^{-1}\mathbf{X}_1'\mathbf{X}_1 Var(\hat{\boldsymbol{\beta}}_1)\mathbf{X}_1'\mathbf{X}_1(\mathbf{X}_1'\mathbf{X}_1)^{-1}
$$
$$
+ (\mathbf{X}_1'\mathbf{X}_1)^{-1}\mathbf{X}_1'\mathbf{X}_2 Var(\hat{\boldsymbol{\beta}}_2, \hat{\boldsymbol{\beta}}_1)\mathbf{X}_1'\mathbf{X}_1(\mathbf{X}_1'\mathbf{X}_1)^{-1}
$$
$$
+ (\mathbf{X}_1'\mathbf{X}_1)^{-1}\mathbf{X}_1'\mathbf{X}_1 Var(\hat{\boldsymbol{\beta}}_1, \hat{\boldsymbol{\beta}}_2)\mathbf{X}_2'\mathbf{X}_1(\mathbf{X}_1'\mathbf{X}_1)^{-1}
$$
$$
+ (\mathbf{X}_1'\mathbf{X}_1)^{-1}\mathbf{X}_1'\mathbf{X}_2 Var(\hat{\boldsymbol{\beta}}_2)\mathbf{X}_2'\mathbf{X}_1(\mathbf{X}_1'\mathbf{X}_1)^{-1}
$$
$$
- \sigma_e^2 (\mathbf{X}_1'\mathbf{X}_1)^{-1}\mathbf{X}_1'\mathbf{X}_1(\mathbf{X}_1'\mathbf{X}_1)^{-1}
$$
$$
Var(\overline{\hat{\mathbf{u}} - \mathbf{u}}) = Var(\hat{\boldsymbol{\beta}}_1) + (\mathbf{X}_1'\mathbf{X}_1)^{-1}\mathbf{X}_1'\mathbf{X}_2 Var(\hat{\boldsymbol{\beta}}_2)\mathbf{X}_2'\mathbf{X}_1(\mathbf{X}_1'\mathbf{X}_1)^{-1}
$$
$$
+ (\mathbf{X}_1'\mathbf{X}_1)^{-1}\mathbf{X}_1'\mathbf{X}_2 Var(\hat{\boldsymbol{\beta}}_2, \hat{\boldsymbol{\beta}}_1)
$$
$$
+ Var(\hat{\boldsymbol{\beta}}_1, \hat{\boldsymbol{\beta}}_2)\mathbf{X}_2'\mathbf{X}_1(\mathbf{X}_1'\mathbf{X}_1)^{-1} - \sigma_e^2 (\mathbf{X}_1'\mathbf{X}_1)^{-1}
$$

Thus in this scenario, $PEVMean = Var(\hat{\boldsymbol{\beta}}_1) + (\mathbf{X}_1'\mathbf{X}_1)^{-1}\mathbf{X}_1'\mathbf{X}_2 Var(\hat{\boldsymbol{\beta}}_2)\mathbf{X}_2'\mathbf{X}_1(\mathbf{X}_1'\mathbf{X}_1)^{-1} + (\mathbf{X}_1'\mathbf{X}_1)^{-1}\mathbf{X}_1'\mathbf{X}_2 Var(\hat{\boldsymbol{\beta}}_2, \hat{\boldsymbol{\beta}}_1) + Var(\hat{\boldsymbol{\beta}}_1, \hat{\boldsymbol{\beta}}_2)\mathbf{X}_2'\mathbf{X}_1(\mathbf{X}_1'\mathbf{X}_1)^{-1} - \sigma_e^2 (\mathbf{X}_1'\mathbf{X}_1)^{-1}$ as shown above.

Additional files

> **Additional file 1: Figure S1.** A pdf file containing figures showing the differences in PEVMean between when **H** as opposed to **A** was used to model $Var(\mathbf{u})$. First column is diagonal elements, second column is off-diagonal elements. The red line indicates where the element of PEVMean was equal if either **H** and **A** was used.
>
> **Additional file 1: Figure S2.** A pdf file containing figures showing the relationship between flock harmonic mean and the CR when flock correlation is below 0.01 and **A** was used. The left hand side is model 2, the right side is model 3.
>
> **Additional file 1: Figure S3.** A pdf file containing figures showing the relationship of the correction factor and CR between Models 3 and 4 when **A** was used. The first column is Correction factor. The second column is CR. The red line on second column is equality.

Authors' contributions

JH derived the equations, wrote and ran the code and drafted the manuscript. JH, ML and KD interpreted the results. ML and KD revised, improved the manuscript and contributed to the design of the study. All authors read and approved the final manuscript.

References

1. Campbell AW, Knowler K, Behrent M, Jopson NB, Cruickshank G, McEwan JC, et al. The alliance central progeny test: preliminary results and future directions. Proc N Z Soc Anim Prod. 2003;63:197–200.
2. Young MJ, Newman SA. SIL-ACE-increasing access to genetic information for sheep farmers. Proc N Z Soc Anim Prod. 2009;69:153–54.
3. Foulley JL, Bouix J, Goffinet B, Elsen JM. In: Gianola D, Hammond K, editors. Advances in statistical methods for genetic improvement of livestock, Chap 13. Berlin: Springer; 1990. p. 277–308.
4. Foulley J, Hanocq E, Boichard D. A criterion for measuring the degree of connectedness in linear models of genetic evaluation. Genet Sel Evol. 1992;24:315–30.
5. Laloë D. Precision and information in linear models of genetic evaluation. Genet Sel Evol. 1993;25:557–76.
6. Laloë D, Phocas F, Ménissier F. Considerations on measures of precision and connectedness in mixed linear models of genetic evaluation. Genet Sel Evol. 1996;28:359–78.
7. McLean RA, Sanders WL, Stroup WW. A unified approach to mixed linear models. Am Stat. 1991;45:54–64.
8. Kerr RJ, Dutkowski GW, Jansson G, Persson T, Westin J. Connectedness among test series in mixed linear models of genetic evaluation for forest trees. Tree Genet Genomes. 2015;11:67.
9. Searle SR. Linear models. New York: Wiley; 1971.
10. Henderson CR. Applications of linear models in animal breeding. Guelph: University of Guelph; 1984.

11. Fouilloux MN, Clément V, Laloë D. Measuring connectedness among herds in mixed linear models: from theory to practice in large-sized genetic evaluations. Genet Sel Evol. 2008;40:145–59.

12. Kennedy BW, Trus D. Considerations on genetic connectedness between management units under an animal model. J Anim Sci. 1993;71:2341–52.

13. Kuehn LA. Implications of connectedness in the genetic evaluation of livestock. PhD thesis, Virginia Polytechnic Institute and State University. 2005.

14. Kuehn LA, Lewis RM, Notter DR. Managing the risk of comparing estimated breeding values across flocks or herds through connectedness: a review and application. Genet Sel Evol. 2007;39:225–47.

15. Lewis RM, Crump RE, Simm G, Thompson RR. Assessing connectedness in across-flock genetic evaluations. In: Proceedings of the British society of animal science annual meeting, 23–25 March 1998; Scarborough. 1999. p. 121.

16. Mathur PK, Sullivan BP, Chesnais JP. Measuring connectedness: concept and application to a large industry breeding program. In: Proceedings of the 7th world congress on genetics applied to livestock production, 19–23 August 2002; Montpellier; 200.

17. Sorensen DA, Kennedy B. The use of the relationship matrix to account for genetic drift variance in the analysis of genetic experiments. Theor Appl Genet. 1983;66:217–20.

18. Roso VM. Genetic evaluation of multi-breed beef cattle.PhD thesis, University of Guelph; 2004.

19. Roso VM, Schenkel FS, Miller SP. Degree of connectedness among groups of centrally tested beef bulls. Can J Anim Sci. 2004;84:37–47.

20. Holmes JB, Auvray B, Newman SA, Dodds KG, Lee MA. A comparison of genetic connectedness measures using data from the NZ sheep industry. Proc Assoc Adv Breed Genet. 2015;21:469–72.

21. Meuwissen T, Luo Z. Computing inbreeding coefficients in large populations. Genet Sel Evol. 1992;24:305–13.

22. VanRaden PM. Efficient methods to compute genomic predictions. J Dairy Sci. 2008;91:4414–23.

23. Aguilar I, Misztal I, Johnson DL, Legarra A, Tsuruta S, Lawlor TJ. Hot topic: A unified approach to utilize phenotypic, full pedigree, and genomic information for genetic evaluation of holstein final score. J Dairy Sci. 2010;93:743–52.

24. Gogel BJ, Gilmour AR, Welham SJ, Cullis BR, Thompson R. ASReml update what's new in release 4.1.2015. https://www.vsni.co.uk/resources/documentation/asreml-user-guide/.

25. R Core Team. R: A Language and Environment for Statistical Computing. Vienna: R Foundation for Statistical Computing; 2013. R Foundation for Statistical Computing. http://www.R-project.org/.

26. Loy A, Hoffman H. Diagnostic tools for hierarchical linear models. WIREs Comput Stat. 2013;5:48–61.

27. Nakagawa S, Schielzeth H. A general and simplemethod for obtaining R^2 from generalized linear mixed-effects models. Meth Ecol Evol. 2013;4:133–42.

28. Edwards LJ, Muller KE, Wolfinger RD, Qaqish BF, Schabenberger O. An R^2 statistic for fixed effects in the linear mixed model. Stat Med. 2008;27:6137–57.

29. Henderson CR, Kempthorne O, Searle SR, von Krosigk CM. The estimation of enivironmental and genetic trends from records subject to culling. Biometrics. 1959;15:192–218.

14

Thermal sensitivity of growth indicates heritable variation in 1-year-old rainbow trout (*Oncorhynchus mykiss*)

Matti Janhunen[1]*, Juha Koskela[2], Nguyễn Hữu Ninh[3], Harri Vehviläinen[1], Heikki Koskinen[4], Antti Nousiainen[4] and Ngô Phú Thỏa[5]

Abstract

Background: Rainbow trout is an important aquaculture species, which has a worldwide distribution across various production environments. The diverse locations of trout farms involve remarkable variation in environmental factors such as water temperature, which is of major importance for the performance of fish. Thus, robust fish that could thrive under different and suboptimal thermal conditions is a desirable goal for trout breeding. Using a split-family experimental design (40 full-/half-sib groups) for a rainbow trout population derived from the Finnish national breeding program, we studied how two different rearing temperatures (14 and 20 °C) affect feed intake, growth rate and feed conversion ratio in 1-year-old fish. Furthermore, we quantified the additive genetic (co-)variation for daily growth coefficient (DGC) and its thermal sensitivity (TS), defined as the slope of the growth reaction norm between the two temperatures.

Results: The fish showed consistently lower feed intake, faster growth and better feed conversion ratio at the lower temperature. Heritability of TS of DGC was moderate (h^2_{TS} = 0.24). The co-heritability parameter derived from selection index theory, which describes the heritable variance of TS, was negative when the intercept was placed at the lower temperature (−0.28). This resulted in moderate accuracy of selection. At the higher temperature, co-heritability of TS was positive (0.20). The genetic correlation between DGC and its TS was strongly negative (−0.64) when the intercept was at the lower temperature and positive (0.38) but not significantly different from zero at the higher temperature.

Conclusions: The considerable amount of genetic variation in TS of growth indicates a potential for selection response and thus for targeted genetic improvement in TS. The negative genetic correlation between DGC and its TS suggests that selection for high growth rate at the lower temperature will result in more temperature-sensitive fish. Instead, the correlated response of TS is less pronounced if the selection for a higher DGC occurred at the higher temperature. It seems possible to control the correlated genetic change of TS while selecting for fast growth across environments, especially if measurements from both environments are available and breeding values for reaction norm slope are directly included in the selection index.

Background

Different genotypes, which are typically referred to as sib-groups, strains or populations, may differ in their average performance response to environmental variables. In wild populations, an organism's ability to modify its phenotype in response to environmental changes (termed phenotypic plasticity) can itself be an adaptive life-history trait, which is subject to natural selection [1–4]. Phenotypic plasticity is considered synonymous to macro-environmental sensitivity, which is a more commonly used term in the animal breeding context [5]. For animal breeders, macro-environmental sensitivity is an important aspect due to its association with the animals' performance across production environments, and with their robustness (stability) and welfare [6–9].

For any measurable phenotypic trait, the macro-environmental sensitivity of a genotype can be illustrated as

*Correspondence: matti.janhunen@luke.fi
[1] Biometrical Genetics, Natural Resources Institute Finland (Luke), Myllytie 1, 31600 Jokioinen, Finland
Full list of author information is available at the end of the article

the response function with environmental change [10]. Assuming a linear reaction norm, the degree of sensitivity for a genotype can be quantified by the regression slope of a genotype's performance across an environmental gradient [11, 12]. The existence of macro-environmental sensitivity for a given trait is indicated by slopes that deviate from zero, whereas flat reaction norms across the environmental gradient axis reflect stability of the trait. Since the reaction norms also depict the extent of re-ranking among genotypes and the change in additive genetic variance with the environment (i.e., two forms of genotype × environment interaction) they can provide information about the capacity of populations and species to adapt to environmental variability [13].

The rainbow trout, *Oncorhynchus mykiss* (Walbaum), is an example of a globally important aquaculture species, which is distributed across various production environments and systems, which range from offshore net cages to land-based re-circulation facilities. The diverse geographical locations of rainbow trout farms may involve considerable variation in many abiotic (e.g., water temperature, salinity, and photoperiod) and biotic (quality of feed, pathogens and parasites) factors, which are of major importance for the performance of fish. High growth capacity may be considered worldwide as the single most economically important trait to be improved by selective breeding [14], but the capacity of fish to express the selected growth potential under variable or suboptimal environmental conditions may be constrained. Therefore, a more robust fish material with stabile growth would be an eligible product for breeding under variable environmental conditions.

Being native to cool, temperate regions of the northern hemisphere, the rainbow trout, like all other salmonids, is adapted to relatively low water temperatures [15, 16]. Stability of growth is of special importance in trout farming areas, where rearing temperatures remain constantly high or where strong seasonal warming occurs. Furthermore, due to global warming, it is likely that there will be an increasing demand in the fish farming sector for populations of more heat-tolerant trout in the future. To assess whether thermal sensitivity (TS) of growth has the potential to be changed by selection, an estimate of the additive genetic component in the slopes of reaction norms is needed. The existence of genetic variation in growth responses as the temperature changes would enable the development of more temperature-tolerant or locally-adapted populations for different thermal conditions.

In this study, we first investigated at a general (population) level how two different rearing temperatures (14 °C, namely 'low', and 20 °C, namely 'high') influence feed intake, growth and feed conversion ratio in 1-year-old rainbow trout. Second, by using a split-family design of the experiment, we quantified the additive genetic (co-) variation of growth rate (daily growth coefficient, DGC) and its TS, the latter trait being defined as the slope of the reaction norm between the two temperature conditions.

Methods
Study material
The fish used in this study were derived from the Finnish national breeding program that is maintained at the Tervo fish farm (breeding nucleus) by the Natural Resource Institute Finland (Luke). The phenotypic data comprised 800 individuals from 40 families, which were created in April 2013 using a partial factorial mating design for 35 sires and 26 dams. Each sire was mated to an average of 1.1 dams (ranging from 1 to 3) and each dam to an average of 1.5 sires (ranging from 1 to 3). The average number of offspring was 22.9 per sire (ranging from 20 to 60) and 30.8 per dam (ranging from 20 to 60). The parental fish were selected using a multi-trait selection index with the main weight on improved growth (50% of the index). The pedigree file included 1661 individuals and nine generations tracing back to the base population established in 1989 and 1990 (see Additional file 1).

Rearing protocol
In this study, the protocols used were approved by the FGFRI Animal Care Committee, Helsinki, Finland.

The first 6 months of rearing took place in the breeding nucleus, where the full-sib families were reared separately in round 150-L indoor tanks until tagging. Variation in rearing temperature followed variation in ambient waterway throughout that period (ranging from 0 to 20 °C from the start of hatching until the start of id-tagging). During the period between January 10 and 21 2014, 25 randomly chosen fish from each studied family (73.6 ± 14.4 g, mean weight ± SD) were individually tagged with passive integrated transponders (Biomark, Inc., Boise, Idaho, USA). The tagged fish were transported into the communal pool at the Laukaa fish farm, where they were reared under ambient temperature (1–10 °C) and light conditions (day length 16.30–21.30 h during the last month prior to the experiment) until start of the experiment. In June 2014, 20 tagged fish per family were randomly sampled for the temperature trial. The rearing temperatures were gradually increased to the experimental temperatures (14 and 20 °C) in the course of 3 days. To construct a split-family design, each of the 40 families was first randomly split into two groups to be reared at low and high temperatures. These groups were evenly distributed over 4 + 4 (low temperature) and 4 + 4 (high temperature) round 0.4-m^3 green plastic tanks (two replicate tanks per family). In total, the temperature trial began with a total of 800 fish, each tank containing 50 fish (ten families and five fish from each family).

The trial was conducted from June 3 to August 12 2014. The fish were fed ad libitum 6 h per day (4.00 am to 10.00 am) using belt feeders with commercial trout diet (Raisioagro Ltd, Finland Vital pro LP; chemical composition given by the manufacturer 3.5/5.0 mm; crude protein 43.0/40.0%, crude fat 28.0/30.0%, crude fibre 1.5/1.5%, ash 6.5/6% and gross energy 24.4/24 MJ kg^{-1}). From days 1 to 10, the fish were fed with 3.5-mm pellets, followed by a mixture (1:1) of 3.5- and 5.0-mm pellets from day 11 to 20, and thereafter with 5.0-mm pellets until the end of trial. During the experiment, daily feeding amount was increased so that the share of waste feed ranged from 0 to 35% of the level of daily feed. The numbers of uneaten pellets were collected at the tank outlet in a box with a mesh bottom. The daily number of waste pellets was calculated, and their weight was estimated by multiplying the number of waste pellets by the air dry weight of a pellet. Before calculations, five 100-pellet subsamples were taken from each of the diets to measure air dry weight of pellets. The daily intake of a tank's population was calculated as the difference in weight between the fed and waste feed. Tanks of the low-temperature group were supplied with fresh lake water and tanks of the high-temperature groups were supplied with water via semi-intensive recirculating aquaculture systems (RAS; flow rate of makeup water 4–6 m^3 kg^{-1} feed). Pure oxygen was added to incoming water for both temperature groups to improve water oxygen content and baking soda was added to the RAS to maintain the pH between 6.7 and 7.0.

During the experiment, the water temperature was automatically recorded hourly (low-temperature group 14.1 ± 1.0 °C and high-temperature group 20.4 ± 1.8 °C; mean ± SD). Water oxygen saturation (%) was recorded once every second week (low-temperature/high-temperature; tank inlet: 96.5 ± 7.8/105.7 ± 4.9, tank outlet: 78.6 ± 6.8–83.3 ± 7.1/82.0 ± 3.5–86.8 ± 5.2) and other water quality parameters were recorded weekly (high temperature pH 6.9 ± 0.1, total ammonia mg L^{-1} ($NH_3 + NH_4$) 0.05 ± 0.04, un-ionized ammonia mg L^{-1} (NH_3) <0.001, nitrite mg L^{-1} (NO_2) 0.07 ± 0.01, nitrate mg L^{-1} (NO_3) 4.45 ± 0.7). A 24-h white light was provided with led lamps on the tank cover.

Measurements and calculations
Individual tag number and body weight (to the nearest g) were recorded at the beginning (129 ± 28 g; mean ± SD, $n = 800$ fish) and end of the trial (516 ± 98 g, $n = 785$). Fifteen fish died during the trial, thus only the initial body weight was available for these. Daily growth coefficients (DGC, % day^{-1}) of 785 fish were calculated as [17]:

$$DGC = \left[\left(BW_2^{1/3} - BW_1^{1/3} \right)/t \right] \times 100,$$

where BW_1 and BW_2 are the body weight of the fish at the start and end of the experiment, and t is the duration of the experiment (69–70 days) (see Additional file 2). Unlike specific growth rate (SGR), another widely used measure of fish growth rate, the DGC is independent of fish body weight and time interval between weighings at a given temperature [17]. This was also validated for rainbow trout [18].

The mean feed intake of a tank's population per day (FI_{mean}, g day^{-1}) was calculated as $FI_{cum}/t1$, where FI_{cum} is cumulative feed intake (g) of a tank's population during the period of feed intake measurements divided by the number of measurement days (t1 = 57d). The relative feed intake (FI % biomass^{-1} day^{-1}) was calculated as follows: $100 \times FI_{mean}/[(biomass_1 + biomass_2)/2]$, where biomass$_1$ and biomass$_2$ are the initial and final tank biomasses (g), respectively (see Additional file 3). Feed conversion ratio (FCR) was calculated as $FI_{mean} \times t/(biomass_2 - biomass_1)$.

Statistical analyses
The difference in DGC means between temperature treatments was tested for individual data using restricted maximum likelihood method in SAS® 9.4 (MIXED procedure; SAS® Institute, Cary, NC, USA). The model used was:

$$y_{ijk} = treatment_j + tank(treatment)_k + e_{ijk}, \quad (1)$$

where y is the observation of the ith individual, treatment$_j$ is the fixed effect of temperature treatment ($j = 1$–2), tank$_j$ is the random effect of rearing tank during the trial ($k = 1$–16), nested within treatment, and e_{ijk} is the random error term. Error variances were modelled separately for each temperature condition. In addition, degrees of freedom for the test of the fixed effect were corrected using the method of Kenward and Roger [19].

For the relative feed intake and FCR, tank population values were used as observations ($n = 8$ per treatment group) and the analysis of variance (ANOVA) was used to compare the differences in means between the treatment groups. No covariate was used in these models.

Genetic (co)variance of TS (regression slope) for DGC was estimated using a linear random regression model (also termed as a reaction norm model). (Co)variance components were estimated by restricted maximum likelihood in ASReml 3.0 [20]. Approximate standard errors were calculated with ASReml according to Fisher et al. [21]. The linear random regression model was as follows:

$$y_{hij} = \beta_{int} + \beta_{sl}X_h + a_{i,int} + a_{i,sl}X_h + e_{hij}, \quad (2)$$

where β_{int} is the fixed regression coefficient for the population intercept (int) and β_{sl} is the overall fixed regression slope (sl) of the trait on the h-th levels of an environmental gradient X_h. X_h is the regressor for the environments in which the intercept was placed either on the low or high temperature environment (at $X_h = 0$). The value of X_h was 6 for high temperature and -6 for low temperature when these environments were not used at the intercept. The scale of X is equivalent to the difference in experimental temperatures, applying a unit of 1 °C. The values of 0 and 6 (or -6) were used instead of the actual temperature values (14 and 20 °C) in order to have an appropriate interpretation for the intercept. a_i is the random genetic effect of the intercept and slope of reaction norm, $\begin{bmatrix} a, \text{int} \\ a, \text{sl} \end{bmatrix} \sim \text{MVN}[\mathbf{0}, \mathbf{A} \otimes \mathbf{G}]$, where MVN is a multivariate normal distribution, $\mathbf{A}$ is the additive genetic relationship matrix derived from the pedigree traced back to the base population, and $\mathbf{G}$ is the additive genetic covariance matrix: $\mathbf{G} = \begin{bmatrix} \sigma_{a,\text{int}}^2 & \sigma_{a,\text{int,sl}} \\ \sigma_{a,\text{int,sl}} & \sigma_{a,\text{sl}}^2 \end{bmatrix}$, where $\sigma_{a,\text{int}}^2$ and $\sigma_{a,\text{sl}}^2$ are the additive genetic variances of the intercept and slope, respectively, and $\sigma_{a,\text{int,sl}}$ is the additive genetic covariance between the intercept and slope. $e \sim N\left(\mathbf{0}, \begin{bmatrix} \mathbf{I}\sigma_{e_1}^2 & 0 \\ 0 & \mathbf{I}\sigma_{e_2}^2 \end{bmatrix}\right)$ is the random residual effect of individual i in environment h where $\mathbf{I}$ is the identity matrix with a different residual variance for each environment. In addition, the random term $\text{tank}_k \times \text{fullsib}_l$, accounting for the interaction effect of experimental tank and full-sib family (modelled without the effect on the slope; $k = 1$–8 at low temperature and 11–18 at high temperature, $l = 1$–40), was tested. This variance parameter took the permanent environment effects into

and another five sires with close to zero EBV for the slope (the least sensitive) for drawing the reaction norms. Since there were only two environments, the EBV of DGC for the high temperature environment could be derived from a simple equation:

$$\text{EBV}_{\text{DGC,highT}} = \text{EBV}_{\text{int,lowT}} + 6 \times \text{EBV}_{\text{sl}}. \quad (3)$$

The genetic values of the slope are multiplied by 6 to adjust the reaction norms to the scale of X (change of 6 °C).

For the intercept of the reaction norms, heritability (h_{int}^2) was calculated as: $h_{\text{int}}^2 = \widehat{\sigma}_{a,\text{int}}^2 / \widehat{\sigma}_{P,\text{int}}^2$, where $\widehat{\sigma}_{P,\text{int}}^2$ is the phenotypic variance of DGC in the intercept environment when $X = 0$ (equal to the sum of additive genetic and residual variance in the intercept environment: $\widehat{\sigma}_{a,\text{int}}^2 + \widehat{\sigma}_{e,\text{int}}^2$).

Because there is no phenotypic variance for the slope, the strict sense heritability cannot be calculated. Therefore, two alternative parameters were used to describe the genetic characteristics of TS. Following Sae-Lim et al. [23], the heritability for TS (h_{TS}^2) was calculated as:

$$h_{\text{TS}}^2 = \frac{\widehat{\sigma}_{a,\text{sl}}^2 \times \widehat{\sigma}_{a,X}^2}{\widehat{\sigma}_{P,\text{Total}}^2}, \quad (4)$$

where $\widehat{\sigma}_{a,\text{sl}}^2 \times \widehat{\sigma}_{a,X}^2$ is the additive genetic variance of the slope multiplied by the variance of X, respectively. $\widehat{\sigma}_X^2$ is equal to 18 in this study, since the values of X are 0 and 6. The standardized numerator in Eq. (4) is equivalent to the variance of the genotype by environment (GxE) interaction, which is independent from the different scales of an environmental variable X. The denominator $\widehat{\sigma}_{P,\text{Total}}^2$ was defined as follows:

$$\widehat{\sigma}_{P,\text{Total}}^2 = \left[\frac{(n_{\text{lowT}} - 1)\widehat{\sigma}_{P_{\text{DGC,lowT}}}^2 + (n_{\text{highT}} - 1)\widehat{\sigma}_{P_{\text{DGC,highT}}}^2 + n_{\text{lowT}}n_{\text{highT}}\left(\overline{G}_{\text{lowT}} - \overline{G}_{\text{highT}}\right)^2 / n_{\text{lowT}} + n_{\text{highT}}}{n_{\text{lowT}} + n_{\text{highT}} - 1} \right],$$

account, which were caused by different rearing tanks between and within families. However, based on the likelihood ratio test, inclusion of the $\text{tank}_k \times \text{fullsib}_l$ term did not affect the fit of the model ($\chi^2 = 0.001$, $p = 0.486$). Therefore, the results are only presented for the models in which this variance parameter was omitted.

Both the magnitude and sign of a genetic correlation between the intercept and slope, as well as the genetic variance of the trait, depend on the environment for which the intercept is defined [22]. Therefore, the random regression model was run twice, either with low ($X_{h_1} = 0$) or high temperature treatment ($X_{h_2} = 0$) as the intercept environment. The covariance between estimated breeding values (EBV) of DGC at intercept (int) and slope (sl) was graphically illustrated by choosing five sires with the highest absolute EBV (i.e., genetically the most sensitive sires)

where n is the number of individuals with a record for an animal trait, $\widehat{\sigma}_{P_{\text{DGC}}}^2$ is the estimated phenotypic variance of the trait and $\overline{G}$ is the raw phenotypic mean of DGC. The denominator was derived from Scheiner's approach, where the total phenotypic variance across environments was calculated from an analysis of variance [24]. However, it is important to note that $\widehat{\sigma}_{P,\text{Total}}^2$ is not the phenotypic variance of TS, and thus h_{TS}^2 is a descriptive rather than a predictive parameter [24]. The definition of heritability in Eq. (4) does not correspond with the conventional definition of heritability, which is the regression of breeding value on phenotype.

Following Sae-Lim et al. [23], an alternative measure that is called co-heritability was defined on the basis of selection index principles. Co-heritability is expressed as the regression coefficient (b) of the breeding value of slope on the phenotype P and defines the heritable genetic variance of TS of DGC when the selection criterion is DGC in one environment. The phenotypic variance (σ_P^2) of a trait is:

$$\sigma_P^2 = \sigma_{a,\text{int}}^2 + 2X\sigma_{a,\text{int,sl}} + X^2\sigma_{a,\text{sl}}^2 + \sigma_e^2, \tag{5}$$

Co-heritability can vary in magnitude and have both positive and negative values, depending on which environment is set as intercept environment ($X = 0$). The sign of the co-heritability explains the change in correlated response of TS when mass selection for higher phenotypic values of DGC is practiced in one environment [25]. Here, the selection on DGC was assumed to be performed either at low or high temperature (intercept environment; $X = 0$), which gives the co-heritability b in the following equation:

$$b = \frac{6\widehat{\sigma}_{a,\text{int,sl}}}{\widehat{\sigma}_{a,\text{int}}^2 + \widehat{\sigma}_{e,\text{int}}^2} = \frac{6\widehat{\sigma}_{a,\text{int,sl}}}{\widehat{\sigma}_{P_h}^2}, \tag{6}$$

where $\widehat{\sigma}_{P_h}^2$ is the phenotypic variance of DGC in the selection environment h. Co-heritability is predictive for response to selection.

The genetic correlation between intercept and slope $(r_{G(\text{int,sl})})$ was calculated as:

$$r_{G(\text{int,sl})} = \frac{\widehat{\sigma}_{a\text{int,sl}}}{\sqrt{\widehat{\sigma}_{a,\text{int}}^2 \times \widehat{\sigma}_{a,\text{sl}}^2}}. \tag{7}$$

Finally, the accuracy (r_{IH}) of EBV for TS when DGC is used as a selection criterion in one of the environments is equal to:

$$r_{\text{IH}} = \frac{\widehat{\sigma}_{a,\text{int,sl}} + X\widehat{\sigma}_{a,\text{sl}}^2}{\widehat{\sigma}_P\widehat{\sigma}_{a,\text{sl}}}, \tag{8}$$

where σ_P is the phenotypic standard deviation and $\sigma_{a,\text{sl}}$ is the slope standard deviation. Equation (4) is equivalent to that derived by Kolmodin and Bijma [25].

Results

Means of growth rate, feed intake and feed conversion ratio

The low-temperature group had slightly but significantly higher DGC means than the high-temperature group (Table 1). For 25 of the 40 families, the raw (uncorrected) DGC mean was higher at the lower temperature (Fig. 1). In contrast, both feed intake (FI) and feed conversion ratio (FCR) means were significantly lower in the low-temperature group (Table 1).

Table 1 Effect of rearing temperature (lowT 14.1 °C and highT 20.4 °C) on daily growth coefficient (DGC), feed intake (FI) and feed conversion ratio (FCR, intake/gain)

Treatment	DGC % day^{-1}	FI % biomass^{-1} day^{-1}	FCR
LowT	4.35 ± 0.63	1.66 ± 0.05	0.88 ± 0.01
HighT	4.19 ± 0.53	1.74 ± 0.05	0.97 ± 0.02
F-ratio	5.13	8.40	115.9
df	1, 13.5	1, 14	1, 14
p value	0.041	0.012	< 0.001

df = degrees of freedom

The values are raw phenotypic mean ± S.D. DGC was analysed using data from individual fish, whereas tank values were used as observations for FI and FCR

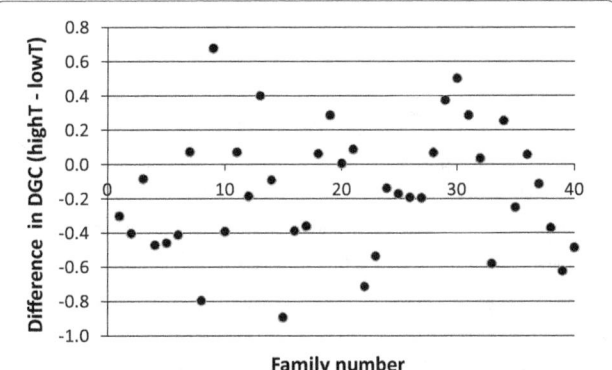

Fig. 1 Difference in daily growth coefficient means for rainbow trout families reared at low (14.1 °C) and high (20.4 °C) temperatures. Families with a negative value grew better at low than at high temperature

Genetic (co)variance of DGC and its thermal sensitivity

The heritability of the slope that defines TS was moderate ($h_{\text{TS}}^2 = 0.24$), which indicates that the additive genetic variation in TS constitutes quite a large proportion of the total phenotypic variation in DGC across environments. The co-heritability for TS was moderately negative (-0.28) when the lower temperature was assigned as the intercept environment. This indicates that a moderate accuracy of selection for TS of growth can be achieved when individual selection for DGC is practiced in a low-temperature environment ($r_{\text{IH}} = 0.44$). Instead, the co-heritability estimate was positive (0.20) when a high-temperature environment was used for the intercept. This resulted in lower accuracy (0.25), compared to that of selection at the lower temperature. For the DGC at the intercept, the heritability estimates were similar and moderate ($h_{\text{int}}^2 = 0.46$) at both temperatures (Table 2). Thus, the heritable

Table 2 Genetic parameters and genetic correlations (±their approximate standard error) between intercept and slope obtained from the random regression models for daily growth coefficient (DGC) when the intercept was placed either in the low or high temperature environment

Parameter	Intercept environment	
	LowT	HighT
$\hat{\sigma}^2_{a,\text{int}}$	0.190 (0.063)	0.130 (0.043)
$\hat{\sigma}^2_{e,\text{int}}$	0.221 (0.041)	0.156 (0.028)
$\hat{\sigma}^2_{a,\text{sl}}$	0.005 (0.002)	0.005 (0.002)
$\hat{\sigma}^2_{P,\text{Total}}$	0.354	0.354
h^2_{int}	0.463 (0.123)	0.455 (0.120)
h^2_{TS}	0.244	0.244
Co-heritability of TS	−0.284 (0.124)	0.197 (0.141)
$r_{G(\text{int,sl})}$	−0.643* (0.147)	0.376 (0.214)

$\hat{\sigma}^2_{a,\text{int}}$ = genetic variance of DGC at the intercept point; $\hat{\sigma}^2_{e,\text{int}}$ = residual variance of DGC at the intercept point; $\hat{\sigma}^2_{a,\text{sl}}$ = genetic variance of the reaction norm slope; $\hat{\sigma}^2_{P,\text{Total}}$ = total phenotypic variance of DGC across environments; h^2_{int} = heritability of DGC at the intercept ($\hat{\sigma}^2_{a,\text{int}}/\hat{\sigma}^2_{P,\text{int}}$), where $\hat{\sigma}^2_{P,\text{int}}$ is the

phenotypic variance of DGC; co-heritability of TS $\left(\frac{6\hat{\sigma}_{a,\text{int,sl}}}{\hat{\sigma}^2_{a,\text{int}}+\hat{\sigma}^2_{e,\text{int}}}\right)$, where $\hat{\sigma}_{a,\text{int,sl}}$ is

the additive genetic covariance between the intercept and slope

h^2_{TS} = heritability of the slope $\left(\frac{\hat{\sigma}^2_{a,\text{sl}}\times\hat{\sigma}^2_{a,X}}{\hat{\sigma}^2_{P,\text{Total}}}\right)$, where $\hat{\sigma}^2_{a,\text{sl}}\times\hat{\sigma}^2_{a,X}$ is the additive

genetic variance of the slope multiplied by the variance of environmental values

X, respectively; $r_{G(\text{int,sl})}$ = genetic correlation between the intercept and slope

$\left(\frac{\hat{\sigma}_{a,\text{int,sl}}}{\sqrt{\hat{\sigma}^2_{a,\text{int}}\times\hat{\sigma}^2_{a,\text{sl}}}}\right)$

* Estimate that is significantly different from 0 (95% CI does not include zero)

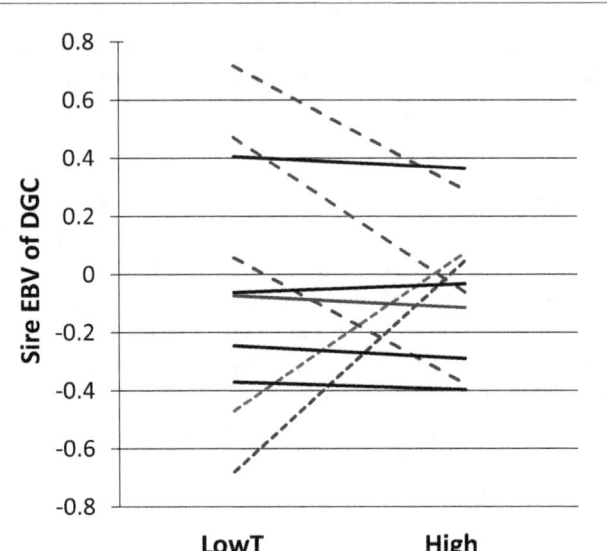

Fig. 2 Genetic reaction norms of ten rainbow trout sires across two temperature environments. Ten sires with the highest absolute EBV (five *dashed lines*) and close to zero EBV (five *solid lines*) for the slope are represented. The lines connect the sire EBV for daily growth coefficient (DGC) across the two temperature environments, when the intercept was placed at the lower temperature ($X = 0$)

potential for growth rate did not change between the two temperature conditions.

The genetic correlation between DGC and its TS was significant and strongly negative (−0.64) when the lower temperature environment was used for the intercept (Table 2). This implies that a high DGC at the lower temperature is genetically associated with increased TS across environments. However, Fig. 2 shows that the genotypes (sires) with steep slope EBV were not consistently those that showed the fastest growth potential in the intercept environment. In fact, some genotypes associated with slow growth also showed considerable sensitivity to thermal change, although in the opposite direction. When the intercept was placed at the higher temperature, the estimated genetic correlation was positive (0.38) although not statistically different from zero (based on the large standard error; Table 2). Hence, the growth potential of genotypes at the higher temperature may not show an association with differences in TS when the individuals are moved to the lower temperature.

Discussion

The temperature difference of 6 °C in our experiment was sufficient to cause substantial variation in the growth reaction norms among 1-year-old rainbow trout families, which indicated heritable differences in their TS. Indeed, the TS of DGC involved a considerable amount of genetic variation, which indicates a potential for response to targeted selection on TS. Both the descriptive parameter h^2_{TS} and the co-heritability, which explain the heritable variance of TS of growth, proved to be moderate. Our finding is not consistent with previous data in the literature, including 18 studies on fish growth traits, which showed that the heritability of macro-environmental sensitivity is generally low [23, 24]. For example, Sae-Lim et al. [23] who used a multigeneration dataset on Finnish rainbow trout did find substantial additive genetic variation in macro-environmental sensitivity of body weight, but the estimated heritability was low (0.07). In their study, the two macro-environments were a freshwater breeding nucleus and a sea test station, which had discrete locations and diverged in several environmental factors, including water salinity and temperature, and rearing system as a whole (earth-bottomed raceways vs. sea net cages, fish density, diet and feeding intensity). Our results support the idea that genetic variation in macro-environmental sensitivity would be smaller than that in the phenotypic value of the trait at the intercept point [24].

As expected, in our study, the rainbow trout showed, on average, lower feed intake, faster growth and better feed conversion ratio at the lower (14 °C) than at the higher rearing temperature (20 °C). The percentage decrease in least square means of DGC was 3.5 from low to high temperature. Under conditions, with a normal oxygen content in the water and a sufficient amount of food provided, the juvenile rainbow trout are known to perform well at temperatures of 14 to 19 °C, the optimum temperature for growth being around 17 °C; temperatures higher than 20 °C cause fast decline in growth rate [15, 16, 26, 27]. Furthermore, in general, feed intake has a higher optimum temperature and feed conversion ratio a lower optimum temperature than growth rate of fish [28]. These facts are likely responsible for the observed differences in feed intake, growth and feed conversion ratio between the experimental temperatures. During the experiment, the water quality parameters that were analyzed i.e. oxygen content, pH and nitrogen compounds were at favorable levels for salmonid aquaculture under both temperature conditions [29–31]. Thus, it is unlikely that other water quality parameters than temperature affected the observed results.

Our results show that the estimates of the genetic parameters for DGC were not dramatically influenced by the temperature environments in which the fish were reared. Environmental stress was reported to both increase and decrease the additive genetic variation in important life-history and morphological traits [32, 33]. On the one hand, the amount of environmentally-induced variation may typically increase under unfavorable conditions, and thus decrease the proportion of genetic variation and in turn, the estimated heritability e.g. [34, 35]. On the other hand, the opposite effect was reported in some animal breeding studies; challenged environments increase the genetic variance of a trait more than the residual variance, which results in higher heritability e.g. [36]. In this study, the heritability of DGC (at the intercept) was similar for the two temperatures tested. Both the genetic and residual variance proved to be larger at the lower temperature, which was presumably a milder environment in terms of growth. One can expect that the difference in heritable potential of growth (mean) manifests itself only at more extreme temperatures above or below the optimum.

Multi-trait models have been used in many studies on rainbow trout to show the presence of G × E interactions in growth [37–41]. Multi-trait and random regression models are equivalent when the dimension of the genetic covariance matrix and the fixed effects included in the models are the same [7, 23]. The genetic correlation of DGC between temperature environments was equal to 0.47 (SE 0.20) when a bivariate model was used with our data (see "Appendix"), which confirms the strong re-ranking of families across the two temperatures tested. The same parameter estimate can also be obtained from the random regression model using the genetic (co) variances. Consequently, selection in either of the temperature environments will presumably result in lower-than-expected genetic gains in the other environment, if the G × E interaction is not taken into account [41–43]. Although the genetic correlation that is estimated from a multi-trait model does express the degree of re-ranking among families, it does not describe how macro-environmental sensitivity of the trait can actually evolve across environments. One advantage of the random regression model is that the genetic parameters for macro-environmental sensitivity of a given trait can be obtained directly, which allows implementation of macro-environmental sensitivity as a trait in the selection index [5, 12, 23]. Yet, an assumption for this in our study is that the slopes, estimated from the two environment points, are linear.

Environmental sensitivity was generally shown to increase in response to selection for high phenotypic values when G × E interaction is present [5, 6, 44]. According to Jinks and Connolly [45], this should be true especially when selection for a high phenotypic value occurs in an environment that produces a phenotype with a higher value compared to another environment (synergistic selection). Correspondingly, selection for decreased environmental sensitivity may generally result in reduced mean productivity in more favorable environments [46]. In this study, the genetic correlation between DGC (at the intercept) and its TS (slope) was markedly negative, when the intercept was placed at the lower temperature. This finding is consistent with the assumption of Jinks and Connolly [45]: selection for fast growth in a more favorable temperature environment should favor increased sensitivity, that is, genotypes having steep negative slopes in reaction norms. However, genetically, the most sensitive genotypes with the steepest slope EBV may not consistently have higher genetic potential for growth at the lower temperature, compared to the least sensitive genotypes with flat slope EBV (Fig. 2). In fact, some of the genotypes with a slow growth at the lower temperature also seem to exhibit pronounced sensitivity to thermal change, but in the positive direction (i.e., growing faster at the higher temperature). Negative genetic relationships between production traits and TS have also been reported in terrestrial farm animals. For example, in pigs, a genetic correlation of −0.5 between carcass weight and sensitivity to heat stress was reported [47]. In dairy cattle, genetic correlations between milk yield and heat tolerance ranged from −0.30 to −0.45 [48, 49], whereas, in sheep, this genetic correlation was equal to −0.8 [50]. The observed negative genetic correlation between DGC and its TS and the presence of strong

G × E interaction suggest that selection decisions should be based on more than one thermal environment only. However, by applying a restricted selection criterion, the appropriate index weights that produce the desired genetic responses in both growth rate and its TS can be obtained [51]. It would then be possible to simultaneously improve the growth rate across environments and constrain the genetic change in TS.

In addition to the negative genetic correlation between DGC and its TS, the estimated co-heritability for TS was also negative when a lower temperature was used as the intercept environment. Co-heritability is an approximate measure of the inheritance of the association between DGC and its TS, when the selection criterion is DGC in one temperature environment. The co-heritability has the same sign as the correlated response to direct selection, and, unlike h_{TS}^2 and genetic correlation, this parameter also reflects the accuracy of selection [52, 53]. Our results are in line with a recent survey on aquaculture studies by Sae-Lim et al. [23], which showed that the growth of rainbow trout in one environment is genetically related to macro-environmental sensitivity across environments. However, the correlated response of TS is less pronounced if selection for improved growth rate occurs at the higher temperature. In this case, the estimated co-heritability was also associated with relatively large standard errors, which suggests that it should be treated with caution. The magnitude of the co-heritability generally increases, irrespective of its sign, with an increase in G × E interaction [23].

In this study, macro-environmental sensitivity of each genotype (fish family) was defined as the difference in DGC between two temperatures. The reaction norm slope is not an individual measure, but its breeding value can only be estimated based on the growth records of relatives in two (macro-)environments. Because the macro-environmental sensitivity is basically a progeny trait, the accuracy of selection is actually higher for the parents than for their offspring (which are used as breeding candidates). Rainbow trout, as many other aquaculture species, produces large families, which effectively contribute to the genetic analysis of macro-environmental sensitivity. Since the co-heritability of TS proved to be moderate, translating this into moderate accuracy of selection, very large family sizes are not required to reach moderate-to-high precision in slope EBV.

For a rainbow trout breeder, a stock performing well across multiple temperatures is the most desirable outcome. The least sensitive families with flat slopes of reaction norms could be selected when the breeding goal is to obtain robust fish that thrive under variable temperature conditions (increased stability). Alternatively, families with positive growth responses at higher (or lower) temperatures can be chosen when developing a locally-adapted population for a certain environment. In the latter case, TS can be viewed rather as an advantageous character to be used by selective breeding when improving the 'fit' between the selected fish and the thermal environment in which they are reared [54]. Either way, it is likely that there will be a high demand for more heat-tolerant populations of rainbow trout in the future since temperatures will continue to increase around the world due to global warming.

This study was undertaken as part of a capacity building project with the Research Institute for Aquaculture No. 1 (RIA-1) in Northern Vietnam where a national breeding program for rainbow trout was recently established from the Finnish broodstock (Research Center for Cold Water Aquaculture Species, RIA-1). Vietnam is estimated to be one of the world's most vulnerable areas for the negative impacts due to climate change. This is the case, in particular, with cold water aquaculture, for which temperature and water availability are the main limiting factors [55]. The fish used in this experiment shared relatedness with the RIA-1's broodstock. Combining our results with the records of fish performance in Vietnam under higher temperatures will enable the assessment of selective breeding possibilities in order to decrease TS in the next breeding generations. This will aid in expanding rainbow trout production to lower latitudes and altitudes with better and more stable water resources, and the fish farming sector to adapt to climate change.

Conclusions

We found that the 1-year-old rainbow trout exhibit substantial genetic variation in growth responses across different rearing temperatures. In terms of growth and feed conversion efficiency, the fish performed better predominantly under the lower (14 °C) than the higher temperature conditions (20 °C). Owing to large additive genetic variation, permanent changes in TS of growth are possible in the studied population. There is a trade-off between growth rate and its TS, since strong selection for faster growth at the lower and more favorable temperature will presumably result in less temperature-tolerant fish. However, the correlated genetic change in TS could be effectively controlled while selecting for high growth across environments, especially if slope EBV are incorporated into the selection index with appropriate weighting.

Authors' contributions

All authors participated in planning the study. MJ, HV, NHN, HK and AN contributed to data collection. MJ and JK performed data analysis. MJ was mainly responsible for drafting the manuscript, and JK, HV, NHN, AN and NPT took part in writing and commenting the text. All authors read and approved the final manuscript.

Author details

[1] Biometrical Genetics, Natural Resources Institute Finland (Luke), Myllytie 1, 31600 Jokioinen, Finland. [2] Aquaculture, Natural Resources Institute Finland (Luke), Survontie 9 A, 40500 Jyväskylä, Finland. [3] Research Institute for Aquaculture No. 3 (RIA-3), Nha Trang, Khanh Hoa, Vietnam. [4] Tervo Fish Farm, Natural Resources Institute Finland (Luke), Huuhtajantie 160, 72210 Tervo, Finland. [5] Research Institute for Aquaculture No. 1 (RIA-1), Dinh Bang, Tu Son, Bac Ninh, Vietnam.

Acknowledgements

This experiment was carried out as a part of the ICI project "Capacity building for the development of selective breeding program in Vietnam, special focus on global change and environmental sustainability". The staffs at the Tervo and Laukaa fish farms provided the expertise to maintain the experiment. MJ would like to thank Panya Sae-Lim for his advice on the genetic analysis in ASReml and Timo Pitkänen for his advice concerning the statistics. Four anonymous referees gave valuable comments on the previous drafts of the manuscript. The financial support for the study was provided by the Ministry for Foreign Affairs of Finland.

Competing interests

The authors declare that they have no competing interests.

Appendix

In a multi-trait model, a trait that is recorded in different environments is treated as separate traits (see Additional file 4). Then, the magnitude of the re-ranking of the genetic groups can be quantified by calculating the genetic correlation (r_G) of the trait in each pair of the environments [42, 56]. A multi-trait animal mixed model was used in this study and run using ASReml 3.0. The bivariate model was as follows:

$$y_{ij} = \mu + a_i + e_{ij},$$

where y_{ij} is the observation of the ith individual for the kth trait (DGC being recorded in two thermal environments), μ is an overall trait mean, a_i is the random additive genetic effect of the ith individual, and e_{ij} is the random residual effect. It was assumed that the random variable a is multi-normally distributed with a mean of 0

and variance $\mathbf{A} \otimes \mathbf{G}$, where $\mathbf{A}$ is the additive genetic relationship matrix derived from the pedigree traced back to the base population and $\mathbf{G}$ is the additive genetic (co)variances matrix. In this study:

$$\mathbf{G} = \begin{bmatrix} \sigma^2_{a,\text{lowT}} & \sigma_{a,\text{lowT},a,\text{highT}} \\ \sigma_{a,\text{lowT},a,\text{highT}} & \sigma^2_{a,\text{highT}} \end{bmatrix},$$

where $\sigma^2_{a,\text{lowT}}$ and $\sigma^2_{a,\text{highT}}$ are the additive genetic variances of DGC measured at low and high temperatures, respectively, and $\sigma_{a,\text{lowT},a,\text{highT}}$ is the additive genetic covariance between low and high temperatures. The residual (co)variance matrix is:

$$\mathbf{R} = \begin{bmatrix} \sigma^2_{e,\text{lowT}} & 0 \\ 0 & \sigma^2_{e,\text{highT}} \end{bmatrix},$$

where $\sigma^2_{e,\text{lowT}}$ and $\sigma^2_{e,\text{highT}}$ are the residual variances at low and high temperatures, respectively. Because each individual fish was present only in one temperature environment, the residual covariance between temperatures was set to 0.

For both DGC traits, the heritability was calculated as:

$$h^2 = \sigma^2_a / \sigma^2_P,$$

where σ^2_P is the phenotypic variance (sum of additive genetic and residual variances), i.e. $\sigma^2_a + \sigma^2_e$.

The genetic correlation (r_G) between DGC measured in two temperature environments was calculated as:

$$r_G = \frac{\sigma_{a,\text{lowT},a,\text{highT}}}{\sqrt{\sigma^2_{a,\text{lowT}} \times \sigma^2_{a,\text{highT}}}},$$

where $\sigma_{a,\text{lowT},a,\text{highT}}$ is the covariance between additive genetic values measured at low and high experimental temperatures, and $\sigma^2_{a,\text{lowT}}$ and $\sigma^2_{a,\text{highT}}$ are the additive genetic variances of DGC measured at low and high temperatures, respectively. The genetic parameters estimated using a bivariate animal model are shown in Table 3.

Table 3 Genetic parameter estimates (± their approximate standard errors) for DGC in two thermal environments using a bivariate animal model

Parameter	DGC $_{\text{lowT}}$	DGC $_{\text{highT}}$
σ^2_a	0.130 (0.043)	0.190 (0.063)
σ^2_e	0.156 (0.028)	0.221 (0.041)
σ^2_P	0.286 (0.026)	0.411 (0.038)
h^2	0.455 (0.120)	0.463 (0.123)
r_G	0.468 (0.197)	

References

1. Berven KA, Gill DE. Interpreting geographic variation in life-history traits. Am Zool. 1983;23:85–97.
2. Via S, Lande R. Genotype-environment interaction and the evolution of phenotypic plasticity. Evolution. 1985;39:505–23.
3. Scheiner SM, Lyman RF. The genetics of phenotypic plasticity. II. Response to selection. J Evol Biol. 1991;4:23–50.
4. Hutchings JA. Old wine in new bottles: reaction norms in salmonid fishes. Heredity (Edinb). 2011;106:421–37.
5. Kolmodin R, Strandberg E, Jorjani H, Danell B. Selection in the presence of a genotype by environment interaction: response in environmental sensitivity. Anim Sci. 2003;76:375–85.
6. Falconer DS. Selection in different environments: effects on environmental sensitivity (reaction norm) and on mean performance. Genet Res. 1990;56:57–70.
7. De Jong G, Bijma P. Selection and phenotypic plasticity in evolutionary biology and animal breeding. Livest Prod Sci. 2002;78:195–214.
8. Ellen ED, Star L, Uitdehaag K, Brom FWA. Robustness as a breeding goal and its relation with health, welfare and integrity. In: Philipsson J, Klopcic M, Reents R, editors. Breeding for robustness in cattle. Wageningen: Wageningen Academic Publishers; 2009. p. 45–55.
9. Rauw WM, Gomez-Raya L. Genotype by environment interaction and breeding for robustness in livestock. Front Genet. 2015;6:310.
10. Simms EL. Defining tolerance as a norm of reaction. Evol Ecol. 2000;14:563–70.
11. De Jong G. Quantitative genetics of reaction norms. J Evol Biol. 1990;3:447–68.
12. Sae-Lim P, Gjerde B, Nielsen HM, Mulder H, Kause A. A review of genotype-by-environment interaction and micro-environmental sensitivity in aquaculture species. Rev Aquacult. 2016. doi:10.1111/raq.12098.
13. Ghalambor CK, McKay JK, Carroll SP, Reznick DN. Adaptive versus non-adaptive phenotypic plasticity and the potential for contemporary adaptation in new environments. Funct Ecol. 2007;21:394–407.
14. Sae-Lim P, Komen H, Kause A, van Arendonk JAM, Barfoot AJ, Martin KE, et al. Defining desired genetic gains for rainbow trout breeding objective using analytic hierarchy process. J Anim Sci. 2012;90:1766–76.
15. Jobling M. Temperature tolerance and the final preferendum-rapid methods for the assessment of optimum growth temperatures. J Fish Biol. 1981;19:439–55.
16. Hokanson KEF, Kleiner CF, Thorslund TW. Effects of constant temperatures and diel temperature fluctuations on specific growth and mortality rates and yield of juvenile rainbow trout (*Salmo gairdneri*). J Fish Res Board Can. 1977;34:639–48.
17. Bureau DP, Azevedo PA, Tapia-Salazar M, Cuzon G. Pattern and cost of growth and nutrient deposition in fish and shrimp: Potential implications and applications. In: Cruz-Suárez LE, Ricque-Marie D, Tapia-Salazar M, Olvera-Novoa MA, Civera-Cerecedo R, editors. Avances en Nutrición Acuícola V. Memorias del V Simposium Internacional de Nutrición Acuícola: 19–22 November 2000; Mérida. 2000. p. 112–40.
18. Kaushik SJ. Nutritional bioenergetics and estimation of waste production in non-salmonids. Aquat Living Resour. 1998;11:211–7.
19. Kenward MG, Roger JH. Small sample inference for fixed effects from restricted maximum likelihood. Biometrics. 1997;53:983–97.
20. Gilmour AR, Gogel BJ, Cullis BR, Thompson R. ASReml user guide release 3.0. Hemel Hempstead: VSN International Ltd; 2009.
21. Fischer TM, Gilmour AR, Werf JHW. Computing approximate standard errors for genetic parameters derived from random regression models fitted by average information REML. Genet Sel Evol. 2004;36:363–9.
22. Van Tienderen PH, Koelewijn HP. Selection on reaction norms, genetic correlations and constraints. Genet Res. 1994;64:115–25.
23. Sae-Lim P, Mulder H, Gjerde B, Koskinen H, Lillehammer M, Kause A. Genetics of growth reaction norms in farmed rainbow trout. PLoS One. 2015;10:e0135133.
24. Scheiner SM. Genetics and evolution of phenotypic plasticity. Annu Rev Ecol Syst. 1993;24:35–68.
25. Kolmodin R, Bijma P. Response to mass selection when the genotype by environment interaction is modelled as a linear reaction norm. Genet Sel Evol. 2004;36:435–54.
26. Wurtsbaugh WA, Davis GE. Effects of temperature and ration level on the growth and food conversion efficiency of rainbow trout. Salmo gairdneri Richardson. J Fish Biol. 1977;11:87–98.
27. Mäkinen T. Effect of temperature and feed ration on energy utilization in large rainbow trout, *Oncorhynchus mykiss* (Walbaum). Aquacult Res. 1994;25:213–32.
28. Jobling M. Fish bioenergetics. London: Chapman and Hall; 1994.
29. Fivelstad S, Schwartz J, Stromsnes H, Olsen AB. Sublethal Effects and safe levels of ammonia in seawater for Atlantic Salmon postsmolts (*Salmo Salar* L). Aquacult Eng. 1995;14:271–80.
30. Wedemeyer GA. Effect of rearing conditions on the health and physiological quality of fish in intensive culture. In: Iwama GK, Pickering AD, Sumpter JP, Schreck CB, editors. Fish stress and heath in aquaculture. Cambridge: Cambridge University Press; 1997. p. 35–72.
31. Timmons MB, Ebeling JM, Wheaton FW, Summerfelt ST, Vinci BJ. Recirculation aquaculture systems. 2nd Ed. NRAC Publications No. 01-002. Ithaca: Cayuga Aqua Ventures; 2002.
32. Hoffmann AA, Merilä J. Heritable variation and evolution under favourable and unfavourable conditions. Trends Ecol Evol. 1999;14:96–101.
33. Charmantier A, Garant D. Environmental quality and evolutionary potential: lessons from wild populations. Proc Biol Sci. 2005;272:1415–25.
34. Uller T, Olsson M, Ståhlberg F. Variation in heritability of tadpole growth: an experimental analysis. Heredity (Edinb). 2002;88:480–4.
35. Janhunen M, Piironen J, Peuhkuri N. Parental effects on embryonic viability and growth in Arctic charr *Salvelinus alpinus* at two incubation temperatures. J Fish Biol. 2010;76:2558–70.
36. Herrero-Medrano JM, Mathur PK, ten Napel J, Rashidi H, Alexandri P, Knol EF, et al. Estimation of genetic parameters and breeding values across challenged environments to select for robust pigs. J Anim Sci. 2015;93:1494–502.
37. Fishback AG, Danzmann RG, Ferguson MM, Gibson JP. Estimates of genetic parameters and genotype by environment interactions for growth traits of rainbow trout (*Oncorhynchus mykiss*) as inferred using molecular pedigrees. Aquaculture. 2002;206:137–50.
38. Kause A, Ritola O, Paananen T, Wahlroos H, Mäntysaari EA. Genetic trends in growth, sexual maturity and skeletal deformations, and rate of inbreeding in a breeding programme for rainbow trout (*Oncorhynchus mykiss*). Aquaculture. 2005;247:177–87.
39. Pierce LR, Palti Y, Silverstein JT, Barrows FT, Hallerman EM, Parsons J. Family growth response to fishmeal and plant-based diets shows genotype × diet interaction in rainbow trout (*Oncorhynchus mykiss*). Aquaculture. 2008;278:37–42.
40. Le Boucher R, Quillet E, Vandeputte M, Lecalvez JM, Goardon L, Chatain B, et al. Plant-based diet in rainbow trout (*Oncorhynchus mykiss* Walbaum): are there genotype-diet interactions for main production traits when fish are fed marine vs. plant-based diets from the first meal? Aquaculture. 2011;321:41–8.
41. Sae-Lim P, Kause A, Mulder HA, Martin KE, Barfoot AJ, Parsons JE, et al. Genotype-by-environment interaction of growth traits in rainbow trout (*Oncorhynchus mykiss*): a continental scale study. J Anim Sci. 2013;91:5572–81.
42. Falconer DS. The problem of environment and selection. Am Nat. 1952;86:293–8.
43. Mulder HA, Bijma P. Effects of genotype x environment interaction on genetic gain in breeding programs. J Anim Sci. 2005;83:49–61.
44. van der Waaij EH. A resource allocation model describing consequences of artificial selection under metabolic stress. J Anim Sci. 2004;82:973–81.
45. Jinks JL, Connolly V. Selection for specific and general response to environmental differences. Heredity. 1973;30:33–40.
46. Rosielle AA, Hamblin J. Theoretical aspects of selection for yield in stress and non-stress environment. Crop Sci. 1981;21:943–6.
47. Zumbach B, Misztal I, Tsuruta S, Sanchez JP, Azain M, Herring W, et al. Genetic components of heat stress in finishing pigs: parameter estimation. J Anim Sci. 2008;86:2076–81.
48. Ravagnolo O, Misztal I. Genetic component of heat stress in dairy cattle, parameter estimation. J Dairy Sci. 2000;83:2126–30.
49. Aguilar I, Misztal I, Tsuruta S. Genetic components of heat stress for dairy cattle with multiple lactations. J Dairy Sci. 2009;92:5702–11.

50. Finocchiaro R, van Kaam JB, Portolano B, Misztal I. Effect of heat stress on production of Mediterranean dairy sheep. J Dairy Sci. 2005;88:1855–64.

51. Brascamp E. Selection indices with constraints. Anim Breeding Abstracts. 1984;52:645–54.

52. Falconer DS, Mackay TFC. Introduction to quantitative genetics. 4th ed. Essex: Longman Group Ltd; 1996.

53. Janssens MJJ. Co-heritability: its relation to correlated response, linkage, and pleiotropy in cases of polygenic inheritance. Euphytica. 1979;28:601–8.

54. Lawrence AB, Wall E. Selection for 'environmental fit' from existing domesticated species. Rev Sci Tech. 2014;33:171–9.

55. Institute of Strategy and Policy on Natural Resources and Environment. Viet Nam assessment report on climate change (VARCC). 2009. http://www.unep.org/pdf/dtie/VTN_ASS_REP_CC.pdf. Accessed 27 Sept 2016.

56. Lynch M, Walsh B. Genetics and analysis of quantitative traits. Sunderland: Sinauer Associates Inc; 1998.

15

Higher heritabilities for gait components than for overall gait scores may improve mobility in ducks

Brendan M. Duggan[1*], Anne M. Rae[2], Dylan N. Clements[1] and Paul M. Hocking[1]

Abstract

Background: Genetic progress in selection for greater body mass and meat yield in poultry has been associated with an increase in gait problems which are detrimental to productivity and welfare. The incidence of suboptimal gait in breeding flocks is controlled through the use of a visual gait score, which is a subjective assessment of walking ability of each bird. The subjective nature of the visual gait score has led to concerns over its effectiveness in reducing the incidence of suboptimal gait in poultry through breeding. The aims of this study were to assess the reliability of the current visual gait scoring system in ducks and to develop a more objective method to select for better gait.

Results: Experienced gait scorers assessed short video clips of walking ducks to estimate the reliability of the current visual gait scoring system. Kendall's coefficients of concordance between and within observers were estimated at 0.49 and 0.75, respectively. In order to develop a more objective scoring system, gait components were visually scored on more than 4000 pedigreed Pekin ducks and genetic parameters were estimated for these components. Gait components, which are a more objective measure, had heritabilities that were as good as, or better than, those of the overall visual gait score.

Conclusions: Measurement of gait components is simpler and therefore more objective than the standard visual gait score. The recording of gait components can potentially be automated, which may increase accuracy further and may improve heritability estimates. Genetic correlations were generally low, which suggests that it is possible to use gait components to select for an overall improvement in both economic traits and gait as part of a balanced breeding programme.

Background

Increases in growth rate and breast muscle mass which have been achieved through selective breeding of poultry have been associated with welfare problems, notably an increased incidence of poor gait (which includes 'leg weakness') [1–5]. Birds with leg weakness may suffer pain and have difficulty reaching food and water [1, 6–8], which lead to economic losses for the producer and possible starvation for the animals. Gait problems were first reported in turkeys and broiler chickens [9, 10], although early studies focussed mainly on the emergence of skeletal leg defects rather than gait itself [10, 11]. Poor gait has since been observed in other heavy meat-producing birds [3, 12–15]. Although in Pekin ducks poor gait has not been reported as extensively, there is concern that gait problems may appear in the future if selection for production traits continues along its current trajectory, mirroring their emergence in other poultry species. It is important to consider that while gait problems may be associated with pain, sub-optimal gait may also be simply a functional consequence of an altered morphology in lines which have been heavily selected for increased muscle mass [16, 17].

Traditionally, in chickens and ducks, poor gait is assessed and selected against by using a visual gait score [9, 18], which is an ordinal score given to each bird based on a visual assessment of how that individual

*Correspondence: Brendan.Duggan@roslin.ed.ac.uk
[1] The Roslin Institute and Royal (Dick) School of Veterinary Studies, University of Edinburgh, Easter Bush, Midlothian EH25 9RG, UK
Full list of author information is available at the end of the article

walks. Although efforts have been made to refine the visual gait score [19], it remains a subjective measure of walking ability and thus is prone to error. Previous studies have found relatively moderate kappa coefficients (a measure of agreement between observers) between 0.6 and 0.8 in ducks and chickens [14, 20]. This may suffice for flock-level welfare assessments but is below the accuracy required for selection. An EU report on the welfare of broiler chickens acknowledges the subjective nature of the gait scoring system and highlights the need to develop a more objective system of assessing gait [21].

Gait is a complex trait that requires the integration of sensory input, balance, conformation and fine motor control, and heritability estimates for poultry gait tend to be low [22–24]. Similarly low heritability estimates have been published for visual gait scores in other species [25]. In addition, as the visual assessment of gait is a subjective measure [19], heritability estimates may be low, which limits potential genetic progress when selecting for such a trait. Attempts have been made to circumvent this problem of low heritability estimates by focusing selection on objectively measured traits such as tibial dyschondroplasia or bone deformity [26], although it remains unclear how these phenotypes affect the overall walking ability of birds. However, some gait components, such as step width, will certainly affect the overall walking ability of an animal and have not as yet been genetically evaluated.

The aim of this study was to estimate the reliability, heritability and genetic parameters of the visual gait score which is currently used in Pekin ducks and to compare this to heritability estimates for particular components of gait. It was hypothesised that these components of gait may be more heritable than the overall gait score. This was previously found to be the case in dairy cattle [25]. Components were chosen for ease of measurement as well as for their hypothesised influence on overall gait. This study focusses on two gait components: step width, which influences balance during the stride, and body roll, which is a proxy for medio-lateral centre of mass movement during walking. There may be other components of gait which are more central to the overall movement of the bird but we chose those due to their ease of measurement. The components were also chosen on the basis of our previous findings that poultry lines selected for breast muscle mass ambulate with a wider step width and at a slower velocity (which is likely to increase body roll for a given step width) [27]. The purpose of this study was to ascertain the suitability of selecting for gait components, rather than to identify which components, in particular, should become the focus of future selection programmes.

Methods
Assessment of gait score
In order to assess the reliability of the standard visual gait score in ducks, seven-week-old Pekin ducks were scored for gait by four industry gait scorers. Scorers were shown three video sequences of 36 birds walking over a runway. The video camera (Microsoft LifeCam Studio, recording at 30 frames per second) was placed behind each bird at a height of 15 cm. The video sequence contained 144 walks–four walks (including one duplicate) for each bird. Each walk lasted approximately 3 s in order to replicate the high throughput of birds during assessments on breeding farms. Scorers were asked to rate each walk with a score of 1 (very poor gait) to 5 (perfect gait). None of the scorers were informed that the sequences contained duplicate recordings or multiple walks from the same birds. Agreement between and within scorers was assessed by using Kendall's coefficient of concordance and the Minitab software (Minitab version 17, Minitab Inc.).

Measurement of gait components
Over the course of eight weeks, on one day per week, over 5000 Pekin ducks were visually scored for gait. On average, 650 birds were visually scored during each week. Two breeding lines (A and B) of Pekin duck were used, alternating each week. In total, data was collected from four hatches of each line (a different hatch was measured each week). These breeding lines are grandparent stock of the standard Cherry Valley commercial hybrid duck. Line A forms part of the maternal grandparent stock and Line B forms part of the paternal grandparent stock. All birds were hatched in the same hatchery and raised according to the Cherry Valley published guidelines. Water and feed (standard industry rations) were provided ad libitum. The photoperiod was 23 h light on day 1, reducing by 1 h per day until day 6 when the photoperiod was 18 h of light per day and this was maintained to the end of the trial. Phenotypic data collection for various traits was carried out on a breeding company farm by experienced members of staff. All phenotypic measurements took place at a single measurement station on the same breeding farm. After corralling birds at six weeks of age into a small area adjacent to the measurement station, each bird was weighed and its (ultrasonic) breast muscle depth was recorded. The birds were subsequently placed on a custom-built walkway (1.2-m wide and 4.8-m long) and allowed to walk away at their own pace, during which time each bird's overall gait and gait components were scored (during normal selection procedures, birds are gait scored while walking over loose straw bedding). The walkway consisted of a wooden base (6-mm

thick plywood) which was covered by a sheet of 7-mm green artificial turf in order to provide grip and to create a contrast so as to make the birds' feet easier to see. Perspex sheeting (30-cm high) was fixed to the sides of the walkway to ensure that the birds walked straight to the end of the walkway. Gait was assessed using a visual gait score (which forms part of the company's routine phenotypic measurement). Gait scores for Lines A and B were recorded by two different members of staff (each line was scored by only one individual), both of whom were experienced at scoring gait. The visual gait score used by the breeding company spans a 1 to 5 scale, with 1 representing a bird which is markedly lame and 5 representing perfect gait. The score for a bird was downgraded if, when walking, that individual displayed bowed or splayed legs, medially or laterally rotated feet, or if the angle of the back to the floor was outside the 35 to 65 degree range. Birds which were lame, immobile or walked on their hocks were given a score of 1. Most ducks were assigned scores between 2 and 4 (in this trial, 1% were given a gait score of 1; 29% a score of 2; 61% a score of 3 and 8% a score of 4).

In addition to the overall visual gait score, two gait components (step width and body roll) were recorded simultaneously by one of the authors (BMD). The same author scored components of gait for both lines. Step width was scored visually as the estimated distance (perpendicular to the direction of travel) between the most posterior parts of the feet on a 1 to 3 scale, a score of 1 denoting the feet as being very close together (or overlapping) and a score of 3 denoting that the feet were widely spaced during walking. Body roll (also on a 1 to 3 scale) was recorded as the degree of rolling of the shoulders during walking. This was considered an approximation of medio-lateral centre of mass movement since the position of centre of mass was impossible to ascertain visually. This trait was deemed important because the degree of medio-lateral movement of the centre of mass can affect the birds' balance. Birds which display greater variation in centre of mass position during walking may be at greater risk of stumbles or falls. A score of 1 represented very little rolling of the shoulders, whereas a score of 3 was given to birds which rolled their shoulders to a large degree while walking. The repeatability for both gait component scores was assessed in a small trial at the beginning of this study and deemed to be satisfactory, although no larger scale repeatability test using video was carried out as was the case for the standard gait score. Birds which moved too quickly or too slowly to reliably score gait components were treated as missing values. Hence, gait components were recorded on 4252 of the 5251 birds that were phenotypically measured (Table 2). Among the birds measured, 5% were

given a step width score of 1, 79% were given a score of 2 and 16% were given a score of 3. For body roll, 9% were scored 1, 74% were given a score of 2 and 17% were given a score of 3. In addition to standard phenotypic measures of breast depth and body mass, feed conversion ratios (FCR) for each bird were calculated by automated measurement of each bird's individual feed intake and body mass. Data collected at the phenotypic measurement station was collated with information of the FCR of each bird. The pedigree of all birds was known, stretching back 15 generations.

This study was approved by the Veterinary Ethical Review Committee at the University of Edinburgh.

Genetic analysis

Variance components resulting from univariate and bivariate mixed models of restricted maximum likelihoods were used to estimate heritability of the visual gait score and the gait component scores as well as to calculate the genetic correlations between traits using ASReml (ASReml-W, version 3, VSN International Ltd.). Six traits were analysed using the following model, which included fixed effects of sex and hatch and random effects of animal, pen and the permanent environment effect of the dam. The model terms were:

$$\mathbf{y} = \mathbf{Xb} + \mathbf{Za} + \mathbf{Vp} + \mathbf{Wd} + \mathbf{e},$$

where $\mathbf{y}$ is the vector of trait measurements, $\mathbf{b}$ is a vector of the fixed effects accounting for the interaction between the hatch and the sex of each bird, $\mathbf{a}$ the vector of additive genetic effects, $\mathbf{p}$ is a vector of the pen effects, $\mathbf{d}$ is the vector of permanent environmental effects of the dam and $\mathbf{e}$ is the vector of residuals. $\mathbf{X}$, $\mathbf{Z}$, $\mathbf{V}$ and $\mathbf{W}$ are incidence matrices which relate the vectors $\mathbf{b}$, $\mathbf{a}$, $\mathbf{p}$ and $\mathbf{d}$ with $\mathbf{y}$. The variance/covariance structure was assumed to be:

$$V\begin{bmatrix} \mathbf{a} \\ \mathbf{p} \\ \mathbf{d} \\ \mathbf{e} \end{bmatrix} \begin{bmatrix} \mathbf{A} \otimes \mathbf{G} & \mathbf{0} & \mathbf{0} & \mathbf{0} \\ \mathbf{0} & \mathbf{I} \otimes \mathbf{P} & \mathbf{0} & \mathbf{0} \\ \mathbf{0} & \mathbf{0} & \mathbf{I} \otimes \mathbf{C} & \mathbf{0} \\ \mathbf{0} & \mathbf{0} & \mathbf{0} & \mathbf{I} \otimes \mathbf{R} \end{bmatrix},$$

where $\mathbf{A}$ and $\mathbf{I}$ are the additive genetic relationship matrix and identity matrix, respectively. $\mathbf{G}$, $\mathbf{P}$, $\mathbf{C}$ and $\mathbf{R}$ represent the variance–covariance matrices of additive genetic effects, pen effects, permanent environmental effects of the dam and residual effects, respectively. A multinomial qualifier (with link functions between the observed and underlying scale) was not used as part of the model due to issues with convergence, probably due to limitations of the data structure and size of categorical traits. Residuals for these traits were normally and independently distributed. The pedigree and data structures are summarized in Tables 1 and 2, respectively.

Table 1 Pedigree structure for Lines A and B

Line	Individuals in pedigree	Generations in pedigree	Sires	Sires of sires	Dams of sires	Dams	Sires of dams	Dams of sires
A	120,031	15	1078	364	577	4039	663	1418
B	81,765	15	1078	377	535	3622	699	1349

Figures represent numbers of individuals

Table 2 Means (and standard deviations) for all traits measured in Lines A and B

Line	Number of phenotyped males	Number of phenotyped females	Gait score	Step width	Body roll	Finish weight (g)	Breast depth (mm)	Test FCR
A	1375	1254	2.80 (0.66) [0]	2.13 (0.46) [229]	2.08 (0.53) [230]	3760 (290) [0]	152 (15.3) [0]	1.90 (0.17) [887]
B	1342	1280	2.70 (0.56) [1]	2.10 (0.43) [269]	2.06 (0.47) [271]	3362 (297) [0]	146 (16.7) [0]	2.02 (0.23) [69]

Phenotypes were recorded at six weeks of age. Standard deviations and numbers of missing values for each trait are presented in round and square parentheses, respectively

Results

Kendall's coefficient of concordance, calculated between four experienced observers who scored gait in short video clips, was equal to 0.49 (df = 132, p < 0.001). The Kendall's coefficient of concordance within observers (scoring duplicate videos) was equal to 0.75 (df = 135, p < 0.001). No clear observer drift effect was detected, i.e. scorers deviated to a similar degree when scoring the first 60 walks compared to the last 60.

Heritability estimates with genetic and phenotypic correlations for Lines A and B are in Tables 3 and 4, respectively. The heritability estimates of the standard gait score were low and standard errors in the female line were high. Estimated heritabilities for body roll and gait score were similar whereas for step width they were higher. Estimated heritabilities for economic traits (finish weight, breast depth and FCR) were generally moderate.

Table 3 Heritability estimates and correlations for gait and other major economic traits in Line A

Trait	Gait score	Step width	Body roll	Finish weight	Breast depth	Test FCR
Gait score	**0.061 (0.055)**	−0.346 (0.202)	−0.690 (0.146)	−0.703 (0.373)	−0.374 (0.319)	0.095 (0.303)
Step width	−0.162 (0.034)	**0.238 (0.074)**	0.561 (0.227)	0.217 (0.167)	0.066 (0.165)	−0.111 (0.181)
Body roll	−0.337 (0.025)	0.282 (0.029)	**0.079 (0.034)**	0.160 (0.215)	−0.033 (0.222)	−0.379 (0.218)
Finish weight	−0.039 (0.030)	0.069 (0.034)	0.020 (0.029)	**0.274 (0.091)**	0.452 (0.145)	0.609 (0.135)
Breast depth	0.056 (0.040)	0.092 (0.028)	0.065 (0.037)	0.439 (0.028)	**0.15 (0.074)**	0.205 (0.172)
FCR	0.1226 (0.037)	0.007 (0.036)	−0.037 (0.032)	0.067 (0.036)	0.079 (0.031)	**0.272 (0.096)**

Heritability estimates are in bold italics; genetic correlations are listed above the diagonal and phenotypic correlations are in italics, below the diagonal. Standard errors for all estimates are in parentheses

Table 4 Heritability estimates and correlations for gait and other major economic traits in Line B

Trait	Gait score	Step width	Body roll	Finish weight	Breast depth	Test FCR
Gait score	**0.115 (0.058)**	0.138 (0.199)	−0.506 (0.170)	0.126 (0.176)	−0.022 (0.186)	0.442 (0.136)
Step width	−0.016 (0.028)	**0.166 (0.058)**	0.571 (0.155)	0.029 (0.150)	−0.326 (0.151)	−0.156 (0.160)
Body roll	−0.156 (0.028)	0.314 (0.023)	**0.112 (0.047)**	−0.164 (0.163)	0.059 (0.173)	−0.136 (0.175)
Finish weight	0.186 (0.025)	0.048 (0.027)	0.010 (0.025)	**0.401 (0.090)**	0.230 (0.112)	0.303 (0.127)
Breast depth	0.074 (0.024)	−0.034 (0.025)	0.046 (0.024)	0.390 (0.024)	**0.295 (0.046)**	0.077 (0.140)
FCR	0.071 (0.026)	−0.016 (0.027)	0.004 (0.026)	−0.079 (0.028)	−0.074 (0.025)	**0.294 (0.048)**

Heritability estimates are in bold italics; genetic correlations are listed above the diagonal and phenotypic correlations are in italics, below the diagonal. Standard errors for all estimates are in parentheses

Phenotypic correlations between traits varied between lines. Generally, phenotypic correlations between gait traits and economic traits were very low and correlations between economic traits were also low, with the exception of finish weight and breast depth (Tables 3 and 4). Since in this study, relatively small sample sizes were used, estimates of genetic correlations between traits were associated with relatively high standard errors. Most genetic correlations between gait traits and economic traits were not significant (p > 0.05), with the exception of Line B, where significant genetic correlations were observed between step width and breast depth (t = 2.16, p < 0.05), and between gait score and FCR (t = 3.26, p < 0.01). The standard gait score had moderate to good genetic correlations with body roll (−0.51 to −0.69). Genetic correlations between gait score and step width were not significant. The significant genetic correlations between economic traits were moderate (0.23 to 0.61).

Discussion

Gait problems are a major animal welfare issue facing modern poultry in intensive production systems. Our results suggest that a more targeted approach to assessing gait by focussing on gait components has the potential to improve progress in selecting for better gait in breeding birds.

The pilot study that involved a limited amount of data suggests that the current visual gait scoring system, while showing some level of agreement between scorers, may not be optimal for long-term use in breeding programmes, but can be improved. The Kendall's coefficient of concordance suggests that low concordance exists between scorers. Indeed, when scoring video clips of the same walks (using the standard visual gait score described above), all four scorers agreed 28% of the time and three of the four scorers agreed 74% of the time. Individual scorers failed to allocate the same score to two duplicate walks 26% of the time. Some of these inconsistencies may be due to the short duration of each video recording. Short recordings were chosen in order to replicate conditions during assessments on farm; however for certain birds on farm, the scorer will observe a walk for longer than 3 s before allocating a score for that bird. The viewing angle of the camera, which was chosen to give a clearer view of the birds' gait, is also different from the viewpoint used when scoring during selection on farm, which is from a standing position.

The suboptimal reliability of the visual gait score that was recorded by using these video clips suggests that an alternate and more rigorous method of gait assessment is required to make progress on selection for optimal gait as weight increases. Previous work on gait in cows suggested that assessing components of gait may yield higher

heritability estimates [25]. Certain gait components such as step width and the ratio of double to single support time are known to have changed to a similar extent in both ducks and chickens which have undergone selection for increased body weight and meat yield [27], and selection decisions based on these components may yield greater progress than the current subjective gait scoring system.

This study estimated genetic parameters for components of gait and compared these to those of the overall visual gait score. The heritability of step width was higher than that of the original gait score in both lines and standard errors were approximately the same for both estimates. This is to be expected since the gait score is a subjective measurement based on a visual assessment of overall body movements, without any tangible reference points, whereas step width is a simpler score based on only one aspect of foot placement and therefore one would expect this score to be more objective. In addition, the recorder that measures step width can make use of reference points on the ground to compare successive birds. The heritability of body roll was similar to that of the gait score, probably because unlike step width, the assessment of body roll is a more subjective assessment. Heritability estimates for other economic traits (finish weight, breast depth and FCR) were in the range expected, with some differences observed between lines. For example, the mean estimate for the heritability of body weight in this study (0.34) is in a similar range than the heritabilities of 0.28 to 0.45 which were estimated in recent poultry studies [24, 28–30]. Heritability estimates presented in this study were calculated from only one phenotyped generation; thus, it is expected that these heritabilities would be estimated with more accuracy if more generations had been phenotyped, as is the case within commercial breeding programmes.

Phenotypic correlations between the gait score and production traits were generally low, which suggests that the gait score is indeed a measure of gait, rather than a proxy measure of body mass or breast depth. Phenotypic correlations between the gait score and components of gait were low to moderate, whereas those between each component of gait were generally moderate. Due to the relatively small sample size, genetic correlations were generally associated with relatively large standard errors that were of a similar magnitude to the genetic correlation estimates. The notable exceptions were the genetic correlations between gait score and body roll and between step width and body roll in both Lines A and B. In Line B, breast depth (considered a proxy for pectoral muscle mass) was negatively correlated with step width; continued selection for greater breast depth may result in a narrower step width. The effect of this narrower step width on balance will depend on the degree to which the body's centre of mass moves laterally during gait. Genetic correlations between gait components and production traits were generally low and the data suggest that selection for improved gait will not be compromised by negative responses in economic traits.

These data demonstrate that the visual assessment of gait components during selection is both feasible and yields promising heritability estimates. While some caution must be exercised when interpreting these results (given the presence of categorical traits in the model), the use of gait components holds promise for future progress in selection for improved gait in ducks; since they are simpler traits, the assessment of gait components can be automated, for example by using pressure sensing technology as in Duggan et al. [27]. Automation of measurement has the potential to bring about greater objectivity and to increase breeding success. However, it is important to note that although the gait components that are the focus of this paper can be measured satisfactorily and have reasonable heritability estimates, it is not yet known which components should be selected to improve gait. For example, it could be argued that a wide step width would be beneficial to a bird with large lateral displacement of the centre of mass, whereas a narrow step width would be beneficial to a bird with little lateral centre of mass movement. However, it is also difficult to differentiate cause and effect associations between step width and lateral body movement. A more thorough understanding of how gait components are integrated to perform overall locomotion is therefore necessary before recommendations can be made on which particular gait components should be used in breeding programmes. It is likely that most of the improvement will be achieved using a selection index which combines weighted measurement of various gait components. Indeed, current overall gait scoring methods use a combination of components, which are subconsciously weighted in different ways depending on the observers' opinions of what optimal gait entails. By focussing only on the measurement of gait components, this differential weighting among observers can be avoided.

Conclusions

Scoring overall gait visually is a subjective measure which generally generates low (but useable) heritabilities. We demonstrate that focussing on gait components, rather than overall gait, may result in heritability estimates that are equal to or higher than those of the conventional visual gait score in ducks. The benefit of using components of gait is that their measurement can be automated to generate greater accuracy and easily combined to create an index score of overall gait. Genetic correlations,

while difficult to ascertain, are generally low; therefore it is possible to use gait components to select for an overall improvement in both economic traits and gait as part of a balanced breeding programme.

Authors' contributions
BMD and AMR collected the data. PMH obtained funding for the project. BMD, AMR, DNC and PMH contributed to the design of the study, analysis of data and drafting of the manuscript. All authors read and approved the final manuscript.

Author details
[1] The Roslin Institute and Royal (Dick) School of Veterinary Studies, University of Edinburgh, Easter Bush, Midlothian EH25 9RG, UK. [2] Cherry Valley Farms Ltd., Laceby Business Park, Grimsby Road, Laceby, North Lincolnshire DN37 7DP, UK.

Acknowledgements
We would like to acknowledge Cherry Valley Farms for provision of birds and financial support. Thanks to Ozzie Matika and Tanya Englishby for very useful and helpful comments and feedback. Many thanks to the farm staff at Cherry Valley for assistance with data collection. This work was funded through a Biotechnology and Biological Sciences Research Council Industrial CASE studentship (Grant BB/K501621/1) in collaboration with Cherry Valley Farms. The Roslin Institute is supported by an Institute Core Strategic Grant from the BBSRC.

Competing interests
The authors declare that they have no competing interests.

References
1. Bradshaw RH, Kirkden RD, Broom DM. A review of the aetiology and pathology of leg weakness in broilers in relation to welfare. Avian Poult Biol Rev. 2002;13:45–103.
2. Knowles TG, Kestin SC, Haslam SM, Brown SN, Green LE, Butterworth A, et al. Leg disorders in broiler chickens: prevalence, risk factors and prevention. PLoS One. 2008;3:e1545.
3. Jones TA, Dawkins MS. Environment and management factors affecting Pekin duck production and welfare on commercial farms in the UK. Br Poult Sci. 2010;51:12–21.
4. Paxton H, Daley MA, Corr SA, Hutchinson JR. The gait dynamics of the modern broiler chicken: a cautionary tale of selective breeding. J Exp Biol. 2013;216:3237–48.
5. Farm Animal Welfare Council. Report on the welfare of broiler chickens. 1992.
6. McGeown D, Danbury TC, Waterman-Pearson AE, Kestin SC. Effect of carprofen on lameness in broiler chickens. Vet Rec. 1999;144:668–71.
7. Caplen G, Colborne GR, Hothersall B, Nicol CJ, Waterman-Pearson AE, Weeks CA, et al. Lame broiler chickens respond to non-steroidal anti-inflammatory drugs with objective changes in gait function: a controlled clinical trial. Vet J. 2013;196:477–82.
8. Danbury TC, Weeks CA, Chambers JP, Waterman-Pearson AE, Kestin SC. Self-selection of the analgesic drug carprofen by lame broiler chickens. Vet Rec. 2000;146:307–11.
9. Kestin S, Knowles TG, Tinch AE, Gregory NG. Prevalence of leg weakness in broiler chickens and its relationship with genotype. Vet Rec. 1992;131:190–4.
10. Nestor KE. Genetics of growth and reproduction in the turkey. 9. Long-term selection for increased 16-week body weight. Poult Sci. 1984;63:2114–22.

11. Mercer JT, Hill WG. Estimation of genetic parameters for skeletal defects in broiler chickens. Heredity (Edinb). 1984;53:193–203.

12. Martrenchar A. Animal welfare and intensive production of turkey broilers. Worlds Poult Sci J. 1999;55:143–52.

13. Abourachid A. Comparative gait analysis in two strains of turkey, *Meleagris gallopavo*. Br Poult Sci. 1991;32:271–7.

14. Makagon MM, Woolley R, Karcher DM. Assessing the waddle: an evaluation of a 3-point gait score system for ducks. Poult Sci. 2015;94:1729–34.

15. Da Costa MJ, Grimes JL, Oviedo-Rondón EO, Barasch I, Evans C, Dalmagro M, et al. Footpad dermatitis severity on turkey flocks and correlations with locomotion, litter conditions, and body weight at market age. J Appl Poult Res. 2014;23:268–79.

16. Duggan BM, Hocking PM, Schwarz T, Clements DN. Differences in hindlimb morphology of ducks and chickens: effects of domestication and selection. Genet Sel Evol. 2015;47:88.

17. Corr SA, Gentle MJ, McCorquodale CC, Bennet D. The effect of morphology on walking ability in the modern broiler: a gait analysis study. Anim Welf. 2003;12:159–71.

18. Kestin SC, Gordon S, Su G, Sorensen P. Relationships in broiler chickens between lameness, liveweight, growth rate and age. Vet Rec. 2001;148:195–7.

19. Garner JP, Falcone C, Wakenell P, Martin M, Mench JA. Reliability and validity of a modified gait scoring system and its use in assessing tibial dyschondroplasia in broilers. Br Poult Sci. 2002;43:355–63.

20. Webster AB, Fairchild BD, Cummings TS, Stayer PA. Validation of a three-point gait-scoring system for field assessment of walking ability of commercial broilers. J Appl Poult Res. 2008;17:529–39.

21. Berg C, Bessei W, Faure JM, Jensen P, Porin F, San Gabriel Closas A, et al. The welfare of chickens kept for meat production (broilers). In Report of the scientific committee in Animal Health and Animal Welfare. Brussels European Commission; 2000.

22. EFSA Panel on Animal Health and Welfare. Scientific opinion on the influence of genetic parameters on the welfare and the resistance to stress of commercial broilers. EFSA J. 2010;8:1666.

23. Whitehead CC, Fleming RH, Julian RJ, Sørensen P. Skeletal problems associated with selection for increased production. In: Muir WM, Aggrey SE, editors. Poultry genetics, breeding and biotechnology. Wallingford: CABI Publishing; 2003. p. 29–52.

24. Kapell DNRG, Hocking PM, Glover PK, Kremer VD, Avendaño S. Genetic basis of leg health and its relationship with body weight in purebred turkey lines. Poult Sci. 2017;. doi:10.3382/ps/pew479.

25. Chapinal N, Sewalem A, Miglior F. Short communication: estimation of genetic parameters for gait in Canadian Holstein cows. J Dairy Sci. 2012;95:7372–6.

26. Kapell DNRG, Hill WG, Neeteson AM, McAdam J, Koerhuis AN, Avendaño S. Twenty-five years of selection for improved leg health in purebred broiler lines and underlying genetic parameters. Poult Sci. 2012;91:3032–43.

27. Duggan BM, Hocking PM, Clements DN. Gait in ducks (*Anas platyrhynchos*) and chickens (*Gallus gallus*): similarities in adaptation to high growth rate. Biol Open. 2016;5:1077–85.

28. Rekaya R, Sapp RL, Wing T, Aggrey SE. Genetic evaluation for growth, body composition, feed efficiency, and leg soundness. Poult Sci. 2013;92:923–9.

29. Bailey RA, Watson KA, Bilgili SF, Avendano S. The genetic basis of pectoralis major myopathies in modern broiler chicken lines. Poult Sci. 2015;94:2870–9.

30. Mignon-Grasteau S, Beaumont C, Poivey JP, de Rochambeau H. Estimation of the genetic parameters of sexual dimorphism of body weight in 'label' chickens and Muscovy ducks. Genet Sel Evol. 1998;30:481–91.

16

Computational strategies for alternative single-step Bayesian regression models with large numbers of genotyped and non-genotyped animals

Rohan L. Fernando[1]* ⊕, Hao Cheng[1], Bruce L. Golden[2] and Dorian J. Garrick[1,3]

Abstract

Background: Two types of models have been used for single-step genomic prediction and genome-wide association studies that include phenotypes from both genotyped animals and their non-genotyped relatives. The two types are breeding value models (BVM) that fit breeding values explicitly and marker effects models (MEM) that express the breeding values in terms of the effects of observed or imputed genotypes. MEM can accommodate a wider class of analyses, including variable selection or mixture model analyses. The order of the equations that need to be solved and the inverses required in their construction vary widely, and thus the computational effort required depends upon the size of the pedigree, the number of genotyped animals and the number of loci.

Theory: We present computational strategies to avoid storing large, dense blocks of the MME that involve imputed genotypes. Furthermore, we present a hybrid model that fits a MEM for animals with observed genotypes and a BVM for those without genotypes. The hybrid model is computationally attractive for pedigree files containing millions of animals with a large proportion of those being genotyped.

Application: We demonstrate the practicality on both the original MEM and the hybrid model using real data with 6,179,960 animals in the pedigree with 4,934,101 phenotypes and 31,453 animals genotyped at 40,214 informative loci. To complete a single-trait analysis on a desk-top computer with four graphics cards required about 3 h using the hybrid model to obtain both preconditioned conjugate gradient solutions and 42,000 Markov chain Monte-Carlo (MCMC) samples of breeding values, which allowed making inferences from posterior means, variances and covariances. The MCMC sampling required one quarter of the effort when the hybrid model was used compared to the published MEM.

Conclusions: We present a hybrid model that fits a MEM for animals with genotypes and a BVM for those without genotypes. Its practicality and considerable reduction in computing effort was demonstrated. This model can readily be extended to accommodate multiple traits, multiple breeds, maternal effects, and additional random effects such as polygenic residual effects.

Background

Two types of equivalent mixed linear models are used for whole-genome analyses in livestock [1]. The first type, which we refer to as marker effects models (MEM), includes random effects ($\boldsymbol{\alpha}$) of marker genotype covariates ($\mathbf{M}_g$) in the model [2, 3]. The second type, which we refer to as breeding value models (BVM), includes the breeding values of the animals, $\mathbf{u}_g = \mathbf{M}_g \boldsymbol{\alpha}$, as a random effect that has a covariance computed from $\mathbf{M}_g$ [1, 2, 4–6] rather than from the pedigree.

It was shown that the BVM can be adapted for what is known as single-step genomic best linear unbiased

*Correspondence: rohan@iastate.edu
[1] Department of Animal Science, Iowa State University, Ames, IA 50011, USA
Full list of author information is available at the end of the article

prediction (SS-GBLUP) that combines information from animals with genotypes and from those without genotypes in a single BLUP analysis [7–9]. However, the SS-GBLUP analysis requires computing the inverse of $\mathbf{G}$, which is the matrix of genomic relationships of the animals with genotypes [8, 9]. When the number N_g of genotyped animals exceeds the number of markers, $\mathbf{G}$ is singular, but a full-rank matrix such as $\mathbf{G}^* = 0.95\mathbf{G} + 0.05\mathbf{A}$, with $\mathbf{A}$ being the pedigree-based relationship matrix might be used in its place. Single-step analyses based on the MEM do not require computing $\mathbf{G}$ or its inverse [10]. Furthermore, Bayesian regression analyses based on the MEM are not limited to assuming a normal prior for $\boldsymbol{\alpha}$, which is implicit in SS-GBLUP; Bayesian regression models can accommodate various priors including the t distribution as in BayesA [3, 11], the double exponential distribution as in Bayesian LASSO [12] or mixtures of the t distribution or the normal distribution [3, 11, 13] as in BayesB or BayesC. However, the MME that correspond to single-step MEM (SS-MEM) types of models contain dense blocks that correspond to the imputed genotypes of animals with missing genotypes [10], and those blocks can be large if many animals have missing genotypes.

Liu et al. [14] developed a single-step method based on the BVM with direct estimation of marker effects (SSME-GBLUP). An advantage of that method over SS-GBLUP is that it does not require computing $\mathbf{G}$ or its inverse. Also, their method can be used for Bayesian regression models [14]. However, the MME for SSME-GBLUP contains expressions that involve the inverse of the pedigree-based relationship matrix, $\mathbf{A}_{gg}$, for the animals with genotypes. This is a dense matrix, and therefore a computational strategy was proposed to avoid computing its inverse but it requires solving a dense system of equations of order N_g within each round of Jacobi or pre-conditioned conjugate gradient (PCG) iteration for solution of the MME or within each round of MCMC sampling for Bayesian inference with models such as BayesA or BayesB [3]. Equation (A1) in Legarra and Ducrocq [15] also present a set of similar MME with marker effects for genotyped animals and breeding values for non-genotyped animals. As with the MME in Liu et al. [14], the advantage of the MME of Legarra and Ducrocq [15] is that they do not require the computation of $\mathbf{G}$ or its inverse but require computing the inverse of $\mathbf{A}_{gg}$. Recently, in some livestock such as dairy cattle, N_g has increased towards a million or more, and thus, solving a dense system of equations of order N_g within each round of iteration will place a heavy burden on SSME-GBLUP in computing time and storage requirements.

The objective of this paper is to present computational strategies for whole-genome analyses based on the SS-MEM that avoid storing large, dense blocks of the MME that involve imputed genotypes. First, we will show this for the MME given in [10]. Second, we will present what we refer to as a hybrid type model (HM) that uses a MEM for the animals with marker genotypes and a BVM for animals without genotypes. The MME that correspond to this model also has dense blocks that correspond to animals with missing genotypes. However, in Bayesian regression analyses based on this hybrid model, storing the dense blocks can be avoided even more efficiently than was the case for the MME given in [10]. Finally, we will present the computer storage and time required for a real application.

Theory

In most genomic analyses, the columns of the matrix $\mathbf{M}_g$ of marker covariates are centered to have zero expectations. This ensures that the vector of breeding values, $\mathbf{u}_g = \mathbf{M}_g\boldsymbol{\alpha}$, has a mean of $\mathbf{0}$. Centering $\mathbf{M}_g$ requires knowing the expected value of the marker covariates for founder animals. Often, these expected values are unknown, but can be incorporated into the model as a location parameter [10, 16]. However, to simplify our presentation without loss of generality we assume that $\mathbf{M}_g$ is a matrix of correctly centered marker covariates.

Marker effects model for single-step Bayesian regression

As in Fernando et al. [10], a MEM for single-step Bayesian regression analyses can be derived from writing the model equation as:

$$\begin{bmatrix} \mathbf{y}_n \\ \mathbf{y}_g \end{bmatrix} = \begin{bmatrix} \mathbf{X}_n \\ \mathbf{X}_g \end{bmatrix}\boldsymbol{\beta} + \begin{bmatrix} \mathbf{Z}_n & \mathbf{0} \\ \mathbf{0} & \mathbf{Z}_g \end{bmatrix}\begin{bmatrix} \mathbf{M}_n\boldsymbol{\alpha} + \boldsymbol{\epsilon} \\ \mathbf{M}_g\boldsymbol{\alpha} \end{bmatrix} + \mathbf{e}, \quad (1)$$

where the vectors and matrices for animals without genotypes are denoted with a subscript n and those for the animals with genotypes with a subscript g. Thus, $\mathbf{y}_n$ and $\mathbf{y}_g$ are the vectors of phenotypic values, $\mathbf{X}_n$ and $\mathbf{X}_g$ are the incidence matrices for the fixed effects, $\boldsymbol{\beta}$, $\mathbf{Z}_n$ and $\mathbf{Z}_g$ are incidence matrices that relate the breeding values of animals, $\begin{bmatrix} \mathbf{M}_n\boldsymbol{\alpha} + \boldsymbol{\epsilon} \\ \mathbf{M}_g\boldsymbol{\alpha} \end{bmatrix}$, to the phenotypic values, $\mathbf{M}_g$ is the matrix of centered marker covariates for animals with genotypes, $\mathbf{M}_n = \mathbf{A}_{ng}\mathbf{A}_{gg}^{-1}\mathbf{M}_g$, is the matrix of imputed marker covariates for animals with missing genotypes, $\boldsymbol{\alpha}$ is the vector of random marker effects, $\boldsymbol{\epsilon}$ is the vector of imputation residuals with null means and covariance matrix proportional to the inverse of $\mathbf{A}^{nn}$, the sub-matrix corresponding to animals with missing genotypes in the inverse of the matrix $\mathbf{A}$ of pedigree-based additive relationships, and $\mathbf{e}$ is a vector of residuals. The matrix of imputed genotypes can be more efficiently computed by solving the sparse system of equations [10]:

$$\mathbf{A}^{nn}\mathbf{M}_n = -\mathbf{A}^{ng}\mathbf{M}_g. \qquad (2)$$

Depending on the prior used for $\boldsymbol{\alpha}$, Model (1) can be used for a range of single-step Bayesian regression analyses, including single-step BLUP, BayesA, BayesB, BayesC or Bayesian LASSO [10]. Those models (1) and their corresponding analyses assume that the breeding values can be adequately explained by the marker covariates. If that assumption does not hold, a polygenic residual with a mean of zero and a covariance matrix that is proportional to $\mathbf{A}$ can be included as an additional effect in the model.

The MME that correspond to Model (1) for BayesC with $\pi = 0$ are:

$$\begin{bmatrix} \mathbf{X}'\mathbf{X} & \mathbf{X}'\mathbf{ZM} & \mathbf{X}'_n\mathbf{Z}_n \\ \mathbf{M}'\mathbf{Z}'\mathbf{X} & \mathbf{M}'\mathbf{Z}'\mathbf{ZM} + \mathbf{I}\frac{\sigma_e^2}{\sigma_\alpha^2} & \mathbf{M}'_n\mathbf{Z}'_n\mathbf{Z}_n \\ \mathbf{Z}'_n\mathbf{X}_n & \mathbf{Z}'_n\mathbf{Z}_n\mathbf{M}_n & \mathbf{Z}'_n\mathbf{Z}_n + \mathbf{A}^{nn}\frac{\sigma_e^2}{\sigma_g^2} \end{bmatrix} \begin{bmatrix} \hat{\boldsymbol{\beta}} \\ \hat{\boldsymbol{\alpha}} \\ \hat{\boldsymbol{\epsilon}} \end{bmatrix} = \begin{bmatrix} \mathbf{X}'\mathbf{y} \\ \mathbf{M}'\mathbf{Z}'\mathbf{y} \\ \mathbf{Z}'_n\mathbf{y}_n \end{bmatrix},$$

$$(3)$$

where $\mathbf{X} = \begin{bmatrix} \mathbf{X}_n \\ \mathbf{X}_g \end{bmatrix}$, $\mathbf{Z} = \begin{bmatrix} \mathbf{Z}_n & 0 \\ 0 & \mathbf{Z}_g \end{bmatrix}$, $\mathbf{M} = \begin{bmatrix} \mathbf{M}_n \\ \mathbf{M}_g \end{bmatrix}$, $\mathbf{y} = \begin{bmatrix} \mathbf{y}_n \\ \mathbf{y}_g \end{bmatrix}$, σ_α^2 is the variance of marker effects, σ_g^2 is the additive genetic variance, and σ_e^2 is the residual variance. These Eq. (3) contain matrix-by-matrix products and matrix-by-vector products involving the dense matrix $\mathbf{M}_n$ of imputed genotypes. We will assume here that $\mathbf{X}'\mathbf{ZM}, \mathbf{M}'\mathbf{Z}'\mathbf{X}$ and $\mathbf{M}'\mathbf{Z}'\mathbf{ZM}$ are small enough to be stored in memory. Below, we present computing strategies for calculations that involve $\mathbf{Z}'_n\mathbf{Z}_n\mathbf{M}_n$ or its transpose without storing these large matrices in memory. If the matrices, $\mathbf{X}'\mathbf{ZM}$ and $\mathbf{M}'\mathbf{Z}'\mathbf{X}$, are large, the computing strategies presented below can also be adapted for calculations that involve these matrices as will be done in our example application.

Computing strategies

First, we will discuss the calculations necessary to apply PCG to (3). Following this, we will discuss how to use (3) to obtain Markov chain Monte-Carlo (MCMC) samples of the location parameters of Model (1) from their full conditional distributions.

Preconditioned conjugate gradient iteration The PCG algorithm is widely used to iteratively solve the MME, e.g., [17, 18]. In each iteration of PCG, the left-hand-side of the MME (LHS-MME) is post-multiplied by a vector. However, the LHS-MME given in (3) contains two dense sub-matrices, $\mathbf{Z}'_n\mathbf{Z}_n\mathbf{M}_n$ and its transpose, that may be too large for storage in memory; the remaining sub-matrices in LHS-MME can be stored in memory either because

they are not too large or because they are sparse. In each round of PCG, $\mathbf{Z}'_n\mathbf{Z}_n\mathbf{M}_n$ needs to be post-multiplied by a vector $\mathbf{q}$ that has the same order as $\boldsymbol{\alpha}$ and the transpose of this matrix by a vector $\mathbf{s}$ that has the same order as $\boldsymbol{\epsilon}$. The first of these products can be done without storing $\mathbf{Z}'_n\mathbf{Z}_n\mathbf{M}_n$ in memory as follows. Post-multiplying both sides of Eq. (2) by $\mathbf{q}$ gives:

$$\mathbf{A}^{nn}\mathbf{M}_n\mathbf{q} = -\mathbf{A}^{ng}\mathbf{M}_g\mathbf{q}$$
$$\mathbf{A}^{nn}\mathbf{x} = \mathbf{b}, \qquad (4)$$

where $\mathbf{x} = \mathbf{M}_n\mathbf{q}$ and $\mathbf{b} = -\mathbf{A}^{ng}(\mathbf{M}_g\mathbf{q})$. Note that for efficient computation, the matrix $\mathbf{M}_g$ is first multiplied by $\mathbf{q}$ and the resulting vector is then premultiplied by the sparse matrix $-\mathbf{A}^{ng}$ to get $\mathbf{b}$. Solving the sparse system (4) gives the product $\mathbf{x} = \mathbf{M}_n\mathbf{q}$ without storing the large dense matrix $\mathbf{M}_n$ in memory, and premultiplying $\mathbf{x}$ by $\mathbf{Z}'_n\mathbf{Z}_n$ gives the first product that is required for PCG. To obtain the second product, note that from Eq. (2),

$$\mathbf{M}'_n = -\mathbf{M}'_g\mathbf{A}^{gn}(\mathbf{A}^{nn})^{-1}. \qquad (5)$$

Thus, the required product $\mathbf{M}'_n\mathbf{Z}'_n\mathbf{Z}_n\mathbf{s}$ can be written as $-\mathbf{M}'_g\mathbf{A}^{gn}(\mathbf{A}^{nn})^{-1}\mathbf{Z}'_n\mathbf{Z}_n\mathbf{s}$. To compute this efficiently, first the product $\mathbf{b} = \mathbf{Z}'_n\mathbf{Z}_n\mathbf{s}$ is obtained. Then, solving the sparse system:

$$\mathbf{A}^{nn}\mathbf{x} = \mathbf{b}, \qquad (6)$$

gives $\mathbf{x} = (\mathbf{A}^{nn})^{-1}\mathbf{Z}'_n\mathbf{Z}_n\mathbf{s}$, where $\mathbf{b}$ and $\mathbf{x}$ have been reused to denote intermediate results in these computations. Next, $\mathbf{x}$ is premultiplied by the sparse matrix $-\mathbf{A}^{gn}$ and the resulting vector is premultiplied by $\mathbf{M}'_g$ to get the second product that is required for PCG. The remaining matrix-by-vector products for PCG can be obtained directly because these matrices are stored in memory.

We will now describe how these matrices and the right hand sides involving $\mathbf{M}_n$ can be computed in order to form the other elements of the MME without storing $\mathbf{M}_n$ in memory.

Consider computing:

$$\mathbf{M}'\mathbf{Z}'\mathbf{ZM} = \mathbf{M}'_n\mathbf{Z}'_n\mathbf{Z}_n\mathbf{M}_n + \mathbf{M}'_g\mathbf{Z}'_g\mathbf{Z}_g\mathbf{M}_g,$$

without storing $\mathbf{M}_n$ in memory. Let $\mathbf{m}'_{n_i}$ denote row i of $\mathbf{Z}_n\mathbf{M}_n$. Then, $\mathbf{M}'_n\mathbf{Z}'_n\mathbf{Z}_n\mathbf{M}_n$ can be written as:

$$\mathbf{M}'_n\mathbf{Z}'_n\mathbf{Z}_n\mathbf{M}_n = \sum_i \mathbf{m}_{n_i}\mathbf{m}'_{n_i}. \qquad (7)$$

Thus, the matrix product $\mathbf{M}'_n\mathbf{Z}'_n\mathbf{Z}_n\mathbf{M}_n$ can be computed without storing $\mathbf{M}_n$ in memory if each row of $\mathbf{Z}_n\mathbf{M}_n$ can be obtained without computing the entire matrix. Rearranging (2), row i of $\mathbf{Z}_n\mathbf{M}_n$ can be computed as:

$$\mathbf{m}'_{n_i} = -\mathbf{e}'_i\mathbf{Z}_n(\mathbf{A}^{nn})^{-1}\mathbf{A}^{ng}\mathbf{M}_g, \qquad (8)$$

where $\mathbf{e}_i'$ is a row vector with 1 in the ith position and 0s elsewhere, and the product $\mathbf{e}_i'\mathbf{Z}_n(\mathbf{A}^{nn})^{-1}$ can be obtained by solving the sparse system:

$$\mathbf{A}^{nn}\mathbf{x} = \mathbf{b}, \qquad (9)$$

where $\mathbf{b} = \mathbf{Z}_n'\mathbf{e}_i$. Note that the solution to (9) gives $\mathbf{x}' = \mathbf{e}_i'\mathbf{Z}_n(\mathbf{A}^{nn})^{-1}$, without having to invert $\mathbf{A}^{nn}$. These row vectors of $\mathbf{Z}_n\mathbf{M}_n$ can also be used to compute $\mathbf{X}_n'\mathbf{Z}_n\mathbf{M}_n$ as:

$$\mathbf{X}_n'\mathbf{Z}_n\mathbf{M}_n = \sum_i \mathbf{x}_i\mathbf{m}_{n_i}', \qquad (10)$$

where $\mathbf{x}_i$ is used here to denote the ith column of $\mathbf{X}_n'$, which is the first term of

$$\mathbf{X}'\mathbf{Z}\mathbf{M} = \mathbf{X}_n'\mathbf{Z}_n\mathbf{M}_n + \mathbf{X}_g'\mathbf{Z}_g\mathbf{M}_g,$$

which is a product of $\mathbf{M}_n$. Similarly, the right-hand-side vector $\mathbf{M}'\mathbf{Z}'\mathbf{y}$ can be written as the sum:

$$\mathbf{M}'\mathbf{Z}'\mathbf{y} = \mathbf{M}_n'\mathbf{Z}_n'\mathbf{y}_n + \mathbf{M}_g'\mathbf{Z}_g'\mathbf{y}_g,$$

which is a product of $\mathbf{M}_n$, and its first term can be computed as:

$$\mathbf{M}_n'\mathbf{Z}_n'\mathbf{y}_n = \sum_i \mathbf{m}_{n_i}y_i, \qquad (11)$$

where y_i is used to denote the ith element of $\mathbf{y}_n$.

Note that computing $\mathbf{m}_{n_i}'$ corresponding to row i of $\mathbf{Z}_n\mathbf{M}_n$ using Eq. (8) can be done independently of its computation for any other row, and thus, the computations in Eqs. (7), (10), and (11) can be easily parallelized.

There are a number of approaches to compute $\mathbf{m}_{n_i}'$ that can be used. One approach for solving Eq. (9) for n less than approximately ten million using a typical workstation computer is to obtain a sparse Cholesky factor of $\mathbf{A}^{nn}$ and directly solve for each $\mathbf{m}_{n_i}'$ using forward and backward substitution. Software libraries exist for obtaining a Cholesky factor of large sparse matrices [19] using multiple threads or general purpose graphics processing units (GPU). Once the factor is obtained, independent threads can be used to solve in parallel from a single memory copy of the factor. Note that the Cholesky factor of $\mathbf{A}^{nn}$ may be denser than $\mathbf{A}^{nn}$, depending upon the nature of the relationships between genotyped and non-genotyped animals. For example, if non-genotyped animals comprise only non-parents, then $\mathbf{A}^{nn}$ is diagonal and solution for $\mathbf{m}_i'$ is trivial. For larger linear systems with non-genotyped parents where the Cholesky factor is too large, indirect solution using high performance methods on GPU is a practical alternative. The PCG algorithm parallelizes well and performs efficiently on GPU.

MCMC sampling Gibbs sampling is a widely used MCMC method for inference with Bayesian regression models, e.g., [3, 20, 21]. One of the most time-consuming tasks in these analyses is single-site sampling of the location parameters from their full-conditional distributions. Let $\boldsymbol{\theta} = \begin{bmatrix} \boldsymbol{\beta} \\ \boldsymbol{\alpha} \\ \boldsymbol{\epsilon} \end{bmatrix}$ denote the location parameters in Model (1). Then, following [22], the full-conditional distribution for θ_i under BayesC with $\pi = 0$ is:

$$\theta_i|\text{ELSE} \sim \text{N}\left(\tilde{\theta}_i, c_{ii}^{-1}\sigma_e^2\right),$$

where ELSE is used to denote all the other parameters in the model and the vector of phenotypes, $\tilde{\theta}_i$ is the solution to:

$$c_{ii}\tilde{\theta}_i = r_i - \mathbf{c}_i'\boldsymbol{\theta} + c_{ii}\theta_i, \qquad (12)$$

c_{ii} is the ith diagonal of the matrix $\mathbf{C}$ that denotes the LHS-MME given in (3), r_i is the right-hand-side element from (3) corresponding to θ_i, and $\mathbf{c}_i'$ is row i of $\mathbf{C}$. However, as mentioned previously, some sub-matrices of the LHS-MME given in (3) are dense and too large to be stored in memory. However, as explained below, the same strategy used to avoid storing these sub-matrices in PCG calculations can also be used here.

Consider computing the full conditional mean and variance for $\theta_i = \alpha_j$. Then c_{ii}, the ith diagonal element from $\mathbf{C}$ is obtained from the jth diagonal of $\mathbf{B} = \mathbf{M}'\mathbf{Z}'\mathbf{Z}\mathbf{M} + \mathbf{I}\dfrac{\sigma_e^2}{\sigma_\alpha^2}$, which can be stored in memory. Similarly, $r_i - \mathbf{c}_i'\boldsymbol{\theta} + c_{ii}\theta_i$ is computed as:

$$r_i - \mathbf{c}_i'\boldsymbol{\theta} + c_{ii}\theta_i = d_j - \mathbf{b}_j'\boldsymbol{\alpha} + b_{jj}\alpha_j,$$

where d_j is element j of the vector

$$\mathbf{d} = \mathbf{M}'\mathbf{Z}'\mathbf{y} - \mathbf{M}'\mathbf{Z}'\mathbf{X}\boldsymbol{\beta} - \mathbf{M}_n'\mathbf{Z}_n'\mathbf{Z}_n\boldsymbol{\epsilon},$$

$\mathbf{b}_j'$ is row j and b_{jj} is the jth diagonal of $\mathbf{B}$. We have already seen how the large, dense matrix $\mathbf{M}_n'\mathbf{Z}_n'\mathbf{Z}_n$ can be multiplied by a vector such as $\boldsymbol{\epsilon}$ without storing this matrix in memory, and this same strategy can be used here to compute $\mathbf{M}_n'\mathbf{Z}_n'\mathbf{Z}_n\boldsymbol{\epsilon}$. The full-conditional distribution for α_j, under BayesC with $\pi = 0$, becomes:

$$\alpha_j|\text{ELSE} \sim \text{N}\left(\tilde{\alpha}_j, b_{jj}^{-1}\sigma_e^2\right),$$

where $\tilde{\alpha}_j$ is the solution to:

$$b_{jj}\tilde{\alpha}_j = d_j - \mathbf{b}_j'\boldsymbol{\alpha} + b_{jj}\alpha_j. \qquad (13)$$

The right-hand-side of this Eq. (13) is also used for calculations that involve variable selection in BayesB and BayesC when $\pi > 0$ [21, 23].

Similarly, to compute full-conditional mean and variance for $\theta_i = \epsilon_j$, c_{ii} is obtained from the jth diagonal of $\mathbf{B}$ that now denotes $\mathbf{B} = \mathbf{Z}_n'\mathbf{Z}_n + \mathbf{A}^{nn}\dfrac{\sigma_e^2}{\sigma_g^2}$, and

$$r_i - \mathbf{c}'_i \boldsymbol{\theta} + c_{ii}\theta_i = d_j - \mathbf{b}'_j \boldsymbol{\epsilon} + b_{jj}\epsilon_j,$$

where d_j is element j of the vector that now denotes:

$$\mathbf{d} = \mathbf{Z}'_n\mathbf{y}_n - \mathbf{Z}'_n\mathbf{X}_n\boldsymbol{\beta} - \mathbf{Z}'_n\mathbf{Z}_n\mathbf{M}_n\boldsymbol{\alpha}.$$

The product $\mathbf{Z}'_n\mathbf{Z}_n\mathbf{M}_n\boldsymbol{\alpha}$ is obtained as described for PCG calculations. Then, the full-conditional distribution for ϵ_j becomes:

$$\epsilon_j|\text{ELSE} \sim \mathrm{N}\left(\tilde{\epsilon}_j, b_{jj}^{-1}\sigma_e^2\right),$$

where $\tilde{\epsilon}_j$ is the solution to

$$b_{jj}\tilde{\epsilon}_j = d_j - \mathbf{b}'_j\boldsymbol{\epsilon} + b_{jj}\epsilon_j.$$

Samples of model effects such as $\boldsymbol{\beta}, \boldsymbol{\alpha}$, and $\boldsymbol{\epsilon}$, or their linear functions that represent breeding values namely $\mathbf{M}_g\boldsymbol{\alpha}$ for genotyped animals or $\mathbf{M}_n\boldsymbol{\alpha} + \boldsymbol{\epsilon}$ for non-genotyped animals can be accumulated as sums and sums of squares to obtain posterior means and prediction error variances. Alternatively, samples of fitted model effects can be written to a file for post-processing.

Hybrid model for single-step Bayesian regression

The large, dense matrix $\mathbf{M}_n$ appears in the MEM given by Model (1). This is avoided here by using a BVM for animals with missing genotypes rather than expressing their breeding values as the sum of the effects of their imputed marker genotypes plus their separate imputation residuals. The advantages of the MEM such as allowing for alternative priors for marker effects are retained by still fitting a MEM but only for animals with genotypes. The hybrid model equation is:

$$\begin{bmatrix} \mathbf{y}_n \\ \mathbf{y}_g \end{bmatrix} = \begin{bmatrix} \mathbf{X}_n \\ \mathbf{X}_g \end{bmatrix}\boldsymbol{\beta} + \begin{bmatrix} \mathbf{0} & \mathbf{Z}_n \\ \mathbf{Z}_g\mathbf{M}_g & \mathbf{0} \end{bmatrix}\begin{bmatrix} \boldsymbol{\alpha} \\ \mathbf{u}_n \end{bmatrix} + \mathbf{e}, \quad (14)$$

with $\mathbf{u}_n = \mathbf{M}_n\boldsymbol{\alpha} + \boldsymbol{\epsilon}$, and thus, this single-step hybrid model (SS-HM) is equivalent to the SS-MEM (1). To construct the MME for this model (14), we need to invert the covariance matrix corresponding to the random effects, namely $\boldsymbol{\Sigma} = \mathrm{Var}\left(\begin{bmatrix} \boldsymbol{\alpha} \\ \mathbf{u}_n \end{bmatrix}\right)$. That inverse can be obtained by first writing the random effects of (14) as:

$$\begin{bmatrix} \boldsymbol{\alpha} \\ \mathbf{u}_n \end{bmatrix} = \begin{bmatrix} \mathbf{I} & \mathbf{0} \\ \mathbf{M}_n & \mathbf{I} \end{bmatrix}\begin{bmatrix} \boldsymbol{\alpha} \\ \boldsymbol{\epsilon} \end{bmatrix}.$$

Then, $\boldsymbol{\Sigma}$ can be written as:

$$\boldsymbol{\Sigma} = \begin{bmatrix} \mathbf{I} & \mathbf{0} \\ \mathbf{M}_n & \mathbf{I} \end{bmatrix}\mathrm{Var}\left(\begin{bmatrix} \boldsymbol{\alpha} \\ \boldsymbol{\epsilon} \end{bmatrix}\right)\begin{bmatrix} \mathbf{I} & \mathbf{M}'_n \\ \mathbf{0} & \mathbf{I} \end{bmatrix}$$

$$= \begin{bmatrix} \mathbf{I} & \mathbf{0} \\ \mathbf{M_n} & \mathbf{I} \end{bmatrix}\begin{bmatrix} \mathbf{I}\sigma_\alpha^2 & \mathbf{0} \\ \mathbf{0} & (\mathbf{A}^{nn})^{-1}\sigma_g^2 \end{bmatrix}\begin{bmatrix} \mathbf{I} & \mathbf{M}'_n \\ \mathbf{0} & \mathbf{I} \end{bmatrix},$$

and its inverse can be obtained as:

$$\boldsymbol{\Sigma}^{-1} = \begin{bmatrix} \mathbf{I} & -\mathbf{M}'_n \\ \mathbf{0} & \mathbf{I} \end{bmatrix}\begin{bmatrix} \mathbf{I}\frac{1}{\sigma_\alpha^2} & \mathbf{0} \\ \mathbf{0} & \mathbf{A}^{nn}\frac{1}{\sigma_g^2} \end{bmatrix}\begin{bmatrix} \mathbf{I} & \mathbf{0} \\ -\mathbf{M}_n & \mathbf{I} \end{bmatrix}$$

$$= \begin{bmatrix} \mathbf{I} & \mathbf{0} \\ \mathbf{0} & \mathbf{0} \end{bmatrix}\frac{1}{\sigma_\alpha^2} + \begin{bmatrix} -\mathbf{M}'_n \\ \mathbf{I} \end{bmatrix}\mathbf{A}^{nn}\frac{1}{\sigma_g^2}\begin{bmatrix} -\mathbf{M}_n & \mathbf{I} \end{bmatrix}$$

$$= \begin{bmatrix} \mathbf{I} & \mathbf{0} \\ \mathbf{0} & \mathbf{0} \end{bmatrix}\frac{1}{\sigma_\alpha^2} + \begin{bmatrix} \mathbf{M}'_n\mathbf{A}^{nn}\mathbf{M}_n & -\mathbf{M}'_n\mathbf{A}^{nn} \\ -\mathbf{A}^{nn}\mathbf{M}_n & \mathbf{A}^{nn} \end{bmatrix}\frac{1}{\sigma_g^2}.$$

Now, using the result $\mathbf{M}_n = \mathbf{A}_{ng}\mathbf{A}_{gg}^{-1}\mathbf{M}_g = -(\mathbf{A}^{nn})^{-1}\mathbf{A}^{ng}\mathbf{M}_g$ [10], in the off-diagonal blocks of the second term, $\boldsymbol{\Sigma}^{-1}$ becomes:

$$\boldsymbol{\Sigma}^{-1} = \begin{bmatrix} \mathbf{I}\frac{1}{\sigma_\alpha^2} + \mathbf{M}'_n\mathbf{A}^{nn}\mathbf{M}_n\frac{1}{\sigma_g^2} & \mathbf{M}'_g\mathbf{A}^{gn}\frac{1}{\sigma_g^2} \\ \mathbf{A}^{ng}\mathbf{M}_g\frac{1}{\sigma_g^2} & \mathbf{A}^{nn}\frac{1}{\sigma_g^2} \end{bmatrix},$$

and then the MME for the HM (14) can be written as:

$$\begin{bmatrix} \mathbf{X}'\mathbf{X} & \mathbf{X}'_g\mathbf{Z}_g\mathbf{M}_g & \mathbf{X}'_n\mathbf{Z}_n \\ \mathbf{M}'_g\mathbf{Z}'_g\mathbf{X}_g & \mathbf{Q} & \mathbf{M}'_g\mathbf{A}^{gn}\frac{\sigma_e^2}{\sigma_g^2} \\ \mathbf{Z}'_n\mathbf{X}_n & \mathbf{A}^{ng}\mathbf{M}_g\frac{\sigma_e^2}{\sigma_g^2} & \mathbf{Z}'_n\mathbf{Z}_n + \mathbf{A}^{nn}\frac{\sigma_e^2}{\sigma_g^2} \end{bmatrix}\begin{bmatrix} \hat{\boldsymbol{\beta}} \\ \hat{\boldsymbol{\alpha}} \\ \hat{\mathbf{u}}_n \end{bmatrix} = \begin{bmatrix} \mathbf{X}'\mathbf{y} \\ \mathbf{M}'_g\mathbf{Z}'_g\mathbf{y}_g \\ \mathbf{Z}'_n\mathbf{y}_n \end{bmatrix},$$

$$(15)$$

where $\mathbf{Q} = \mathbf{M}'_g\mathbf{Z}'_g\mathbf{Z}_g\mathbf{M}_g + \mathbf{I}\frac{\sigma_e^2}{\sigma_\alpha^2} + \mathbf{M}'_n\mathbf{A}^{nn}\mathbf{M}_n\frac{\sigma_e^2}{\sigma_g^2}$. These equations involve $\mathbf{M}_g$ rather than $\mathbf{M}_n$, except in $\mathbf{Q}$, the diagonal block that corresponds to $\hat{\boldsymbol{\alpha}}$, which has dimension equal to the number of marker covariates, often less than 50,000, regardless of the number of genotyped or non-genotyped animals. Furthermore, we assume here that $\mathbf{X}'_g\mathbf{Z}_g\mathbf{M}_g$ and $\mathbf{M}'_g\mathbf{Z}'_g\mathbf{X}_g$ are small enough to be stored in memory.

The only difference between Eq. (15) and the MME given by Equation (A1) in Legarra and Ducrocq [15] is in $\mathbf{Q}$. Using the notation in this paper, the matrix expression $\mathbf{M}'_n\mathbf{A}^{nn}\mathbf{M}_n$ that is present in the $\mathbf{Q}$ is expressed as $\mathbf{M}'_g(\mathbf{A}^{gg} - \mathbf{A}_{gg}^{-1})\mathbf{M}_g$ in that paper [15], which involves the inverse of $\mathbf{A}_{gg}$ that is difficult to compute. However, these two expressions are identical because $(\mathbf{A}^{gg} - \mathbf{A}_{gg}^{-1}) = \mathbf{A}^{gn}(\mathbf{A}^{nn})^{-1}\mathbf{A}^{ng}$ and $\mathbf{M}_n = -(\mathbf{A}^{nn})^{-1}\mathbf{A}^{ng}\mathbf{M}_g$.

Computing strategies

The matrix $\mathbf{M}_n$ of imputed genotypes does not appear alone in the MME (15), but the MME involve rather the matrix product $\mathbf{M}'_n\mathbf{A}^{nn}\mathbf{M}_n$. However, $\mathbf{M}'_n\mathbf{A}^{nn}\mathbf{M}_n$ can be computed efficiently without needing to store the entire $\mathbf{M}_n$ matrix in memory, in situations when the number of genotyped animals is less than the number of non-genotyped animals. To do so, first from Eq. (5) $\mathbf{M}'_n\mathbf{A}^{nn} = -\mathbf{M}'_g\mathbf{A}^{gn}$. Next, column i of $\mathbf{M}_n$ is obtained by solving the sparse system (2) for column i and premultiply it by the sparse matrix $\mathbf{A}^{gn}$. This gives column i of the product $\mathbf{A}^{gn}\mathbf{M}_n$, which has the same size as $\mathbf{M}_g$. The columns of $\mathbf{A}^{gn}\mathbf{M}_n$ can be computed one at a time or in parallel. Premultiplying $\mathbf{A}^{gn}\mathbf{M}_n$ by $-\mathbf{M}_g'$ gives:

$$-\mathbf{M}_g'\mathbf{A}^{gn}\mathbf{M}_n = \mathbf{M}_n'\mathbf{A}^{nn}\mathbf{M}_n. \qquad (16)$$

This needs to be done only once to set up the MME and has order equal to the number of marker genotypes which is often much less than the number of genotyped or non-genotyped animals.

These MME also contain two large, dense sub-matrices, namely $\mathbf{A}^{ng}\mathbf{M}_g$ and its transpose. As described previously, in the PCG iteration and in the Gibbs sampling, these matrices need to be post-multiplied by a vector. When the number of genotyped animals is sufficiently smaller than the number of non-genotyped animals, these matrix-by-vector products can be obtained more efficiently by storing in memory the sparse matrix $\mathbf{A}^{ng}$ and the dense but smaller matrix $\mathbf{M}_g$ rather than their product $\mathbf{A}^{ng}\mathbf{M}_g$. In each round of PCG iteration or Gibbs sampling, the matrix-by-vector product $\mathbf{A}^{ng}\mathbf{M}_g\mathbf{q}$, for example, is obtained by first multiplying the dense matrix $\mathbf{M}_g$ by the vector $\mathbf{q}$ and then premultiplying the result by the sparse matrix $\mathbf{A}^{ng}$. The corresponding calculation for the MEM required solving sparse systems of equations given by Eq. (4) in each round of PCG or Gibbs sampling, in addition to the two matrix-by-vector multiplications that are also required here.

In situations when the number of genotyped animals exceeds the number of non-genotyped animals, using SS-MEM that explicitly involves $\mathbf{M}_n$ in off-diagonal blocks may be competitive with SS-HM.

Application of hybrid model

An example dataset from the American Simmental Association is used to demonstrate the computing effort to obtain PCG samples from (15) and the relative computing effort to obtain MCMC samples for the MME of (15) compared to (3). The vector of phenotypes comprised of 4,934,101 birth weight observations; there were 6,179,960 animals in the pedigree file; 31,453 animals in the pedigree file were genotyped and 23,290 of those had birth weight observations. After filtering marker covariates for low minor allele frequency, 40,214 marker effects were included in the model. There were 399,036 fixed effects, including the herd-year-season effects defined in the same manner as in the routine national evaluation. To keep this presentation that compares the computational effort involved in fitting (3) and (15) simple, our application was limited to a single trait ignoring maternal genetic and permanent environmental effects. Furthermore, we did not include a comparison with SS-GBLUP since that model cannot

accommodate mixture priors for marker effects as used in this example.

The analyses were performed using a workstation built on an ASUS X99E WS motherboard, a Xeon E5-1650V3 3.5 Ghz processor overclocked to 4.2 Ghz, 128 GB of DDR4 ECC RAM at 2133 Mhz and four NVidia Titan X GPU, with 9TB of workspace in a RAID5 configuration comprising four SATA disks. The operating system was Ubuntu 14.04 LTS, and the BOLT software package (http://manual.thetasolutionsllc.com/IntroBolt) built with the CUDA Toolkit 7.5 was used.

The vector $\mathbf{y}$, and matrices $\mathbf{X}, \mathbf{Z}, \mathbf{A}^{nn}, \mathbf{A}^{gn}, \mathbf{A}^{ng}$, and $\mathbf{M}_g$ were built from data files using BOLT tools. Ordering the pedigree file, construction of $\mathbf{A}^{-1}$, including calculation of inbreeding, and its partitioning into blocks representing genotyped and non-genotyped animals took 3 min and required 1.0 Gb of disk storage and 302 Mb of memory. While $\mathbf{A}^{-1}$ was being formed, $\mathbf{y}$, $\mathbf{X}$ and $\mathbf{Z}$ were created in about 10 s and required 38, 78 and 83 Mb of disk storage. When stored in memory, they required 19.7, 59.2 and 59.2 Mb respectively. The matrix $\mathbf{M}_g$ required 4.2 Gb of disk and memory when stored in single precision.

The matrix product $\mathbf{X}_g'\mathbf{Z}_g\mathbf{M}_g$ and its transpose $\mathbf{M}_g'\mathbf{Z}_g'\mathbf{X}_g$ were not explicitly formed, instead computations involving those terms were done in parts as described previously in this paper. The sparse Cholesky decomposition of the 6,148,507 order $\mathbf{A}^{nn}$ matrix took just under 4 min. The imputation of $\mathbf{M}_n$, using forward and backward substitution with the Cholesky factor, and its premultiplication by $\mathbf{A}^{gn}$ took just over 35 min using eight parallel processes. The creation of the matrix products $\mathbf{M}_g'\mathbf{Z}_g'\mathbf{Z}_g\mathbf{M}_g$ and $\mathbf{M}_n'\mathbf{A}^{nn}\mathbf{M}_n$ each took about 20 s using 2 GPU after obtaining the imputed values and required 6.2 Gb of disk storage and memory when stored in single precision.

For the analysis using Eq. (15) the PCG solution of the MME stored in double precision took just under 40 min, using a single GPU and diagonal preconditioning. Because the PCG was performed in double precision just under 18 Gb of memory was required to store all the sub-matrices comprising the left-hand side. The right-hand side required 53Mb of memory. Additional memory for work space of approximately 4 Gb was required for PCG. Convergence was determined by comparing solutions from every 200 rounds of iteration to solutions from 5000 rounds. By 1800 rounds the correlation and regression of solutions with those from 5000 rounds were very close to one (.99 each). The PCG residual value was near 1.1e−05. The PCG solution does not give the posterior mean of the marker effects for a model with mixture priors, but was used to define starting values for MCMC sampling of all the effects in the MME, but using a mixture prior for marker effects.

Starting with the same PCG solution but different random number generator seed values, using 4 parallel chains each drawing 10,500 samples on its own GPU took 70 min to obtain a total of 42,000 Gibbs samples, using $\pi = 0.95$ and known variance ratios in Eqs. (3) and (15). Each of the parallel Gibbs Sampler jobs shared a single copy in shared memory of the left-hand-side matrices, reducing the memory requirements and reading from disk.

Experience has shown that 40,000 samples after burn-in is sufficient to obtain posterior means of breeding values that are stable for the hybrid model and MEM. However, we confirmed this by sampling four additional parallel chains each with length 250,000 samples after a 5000 sample burn. The purpose of these very long chains was to confirm that the 40,000 length post-burn-in chain was sufficient, thus supporting the timings provided here to achieve useful results. The correlation of the posterior means of the breeding values for genotyped animals and non-genotyped animals from the aggregated 40,000 length chain was .99 and 1.0, respectively, with the posterior means from the aggregated 1,000,000 length chain. However, a chain longer that 40,000 may be needed to accurately estimate PEV for animals with intermediate to low accuracies. Because only off-diagonal blocks of the left-hand side are used in the GPU computation for updating the right-hand-sides for each vector of single-site Gibbs samples for β, α or $\mathbf{u}_n$, and the Gibbs samples were obtained using single precision, the entire left-hand side without the diagonal blocks fit on the GPU. This strategy also allowed the GPU to asynchronously update the right-hand-side while the next set of effects was being sampled using the CPU.

The Gibbs sampler was performed using single precision for storage of the left- and right-hand sides, requiring approximately half as much memory as the 18 Gb required for the PCG which was performed in double precision. Additional memory for work space of approximately 2 Gb was required for the Gibbs sampler. The total time required to assemble the left- and right-hand sides, after the matrix components were formed, was just under 3 min. The total job time for all steps, starting with the raw data, to obtain posterior mean estimates of the MCMC samples of marker effects and MCMC samples of breeding values of the genotyped and non-genotyped animals and their prediction error variances (from the posterior variances of their MCMC samples), took approximately 3 h.

The memory required to store $\mathbf{M}_g$ is determined by the product of the number of animals genotyped and the number of marker covariates. A compressed dense format (CBRC) allows this matrix to be 32 times larger than with the double precision version used above, but increased the computing time for PCG in this example by 25%.

An additional Gibbs sampler run was made with the MME of (3) that used Eq. (4), which requires within each iteration, forward and backward solves using the factor of $\mathbf{A}^{nn}$. The time required to obtain one sample of all effects was 2.0 s. Using the MME of (15) required only 0.44 s for each sample of all effects. Accordingly, the hybrid model has considerable advantage over that of [10]. These two computing approaches should give the same estimates of breeding values as they represent equivalent models as explained in the theory section. The correlations between the MCMC-derived estimates of breeding values between the two approaches were 1.0 for non-genotyped animals and over 0.99 for genotyped animals.

Computational performance of Eq. (15) was compared ignoring the genotypes on approximately half the genotyped animals to demonstrate the effect of the proportion of genotyped animals on computing time. This reduced dataset left 15,694 animals with genotype information of which 11,683 had a birth weight observation. The total number of animals in the pedigree file and number of observations on birth weight were the same as before. After filtering the marker covariates for low minor allele frequency, 40,211 marker loci remained. The time necessary to complete the PCG solver was about 3 min less than the 27 min needed for the larger analysis, which had approximately double the number of genotyped animals. The reduction in time necessary to complete the PCG solver was primarily due to reductions in time used for matrix multiplications involving the smaller matrix $\mathbf{M}_g$. The time necessary to obtain the 42,000 Gibbs samples was reduced by about 20% to 1 h. Imputation required 24 instead of 35 min. Creating $\mathbf{M}_g' \mathbf{Z}_g' \mathbf{Z}_g \mathbf{M}_g$ and $\mathbf{M}_n' \mathbf{A}^{nn} \mathbf{M}_n$ required just under 20 s, the same as before. Thus, doubling the proportion of genotyped animals increased the total job time from about 2.5 to 3 h.

Discussion

Fernando et al. [10] introduced a single-step MEM that is equivalent to SS-GBLUP in the special case when all markers are fitted in the model. It has the advantage compared to SS-GBLUP that it can accommodate a wider class of models with different priors including mixture distributions. However, the MME corresponding to that model includes large, dense off-diagonal sub-matrices, $\mathbf{Z}_n' \mathbf{Z}_n \mathbf{M}_n$ and its transpose, between the blocks for marker effects and the imputation residuals. These sub-matrices are prohibitively large from a storage and computational viewpoint when there is a large number of non-genotyped animals. We have shown here that these limitations can be circumvented by representing those sub-matrices as:

$$-\mathbf{Z}_n' \mathbf{Z}_n (\mathbf{A}^{nn})^{-1} \mathbf{A}^{ng} \mathbf{M}_g$$

and its transpose, and by doing matrix multiplication in parts. This is possible for large problems but requires repeated solutions of an equation of the form $\mathbf{A}^{nn}\mathbf{x} = \mathbf{b}$. A similar solution is used in every iteration of SS-GBLUP when an APY inverse is exploited [18]. Nevertheless, the model in [10] is practical for realistic problems as demonstrated. It does not require approximations [18] as in SS-GBLUP when large numbers of animals are genotyped.

Here we have introduced a single-step HM that is equivalent to the MEM in [10] and in a special case equivalent to SS-GBLUP. The HM includes marker effects and breeding values, and the off-diagonal sub matrices comprise the term $\mathbf{A}^{ng}\mathbf{M}_g$. Computations that involve this sub-matrix can be done efficiently in parts without having to solve equations of the form $\mathbf{A}^{nn}\mathbf{x} = \mathbf{b}$.

The off-diagonal sub-matrices in both these models are the same size, the lower off-diagonal matrix being of the order of the number of non-genotyped animals by the number of markers. In SS-HM, this sub-matrix has a more convenient structure for storage and computation than is generally the case for SS-MEM. We have demonstrated its practicality and its considerable reduction in computing effort. This model can be readily extended to accommodate multiple traits, multiple breeds, maternal effects, and additional random effects such as polygenic residual effects.

Authors' contributions
DJG developed the computational strategies for the MEM and also proposed the HM. RLF, HC and DJG derived the MME for the HM. BLG wrote the software and performed all the data analyses. All authors read and approved the final manuscript.

Author details
[1] Department of Animal Science, Iowa State University, Ames, IA 50011, USA. [2] Theta Solutions, LLC, Atascadero, CA 93422, USA. [3] Institute of Veterinary, Animal and Biomedical Sciences, Massey University, Palmerston North, New Zealand.

Acknowledgements
We are grateful to the reviewers of this manuscript for several helpful suggestions and for pointing out the relationship between the MME for the hybrid model (15) and the MME in [A1] of Legarra and Ducrocq [15]. The authors thank the American Simmental Association for sharing their data. This work was supported in part by the US Department of Agriculture, Agriculture and Food Research Initiative National Institute of Food and Agriculture Competitive Grant No. 2015-67015-22947.

Competing interests
DJG and BLG are partners in Theta Solutions LLC that developed the BOLT software used in this paper. The authors declare that they have no competing interests.

References
1. Strandén I, Garrick DJ. Technical note: Derivation of equivalent computing algorithms for genomic predictions and reliabilities of animal merit. J Dairy Sci. 2009;92:2971–5.
2. Fernando RL. Genetic evaluation and selection using genotypic, phenotypic and pedigree information. In: Proceedings of the 6th World Congress on Genetics Applied to Livestock Production: 11–16 January 1998. vol. 26. Armidale; 1998. pp. 329–36.
3. Meuwissen THE, Hayes BJ, Goddard ME. Prediction of total genetic value using genome-wide dense marker maps. Genetics. 2001;157:1819–29.
4. Nejati-Javaremi A, Smith C, Gibson JP. Effect of total allelic relationship on accuracy of evaluation and response to selection. J Anim Sci. 1997;75:1738–45.
5. Habier D, Fernando RL, Dekkers JCM. The impact of genetic relationship information on genome-assisted breeding values. Genetics. 2007;177:2389–97.
6. VanRaden PM. Efficient methods to compute genomic predictions. J Dairy Sci. 2008;91:4414–23.
7. Legarra A, Aguilar I, Misztal I. A relationship matrix including full pedigree and genomic information. J Dairy Sci. 2009;92:4656–63.
8. Christensen OF, Lund MS. Genomic prediction when some animals are not genotyped. Genet Sel Evol. 2010;42:2.
9. Aguilar I, Misztal I, Johnson DL, Legarra A, Tsuruta S, Lawlor TJ. Hot topic: a unified approach to utilize phenotypic, full pedigree, and genomic information for genetic evaluation of Holstein final score. J Dairy Sci. 2010;93:743–52.
10. Fernando RL, Dekkers JCM, Garrick DJ. A class of Bayesian methods to combine large numbers of genotyped and non-genotyped animals for whole-genome analyses. Genet Sel Evol. 2014;46:59.
11. Gianola D, de los Campos G, Hill WG, Manfredi E, Fernando R. Additive genetic variability and the Bayesian alphabet. Genetics. 2009;83:347–63.
12. de los Campos G, Naya H, Gianola D, Crossa J, Legarra A, Manfredi E, et al. Predicting quantitative traits with regression models for dense molecular markers and pedigree. Genetics. 2009;182:375–85.
13. Habier D, Fernando RL, Kizilkaya K, Garrick DJ. Extension of the Bayesian alphabet for genomic selection. In: Proceedings of the 9th world congress on genetics applied to livestock production: 1–6 August 2010. Leipzig 2010.
14. Liu Z, Goddard ME, Reinhardt F, Reents R. A single-step genomic model with direct estimation of marker effects. J Dairy Sci. 2014;97:5833–50.
15. Legarra A, Ducrocq V. Computational strategies for national integration of phenotypic, genomic, and pedigree data in a single-step best linear unbiased prediction. J Dairy Sci. 2012;95:4629–45.
16. Vitezica ZG, Aguilar I, Misztal I, Legarra A. Bias in genomic predictions for populations under selection. Genet Res (Camb). 2011;93:357–66.
17. Strandén I, Lidauer M. Solving large mixed linear models using preconditioned conjugate gradient iteration. J Dairy Sci. 1999;82:2779–87.
18. Masuda Y, Misztal I, Tsuruta S, Legarra A, Aguilar I, Lourenco DAL, et al. Implementation of genomic recursions in single-step genomic best linear unbiased predictor for US Holsteins with a large number of genotyped animals. J Dairy Sci. 2016;99:1968–74.
19. Chen Y, Davis TA, Hager WW, Rajamanickam S. Algorithm 887: CHOLMOD, supernodal sparse Cholesky factorization and update/downdate. ACM Trans Math Softw. 2008;35:22.
20. Habier D, Fernando RL, Kizilkaya K, Garrick DJ. Extension of the Bayesian alphabet for genomic selection. BMC Bioinformatics. 2011;12:186.
21. Fernando R, Garrick D. Bayesian methods applied to GWAS. In: Gondro C, van der Werf J, Hayes B, editors. Genome-wide association studies and genomic prediction. New York: Humana Press; 2013.
22. Sorensen DA, Gianola D. Likelihood, Bayesian, and MCMC methods in quantitative genetics. New York: Springer; 2002.
23. Cheng H, Qu L, Garrick DJ, Fernando RL. A fast and efficient Gibbs sampler for BayesB in whole-genome analyses. Genet Sel Evol. 2015;47:80.

17

A strategy to improve phasing of whole-genome sequenced individuals through integration of familial information from dense genotype panels

Pierre Faux[*] and Tom Druet

Abstract

Background: Haplotype reconstruction (phasing) is an essential step in many applications, including imputation and genomic selection. The best phasing methods rely on both familial and linkage disequilibrium (LD) information. With whole-genome sequence (WGS) data, relatively small samples of reference individuals are generally sequenced due to prohibitive sequencing costs, thus only a limited amount of familial information is available. However, reference individuals have many relatives that have been genotyped (at lower density). The goal of our study was to improve phasing of WGS data by integrating familial information from haplotypes that were obtained from a larger genotyped dataset and to quantify its impact on imputation accuracy.

Results: Aligning a pre-phased WGS panel [~5 million single nucleotide polymorphisms (SNPs)], which is based on LD information only, to a 50k SNP array that is phased with both LD and familial information (called scaffold) resulted in correctly assigning parental origin for 99.62% of the WGS SNPs, their phase being determined unambiguously based on parental genotypes. Without using the 50k haplotypes as scaffold, that value dropped as expected to 50%. Correctly phased segments were on average longer after alignment to the genotype phase while the number of switches decreased slightly. Most of the incorrectly assigned segments, and subsequent switches, were due to singleton errors. Imputation from 50k SNP array to WGS data with improved phasing had a marginal impact on imputation accuracy (measured as r^2), i.e. on average, 90.47% with traditional techniques versus 90.65% with pre-phasing integrating familial information. Differences were larger for SNPs located in chromosome ends and rare variants. Using a denser WGS panel (~13 millions SNPs) that was obtained with traditional variant filtering rules, we found similar results although performances of both phasing and imputation accuracy were lower.

Conclusions: We present a phasing strategy for WGS data, which indirectly integrates familial information by aligning WGS haplotypes that are pre-phased with LD information only on haplotypes obtained with genotyping data, with both LD and familial information and on a much larger population. This strategy results in very few mismatches with the phase obtained by Mendelian segregation rules. Finally, we propose a strategy to further improve phasing accuracy based on haplotype clusters obtained with genotyping data.

Background

Most genotyping technologies provide, for each marker, the combination of marker alleles that are carried by an individual. Haplotype reconstruction for such genotyping data, or phasing, refers to statistical methods that determine which marker alleles were inherited from the same parent and are located on the same homolog. It is an essential step in many applications, including imputation [1], pre-phasing of reference panels [2], estimation of identity-by-descent (IBD) probability for genetic or QTL mapping [3], association analysis (e.g. [4–6]), genomic

---
*Correspondence: pierrefaux@gmail.com
Unit of Animal Genomics, GIGA-R and Faculty of Veterinary Medicine, University of Liège, 4000 Liège, Belgium

selection [7–10], studies of genetic diversity, detection of signatures of selection [11, 12] or the study of the recombination process (e.g. [13]).

Most haplotyping methods rely either on familial information (e.g., [14, 15]), linkage disequilibrium (LD, e.g. [16–19]) or both (e.g., [20]). Methods that rely on heuristics (possibly in combination with familial information) have also proven efficient [21–23]. The use of familial information is particularly important to perform haplotype reconstruction at long distances and is extremely precise with large half-sib families whereas LD-based methods are very effective at short distances. Note that the so-called long-range phasing (LRP) methods achieve haplotype reconstruction at long distances without requiring explicit familial information.

In many populations, including livestock species, whole-genome sequencing (WGS) is applied only to a relatively small sample of individuals, because associated costs remain high. In many cases, unrelated reference individuals are selected to capture as much variation from the population as possible [24]. Therefore, the use of familial information might be of little benefit. Consequently, these datasets are most often phased with LD-based methods only (e.g. [25–27]). The small size of the reference population also impacts the efficiency of these LD-based methods and the inferred haplotypes. Improving the phasing accuracy should positively impact all related applications mentioned above. Large samples from a population, including many relatives of these reference individuals, are genotyped with single nucleotide polymorphism (SNP) arrays. As a result, the quality of haplotype reconstruction with such SNP array data is high due to the use of the available familial information. In addition, more genotyped individuals are available to estimate LD patterns (between SNPs on the array).

The main objective of our study was to determine whether phasing of WGS data of reference individuals using their haplotypes that are obtained with genotyping array data as template (hereafter called "scaffold" as in [1, 28]) is more accurate or not. In addition, we evaluated whether phasing based on LD and familial information has an impact on imputation accuracy. Finally, we suggest several possible improvements of the phasing method.

Methods
Data
Selection of SNPs from WGS data
In the current study, we selected 67 bulls and 24 cows that originated from New-Zealand and were all both genotyped and sequenced at high coverage (15x or more) from a larger WGS dataset that was previously used in [29]. It should be noted that, in this study, our aim was

to assess the phasing accuracy for WGS genotypes called with relatively high confidence and not for low-fold WGS data. Detailed procedures to generate the WGS data, including DNA extraction, sequencing procedure, alignment, quality score recalibration and variant calling were previously described in [29].

This WGS dataset is composed of 36 Holstein–Friesian (six cows and 30 bulls), 24 Jersey bulls and 31 Holstein–Friesian/Jersey crossbred (18 cows and 13 bulls) individuals. Among these 91 animals, 38 parent-offspring pairs were available for which data was available in the WGS dataset for the sire of 30 animals, for the dam of two animals and for both sire and dam of three animals. These parent-offspring relationships span over several generations (up to four generations) and were used to phase offspring with high confidence based on the Mendelian segregation rules.

When evaluating phasing accuracy on real WGS data, the estimated phasing errors do not result only from genuine phasing errors but also from other sources (e.g. assembly or genotype calling errors), which can blur the genuine phasing errors. To reduce as much as possible, the noise due to other sources of errors, we performed a very stringent data filtering to select the so-called trusted variants (high-confidence variants). For the sake of generality, we also performed a more traditional variant filtering for ease of comparison with other studies and to evaluate phasing in more realistic conditions. In this paper, the WGS dataset always refers to the trusted set of variants, unless explicitly specified.

The stringent filtering rules applied to the 22,228,949 SNPs from the original VCF file are described hereafter. In addition to calibration score, we used VCFtools [30] to select bi-allelic SNPs that:

- are present in other available bovine WGS datasets (the 1000 bull genomes [31] run 2, the Belgian Blue cattle and New-Zealand populations used in [29] and a Dutch Holstein pedigree of 415 individuals reported in [32]);
- are present in the datasets of all 91 individuals used here;
- have a MAF higher than 0.01 (i.e. any SNP for which the minor allele occurred only once was discarded);
- did not deviate from Hardy–Weinberg equilibrium ($p > 0.05$).

In this selection, we retained SNPs that displayed correct Mendelian segregation in the WGS Dutch Holstein pedigree based on the following rules: no parent-offspring incompatibilities (e.g., opposite homozygotes), no deviation from Hardy–Weinberg proportions ($p > 0.05$) and no deviation from expected genotypic proportions in offspring of heterozygous parents ($p > 0.05$). In addition, we excluded those markers associated with a low power to detect possible parent-offspring inconsistencies. Application of these filtering steps reduced substantially the number of SNPs but also the level of genotyping errors.

In addition to variant quality, we also removed some genomic regions that may be incorrectly mapped (errors in the genome assembly). Additional errors were detected based on the following evidences: multiple long runs of homozygosity (ROH) that had been detected with the genotyping array data were heterozygous for some segments of the WGS data, excess of double cross-overs in the WGS Dutch Holstein pedigree compared to the array-based haplotypes, and split reads or unexpected distances between mate-pairs in a WGS mate-pair library.

Finally, SNPs that were retained in the genotyping array dataset (see below) but discarded based on the filtering step mentioned just above were re-introduced in the WGS dataset. Application of the complete series of filtering steps resulted in a final list of 5,185,663 SNPs (thereafter referred to as the trusted set of WGS SNPs) that are listed in Additional file 1: Table S1, whereas, application of only the more traditional filtering steps, i.e. SNPs that were bi-allelic, present in the datasets of all 91 animals, showed no deviation from Hardy–Weinberg equilibrium with $p > 0.05$, and had a MAF higher than 0.01 resulted in 13,175,535 SNPs. The latter set was used only for illustrative purposes (comparisons to other studies) and will be referred to as the traditionally filtered WGS data (see Additional file 2: Table S2).

Selection of SNPs from genotyping array
A total of 58,369 animals from Livestock Improvement Corporation (LIC, New Zealand), including the 91 sequenced animals, were genotyped using either the BovineSNP50k (v1 and v2) or the BovineHD genotyping array from Illumina. Only SNPs that were common to the three arrays were retained. We removed SNPs that had a call-rate less than 95%, generated more than 10 Mendelian inconsistencies, were monomorphic or strongly deviated from Hardy–Weinberg equilibrium. In addition, map errors were detected and discarded using LINKPHASE3 [33]. Application of these filters resulted in 37,740 autosomal SNPs. Furthermore, 2455 SNPs that showed more than 4% mismatches between the genotype and WGS data for the 91 individuals were discarded. This final panel of 35,285 phased SNPs will be referred to as genotyping data. As stated above, all the SNPs used in the genotyping data were present in the WGS data.

Phasing methods applied to genotype and WGS data
Phasing of the genotype data using only LD information (GEN-P1)
A first phasing was done for all 58,369 genotyped animals from LIC using SHAPEIT2 [34, 35] and default parameters except for the window size (set to 5 Mb). The originality of this method consists in the possibility to efficiently explore the space of the haplotypes that are consistent with a given genotype. This phasing method is referred to as "GEN-P1" and the results were used as the pre-phase for imputation of the WGS data from the genotyping data using only LD information.

Phasing of the genotype data using both LD and familial information (GEN-P2)
As mentioned above, LINKPHASE3 was used to detect and discard map errors. However, the original purpose of this method is to partially phase the genotypes using Mendelian segregation rules and linkage in half-sibs families. After applying this method to the population of 58,369 animals, further haplotype reconstruction was performed by integrating LD information using DAG-PHASE [20] and Beagle [16]. The resulting haplotypes were therefore inferred with both familial and LD information to the 35,285 SNPs (missing genotypes being imputed by Beagle). This phasing method is referred to as "GEN-P2" and was used as scaffold for phasing the WGS data panel using both LD and familial information.

Phasing of the WGS data using only LD information (WGS-P1)
As for the genotype data, we ran directly SHAPEIT2 on the WGS data. Since the population of WGS animals is relatively small (91 animals), we set the number of conditioning states to the maximum value (182 different haplotypes). The window size was set to 0.5 Mb, as suggested in the SHAPEIT2 documentation for use with sequence data. This phasing is referred to as "WGS-P1" and will also serve as a pre-phasing step for two purposes: (1) for phasing the WGS data using both LD and familial information and (2) as reference for imputation to WGS level using only LD information.

Phasing of the WGS data using both LD and familial information (WGS-P2)
This phasing is also achieved using SHAPEIT2 by using the option "call" instead of "phase". The original aim of this option is to improve genotype calling from low coverage WGS data [28] by applying a technique (haplotype scaffold) that uses the phase of a SNP genotyping array as scaffold. The principle is that the scaffold constraints the space of consistent haplotypes. Each non-overlapping successive segment (at least three sequence SNPs) is then aligned to the scaffold.

In our implementation, the WGS data had a high coverage ($\geq 15x$), thus the genotypes are coded as integers rather than real dosages and the space of the haplotypes that is consistent with a given genotype (and also with the scaffold) is expected to be much smaller than in the case of low-coverage data.

In our specific case, the advantage of this technique was that it aligned the pre-phased WGS data (WGS-P1) to the GEN-P2 phase (i.e. the scaffold). In the latter, LD information was obtained from many more samples than for WGS-P1 (58,369 vs. 91 for WGS-P1, see Table 1 for more details) but above all, GEN-P2 phase was also based on very accurate familial information and thus, it is expected to be correct at a longer range than GEN-P1 phase. This argument was verified beforehand: close to 50% of the SNPs of the genotyping data had a GEN-P1 phase that was in opposite phase to that obtained based on Mendelian segregation rules. Since GEN-P2 phase was based on pedigree information, obviously it was in complete concordance with the phase that was obtained based on Mendelian segregation rules. Thus, it is recommended to use the GEN-P2 as a scaffold to phase the WGS data.

In our study, all SNPs of the genotype data are included in the WGS data, which results in the WGS-P1 segments (defined as consecutive WGS SNPs for which the closest genotyped SNP is the same) that align on the GEN-P2 phase to be at least 1 bp long. On average, these WGS-P1 segments contain ~140 WGS SNPs and their median length is ~53 kb (see more details in Table 2).

Regarding the initial phasing of the WGS data, the number of conditioning states was set to 182 and the window size to 0.5 Mb. The number of Markov chain Monte Carlo (MCMC) iterations was optimized using a subset of parent-offspring pairs and subsequently set to 12 burn-in iterations and 30 main iterations (on which haplotypes are averaged). Twelve pruning stages of four iterations each were used for a more parsimonious haplotype graph, as suggested in the SHAPEIT2 documentation.

Table 1 Importance of the familial information for the 91 animals of the WGS dataset

	Phased with 58,369 genotyped animals	Phased with 91 sequenced animals
Both parents genotyped	23	3
Only one parent genotyped	67	32
At least one offspring genotyped (average number of offspring[a])	80 (178.6)	17 (2.2)

[a] The average number of offspring genotyped is the average number of offspring considering only animals with at least one offspring

Table 2 Size distribution of the WGS segments[a] encompassed by the scaffold (GEN-P2) (number of SNPs, physical length)

		GEN-P2 scaffold
Number of WGS SNPs per segment	Minimum	1
	Average	146.97
	Median	110
	Maximum	2241
Singleton segments[b]	Number	145
	Scaffold proportion (%)	0.41
Physical length of segments in bp	Minimum	1
	Average	67,834.76
	Median	53,507
	Maximum	1,703,836
Physical length of non-singleton segments in bp[b]	Minimum	39
	Average	68,114.66
	Median	53,715

[a] WGS segments being defined as all consecutive WGS SNPs of the trusted set of SNPs for which the closest genotyped SNP is the same

[b] "Singleton segments" refers to segments that contain only one SNP from the scaffold, therefore a scaffold SNP encompassing only itself in the WGS data

Figure 1 provides an overview of all the phasing steps described.

Assessing phasing accuracy of haplotypes WGS-P1 and WGS-P2

Two criteria were computed to assess and compare the accuracy of the WGS-P1 and WGS-P2 phases: proportion of phasing errors and number of switches. To compute these statistics, the WGS data was divided as follows: of the 91 animals included here, 77 were retained in the training set and 14 were removed because they were parents (10 sires and 4 dams) of 30 animals of the 77 training animals (28 with only one parent known and two with both parents known). Phases WGS-P1 and WGS-P2 were then estimated by using the training set only.

For each of the 30 animals with at least one parent known, WGS-P1 and WGS-P2 were subsequently compared with the phase that was based on the Mendelian segregation rules, which correctly phase the SNPs that are heterozygous in the offspring and homozygous in at least one parent. Such SNPs are referred to as "phasable" and across these 30 animals, they represent on average ~15% of the WGS SNPs for the animals with only one sequenced parent and ~26% for those with two sequenced parents.

The proportion of phasing errors is the proportion of mismatches between the Mendelian phasing and the method under evaluation for the phasable SNPs. Each sequence of one or more consecutive mismatches delimits an incorrect segment, regardless of the distance between the SNPs in that sequence. Conversely, each

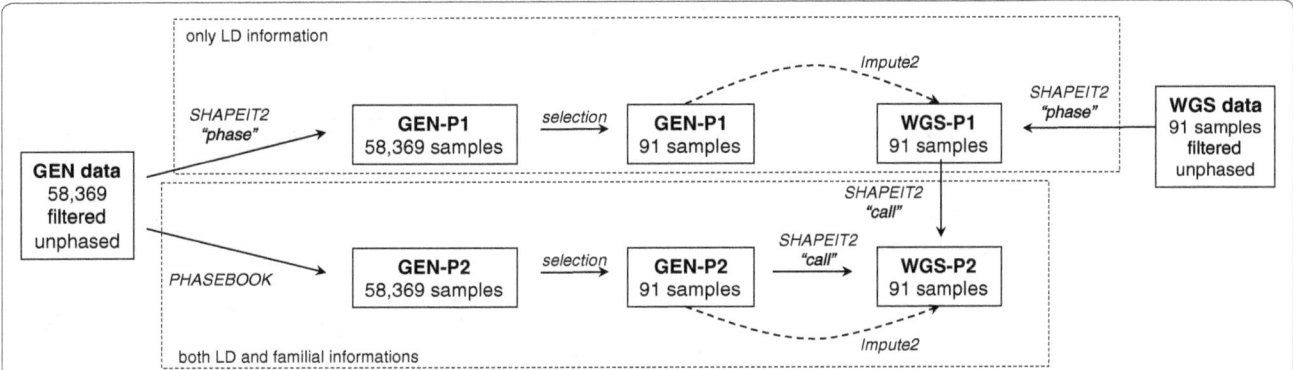

Fig. 1 Flowchart of all phasing and imputation steps. Synoptic view of the two phasing strategies (*P1* with LD information only, *P2* with both LD and familial information) applied to the two datasets (*GEN* 50k dense genotype array data, *WGS* whole-genome sequence data) and the two imputation scenarios

sequence of one or more consecutive matches delimits a correct segment. The number of switches was recorded per animal as the number of times the phase switches from correct to incorrect or conversely. Segment length distribution was also recorded, as well as the number of singleton segments (i.e. segments containing only one phasable SNP).

Assessing the impact of the pre-phasing strategy on accuracy of imputation from genotype data to WGS data

To assess whether a pre-phasing strategy based on both LD and familial information improves or not the accuracy of imputation, we compared two scenarios (see Fig. 1):

1. WGS-I1, imputation using WGS-P1 pre-phased haplotypes, i.e. imputation is performed from GEN-P1 to WGS-P1;
2. WGS-I2, imputation using WGS-P2 pre-phased haplotypes, i.e. imputation is performed from GEN-P2 to WGS-P2.

To evaluate the impact of the pre-phasing strategy on imputation accuracy, a 13-fold cross-validation was performed. The imputation to seven target animals from 84 reference animals was repeated 13 times. Pools of seven animals were randomly chosen without repetition, which resulted finally in 91 imputed animals. Imputation was achieved for all 29 bovine autosomes by using Impute2 [1], with an effective population size set to 200, a number of reference haplotypes set to 168, i.e. twice the number of reference animals, and by applying the option "–allow-large-regions" to impute the entire chromosome at once. For each animal, the result is imputed dosage of both phases.

The following statistics were then obtained for all WGS SNPs by comparing the imputed dosages and observed genotypes of the 91 animals: imputation accuracy r^2, as the squared correlation between imputed dosages and observed genotypes of any WGS SNP, and imputation error rate, as the sum of the residues between imputed dosages and observed genotypes per number of imputed SNP alleles (i.e. twice the number of SNPs).

Results
Phasing accuracy

Proportions of phasing errors, numbers of switches and distributions of length of segments are in Tables 3 and 4 for the trusted set of variants. The results indicate that phasing with LD information only (WGS-P1 phase) leads to random assignment of parental origin: about 50% of SNPs are not correctly phased. Conversely, aligning the WGS-P1 phase on the GEN-P2 phase (relying on familial information), i.e. the WGS-P2 phase, results in accurate inference of the parental origin along each chromosome: 99.62% of the phasable SNPs for the animals in the training set are correctly assigned.

We also observed differences between WGS-P1 and WGS-P2 in terms of number of switches and lengths of segments but they were not as important as those for phasing errors. The WGS-P2 phase presents fewer switches than the WGS-P1 phase, i.e. ~1.2 switches less per chromosome. On average, the distances between consecutive switches are larger for the WGS-P2 phase (3.19 Mb) than for the WGS-P1 phase (3.01 Mb.) We also found that any WGS SNP was located, on average, at 7.8 Mb of the closest switch for the WGS-P2 phase whereas it was only at 6.7 Mb for the WGS-P1 phase (Table 5). In the next section, we assess whether this had an influence on imputation.

Table 3 Statistics of phasing results for the two phasing strategies

	Trusted set of variants				Traditional SNP filtering			
	WGS-P1		WGS-P2		WGS-P1		WGS-P2	
	Average	Median	Average	Median	Average	Median	Average	Median
Proportion of phasing errors								
Per animal	50.95%	50.13%	0.38%	0.32%	50.80%	50.41%	1.10%	1.04%
Number of switches								
Per animal	739.2	631.5	704.5	574	4521	4291	4387.7	4079
Per animal and chromosome	25.49	18.5	24.29	16.5	155.9	105.5	151.3	112

WGS-P1 phased with LD information only, *WGS-P2* phased with both LD and familial information

Figure 2 shows the proportions of segments that are longer than 1, 5, 10 or 20 Mb with both WGS-P1 and WGS-P2, and whether these are correctly or incorrectly phased. Segment lengths that were equal to or longer than 50 Mb (~15% of the genome) were all correctly phased in the case of WGS-P2.

However, the median and maximum segment lengths were greater for the WGS-P1 phase, which is illustrated by the proportion of singleton segments, i.e. they are slightly more numerous for WGS-P2 than for WGS-P1 (respectively, 37.1 and 35.7% of the total number of segments), but about 84% of the singleton segments obtained with WGS-P2 are incorrectly phased. The difference in average segment length between WGS-P1 and WGS-P2 is larger if we consider that only segments below a threshold length are phasing errors: 9.5 versus 11 Mb when discarding singletons and 15 versus 19 Mb when discarding singletons and small segments (maximum 5 phasable SNPs and 5 kb). Discarding singletons and small segments leads to an average length of almost 32 Mb for WGS-P2 segments that were correctly phased.

The results obtained with more traditional variant filtering rules (thus, containing more noise due to errors that do not depend on the phasing method) are in Tables 3 and 6. Compared to the results obtained with the trusted set of variants, we observed more errors. First, correct identification of parental origin drops slightly i.e. to 98.9% of the variants with WGS-P2, whereas parental origin remains randomly assigned with WGS-P1 (Table 3). The proportion of phasing errors increases by a ratio close to the number of SNPs (on average, 2.89 more phasing errors with 2.54 more SNPs). The increase in number of switches (per animal or per animal and per chromosome) is much more pronounced: on average 7.26 more switches than with the stringent set of SNPs (Table 3). When relaxing filters for SNP selection, the size of the segments (whether correctly phased or not) drops substantially from ~3 to ~0.5 Mb for both phases WGS-P1 and WGS-P2, although less in terms of number of SNPs (on average, from 2.38 to 2.85 less SNPs, for phases WGS-P1 and WGS-P2 and for

number of all SNPs or only phasable SNPs, see Table 6). These reductions in overall performances indicate that, with such traditional filtering, many errors remain in the dataset (probably due to errors in the assembly or in the genotype calling), which makes the comparison of methods more difficult. Still, the strategy that relies on familial information results in more accurate phasing: WGS-P1 tends to produce slightly shorter segments than WGS-P2. As for the trusted set of variants, segments with a correctly assigned parental origin are on average about two times longer when phasing relies on familial information (WGS-P2).

Accuracy of imputation of the WGS data

Imputation accuracies (measured as r^2) are in Table 7 for each imputation scenario WGS-I1 (only LD information) and WGS-I2 (both LD and familial information), on both sets of SNPs. Although the scenario that indirectly accounts for familial information (through the use of a scaffold that exploits both familial and LD information) performs better than the other scenario, this difference is small with the trusted set of SNPs: 90.65 for WGS-I2 versus 90.47% for WGS-I1. The overall imputation error rate is 1.70% for WGS-I1 and 1.67% for WGS-I2, averaged per chromosome and animal, i.e. the scenario that indirectly accounts for familial information reduces error rate by ~2% (in relative terms).

However, the difference in imputation accuracy between scenarios is larger for specific classes of SNPs, for which both imputation r^2 are lower. WGS-I2 results in an imputation accuracy (measured as r^2) that is 0.88% higher than that for WGS-I1 for variants with a MAF between 1 and 5%. This difference is mainly due to the rarest SNPs being retained in the WGS dataset (two occurrences of the minor allele). For this particular class of SNPs, the median values of r^2 are 67.47 and 86.78% for WGS-I1 and WGS-I2, respectively.

Both ends of all chromosomes also present lower r^2 and larger differences between methods: on average, r^2 is 2.15 and 0.51% higher for the first and last Mb of each chromosome, respectively, with WGS-I2.

Table 4 Lengths of segments without switches of the trusted set of WGS SNPs for the two phasing strategies[a], whether correctly or wrongly phased or both (all)

	WGS-P1			WGS-P2		
	All	Correct	Wrong	All	Correct	Wrong
Original segments						
Physical length[b]						
Avg	3.01	2.96	3.07	3.19	6.11	84.99 kb
Med	4.58 kb	4.75 kb	4.33 kb	3.38 kb	1.74	1 bp
Max	150.73	150.73	123.75	116.39	116.39	42.76
Proportion of singletons[c]	37.52%	37.53%	37.51%	38.82%	12.18%	67.24%
Number of phasable SNPs per segment						
Avg	1048.45	1041.75	1055.17	1098.05	2119.04	8.39
Med	4	4	4	3	644	1
Max	55,553	55,553	50,217	51,340	51,340	835
Number of SNPs per segment						
Avg	6232.95	6134.89	6331.09	6612.58	12,639.78	179.99
Med	12	13	12	8.5	3641	1
Max	308,884	308,884	240,332	231,051	231,051	85,165
After discarding singletons[c]						
Physical length[b]						
Avg	9.48	9.28	9.67	11.02	19.46	0.36
Med	1.25	1.39	1.12	0.26	6.39	0.01
Max	154.47	154.47	147.3	147.3	147.3	42.76
Number of phasable SNPs per segment						
Avg	3185.72	3163.65	3207.84	3652.87	6524.06	28.54
Med	367	418	314	59	2352	4
Max	67,776	67,776	60,281	67,776	67,776	1452
Number of SNPs per segment						
Avg	19,586.14	19,210.75	19,962.22	22,778.53	40,230.9	748.21
Med	2555	2925.5	2306	523	13,713	15
Max	318,618	318,618	304,742	304,742	304,742	85,165
After discarding segments with less than five phasable SNPs and shorter than 5 kb						
Physical length[b]						
Avg	14.78	14.46	15.11	19.36	31.64	0.72
Med	4.62	4.72	4.51	2.28	19.59	0.06
Max	158.12	158.1	158.12	158.24	158.24	42.76
Number of phasable SNPs per segment						
Avg	4956.66	4911.73	5001.86	6400.99	10,581.41	53.68
Med	1489	1584	1401	522	6580	13
Max	73,348	73,348	60,625	67,776	67,776	1452
Number of SNPs per segment						
Avg	30,549.61	29,916.85	31,186.28	40,033.57	65,412.51	1499.57
Med	9884	10,364	9497.5	4913	41,646	138
Max	327,738	327,706	327,738	327,914	327,914	85,165

A segment is defined as a run of consecutive phasable SNPs without switches

[a] *WGS-P1* phased with LD information only, *WGS-P2* phased with both LD and familial information

[b] Unless specified, all length units are in Mb

[c] "Singleton" refers to segments that contain only one SNP

When relaxing filters for the selection of WGS SNPs (more traditional variant filtering rules), the average imputation accuracy (measured as r^2) drops slightly for both imputation scenarios, but the difference between scenarios is more important than when a more stringent selection is applied: 89.07 for WGS-I2 versus 88.66% for

Table 5 Distance^a between any SNP of the trusted set of WGS SNPs and the closest switch

	WGS-P1	WGS-P2
Average	6.74	7.77
Median	3.49	4.08
Maximum	150.81	98.69

Distances are estimated on 30 animals of the training population

^a In Mb

WGS-I1. This difference is probably due to the classes of rare variants, since they are much more frequent in this dataset (e.g. ~8.5 more SNPs of the rarest class).

Discussion

Integrating familial information in phasing of WGS data results in accurate haplotypes with sparse phasing errors

The main idea of our new strategy is to indirectly use familial and LD information from genotyped populations to improve phasing of a smaller population of whole-genome sequenced reference individuals in a two-step procedure. It should be noted that the strategy is not restricted to WGS data; for instance, phasing of a HD panel can be improved with information from a larger 50k panel. The reasoning is that genotyped populations are larger and thus more familial information (more genotyped parents and more genotyped offspring) is available. For instance, 80 of the 91 animals used in this study have offspring in the genotyped population (178.6 offspring on average, see Table 1). Within the population of animals with sequence data, this number would drop to 17 animals (with 2.2 offspring on average). Moreover, with a larger population, there are more records and a larger variety of haplotypes represented to infer the LD structure. Therefore, haplotype reconstruction in these larger genotyped populations has proven particularly efficient in pedigreed populations and such haplotypes would be good scaffolds (or anchors) to phase the WGS data. Another key point is that we assume that LD-based methods are able to correctly phase segments that are a few Mb long (but not at long range). As long as these correctly phased segments each contain a few SNPs from the lower-density panel, it should be possible to infer their parental origin based on the phased genotype data. Our results prove that these hypotheses are valid for a bovine dataset and that our strategy results in WGS haplotypes being correctly phased along the entire chromosome except for a few small segments (most often singletons).

First, we determined the range of correct phasing with LD-based methods on WGS data. Generally, methods

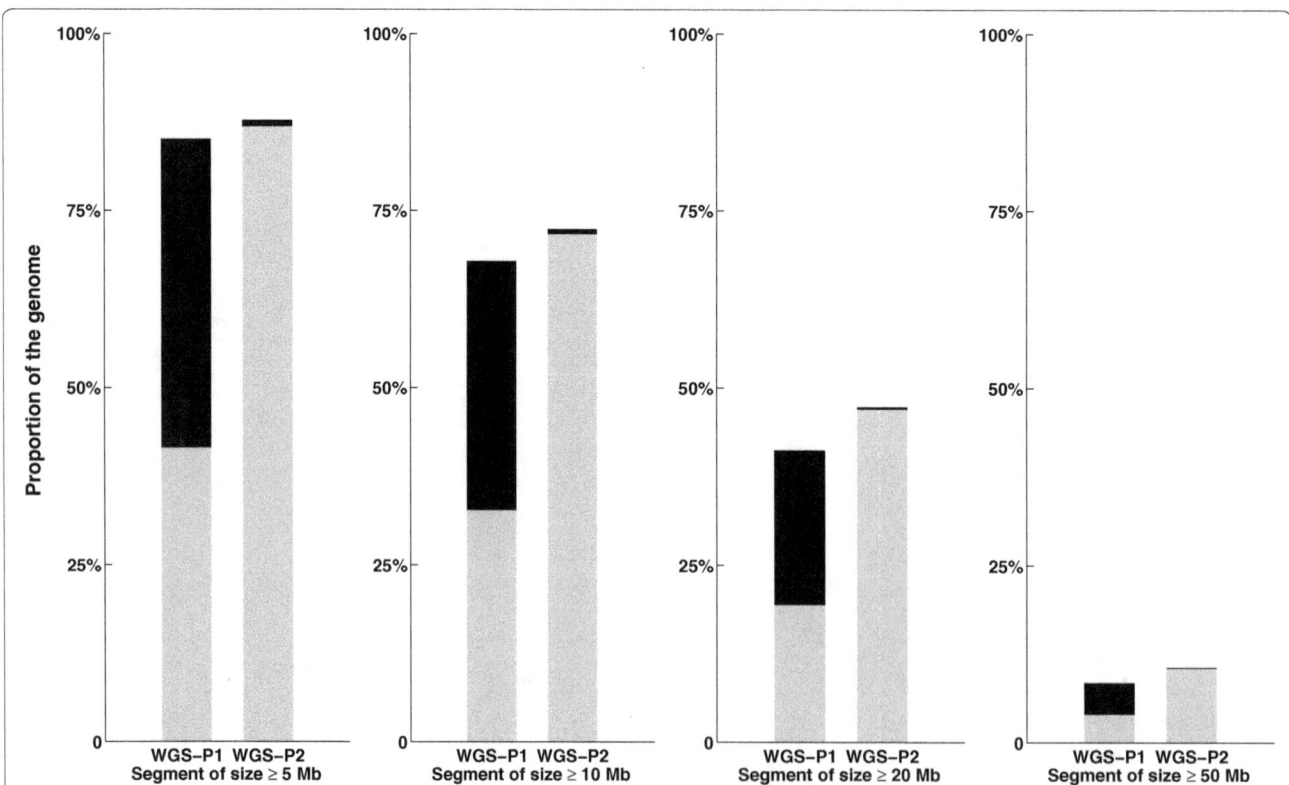

Fig. 2 Proportion of the genome by class of size of phased segments. Proportions of the genome in segments that are longer or equal to 5, 10, 20 or 50 Mb, regardless of whether they are correctly (*grey*) or incorrectly (*black*) phased, when phasing the WGS data using only LD information (WGS-P1) or both LD and familial information (WGS-P2)

Table 6 Lengths of segments without switches obtained with WGS SNPs selected with more traditional filtering rules for the two phasing strategies[a], whether correctly or wrongly phased or both (all)

	WGS-P1			WGS-P2		
	All	Correct	Wrong	All	Correct	Wrong
Original segments						
Physical length[b]						
Avg	0.50	0.49	0.50	0.51	0.99	0.04
Med	346 bp	297 bp	404 bp	396 bp	223.51 kb	1 bp
Max	34.88	34.88	21.33	25.64	25.64	14.65
Proportion of singletons[c]	40.76%	41.05%	40.48%	40.61%	16.11%	65.31%
Number of phasable SNPs per segment						
Avg	373.70	370.72	376.69	384.98	758.49	8.40
Med	2	2	2	2	131	1
Max	29,712	29,712	26,646	32,839	32,839	1813
Number of SNPs per segment						
Avg	2618.11	2593.29	2642.94	2704.68	5179.74	209.22
Med	4	4	4	4	1228.5	1
Max	158,630	158,630	113,469	134,130	134,130	84,929
After discarding singletons[c]						
Physical length[b]						
Avg	1.88	1.87	1.9	1.94	3.64	0.19
Med	0.05	0.05	0.05	0.03	1.04	1.92 kb
Max	63.16	55.98	63.16	85.72	85.72	31.87
Number of phasable SNPs per segment						
Avg	1335.70	1325.27	1346.13	1373.47	2675.79	28.52
Med	14	14	14	10	659	3
Max	74,067	57,000	74,067	97,334	97,334	2787
Number of SNPs per segment						
Avg	9895.56	9823.59	9967.51	10,208.87	19,121.57	1004.46
Med	255	241	266	153	5657	13
Max	325,812	293,893	325,812	437,121	437,121	141,991
After discarding segments with less than five phasable SNPs and shorter than 5 kb						
Physical length[b]						
Avg	4.34	4.31	4.36	4.84	8.84	0.50
Med	0.95	0.95	0.95	0.44	3.52	494.45 kb
Max	121.41	121.41	116.11	121.41	121.41	33.07
Number of phasable SNPs per segment						
Avg	3045.22	3024.33	3066.06	3388.28	6444.96	69.46
Med	318	310.5	325	78	2311	10
Max	110,344	110,344	86,208	112,056	112,056	2793
Number of SNPs per segment						
Avg	22,773.56	22,633.66	22,913.14	25,438.65	46,480.17	2592.66
Med	4951	4939	4971	2206	19,046	254
Max	605,700	605,700	601,045	653,272	653,272	160,715

A segment is defined as a run of consecutive phasable SNPs without switches

[a] WGS-P1: phased with LD information only; WGS-P2: phased with both LD and familial information

[b] Unless specified, all length units are in Mb

[c] "Singleton" refers to segments that contain only one SNP

Table 7 Imputation reliability (measured as r^2 and given in %) for the two scenarios[a] of imputation

	Trusted set of variants						Traditional variant filtering					
	N	WGS-I1[a]		WGS-I2[a]		$D^b_{I2\text{-}I1}$	N	WGS-I1[a]		WGS-I2[a]		$D_{I2\text{-}I1b}$
		Avg r^2	Med r^2	Avg r^2	Med r^2			Avg r^2	Med r^2	Avg r^2	Med r^2	
Overall	5,149,267	90.47	93.63	90.65	93.81	0.18	13,129,937	88.66	93.57	89.07	93.87	0.41
NMA = 2[c]	79,755	56.74	67.47	59.98	86.76	3.24	680,303	63.04	80.94	67.95	96.96	4.91
NMA = 3[c]	78,933	69.10	71.02	70.78	75.35	1.68	510,080	77.28	92.25	79.00	95.49	1.72
0.01 < MAF ≤ 0.05	644,224	77.57	85.82	78.45	87.11	0.88	3,278,384	79.56	91.35	81.01	94.27	1.46
0.05 < MAF ≤ 0.10	673,955	89.15	91.65	89.21	91.81	0.06	2,047,206	89.91	92.82	90.07	93.15	0.16
0.10 < MAF	3,831,088	92.87	94.20	92.95	94.30	0.08	7,804,347	92.15	93.91	92.19	93.96	0.04
First Mb	48,089	85.40	90.90	87.56	92.84	2.15	134,266	83.17	90.10	85.19	92.27	2.01
Last Mb	53,502	87.94	91.55	88.45	92.05	0.51	155,246	85.85	91.26	86.53	91.88	0.68
Between first and last Mb	5,045,959	90.55	93.68	90.70	93.84	0.16	12,840,425	88.75	93.62	89.14	93.91	0.39

[a] WGS-I1: imputation from GEN-P1 to WGS-P1 (using only LD information); WGS-I2: imputation from GEN-P2 to WGS-P2 (using both LD and familial information)

[b] $D_{I2\text{-}I1}$: difference of average r^2

[c] NMA: number of occurrences of the minor allele

that are designed for phasing and imputation in human datasets (e.g. [2, 16, 17]) are used in livestock populations without knowing this information. Here we show, that LD-based methods work quite well, resulting in 3-Mb long correctly phased segments. This average value includes singletons and other very small errors and more than 80% of the genome lies in segments that are larger than 5 Mb (see Fig. 2).

Next, we showed that our strategy improves phasing accuracy: a larger fraction of the genome lies within long correctly phased fragments (more than 75% of the genome lies within segments that are longer than 10 Mb) and fewer switches are observed. However, the main benefit is that the parental origin is correctly inferred across the entire chromosome. The phasing errors are mostly associated to small segments: ~70% of these incorrect segments are singletons and ~81% contain five or less phasable SNPs. An illustration of these results for two animals with different profiles is in Fig. 3, i.e. with our new strategy, the chromosome shown for the first animal is divided into 15 segments (14 switches) and all segments that are assigned an incorrect parental origin contain three or less phasable SNPs (only one for most of them), whereas for the second animal there are many more switches (138) but the size of incorrectly phased segments remains small in general.

We suggest that all LD-based phasing methods should offer the possibility to incorporate external phasing information (such as haplotype information inferred from low-density panels), for instance as scaffold. This is often not possible with software programs that are primarily designed for human genetics studies. Popular rule-based

phasing and imputation methods that are commonly used in animal breeding genetics such as FImpute [23], findhap [36] or AlphaPhase [21] use information from relatives genotyped at lower marker density to phase animals in the reference panel. A recent study [37] compared haplotypes that were obtained from genotyping array data with such methods to those obtained with LD-based methods and found that FImpute [23] achieved a more accurate phasing than other methods when at least one parent was genotyped.

Improvement of phasing accuracy should positively impact all applications using haplotypes. For instance, for the detection of signatures of selection, it is important that haplotypes are not subdivided into smaller segments. Larger correctly phased segments allow to better identify IBD relationships and to better cluster local haplotypes for imputation, association studies and genomic selection. These applications would work nicely for SNPs that are located in the center of segments, thus only SNPs that are closer to the segments' boundaries (closer to switches) would remain problematic. LD-based methods result in many more such switches that might locally impact haplotype-based applications (our results show that our two-step strategy increases the proportion of SNPs that are distantly located from switches). In addition, the presence of singletons (as observed with our new strategy) is often well handled by imputation or haplotype clustering methods that accommodate for genotyping errors.

The major difference between our strategy and LD-based methods is the ability to correctly infer the parental origin along the entire length of chromosomes and we

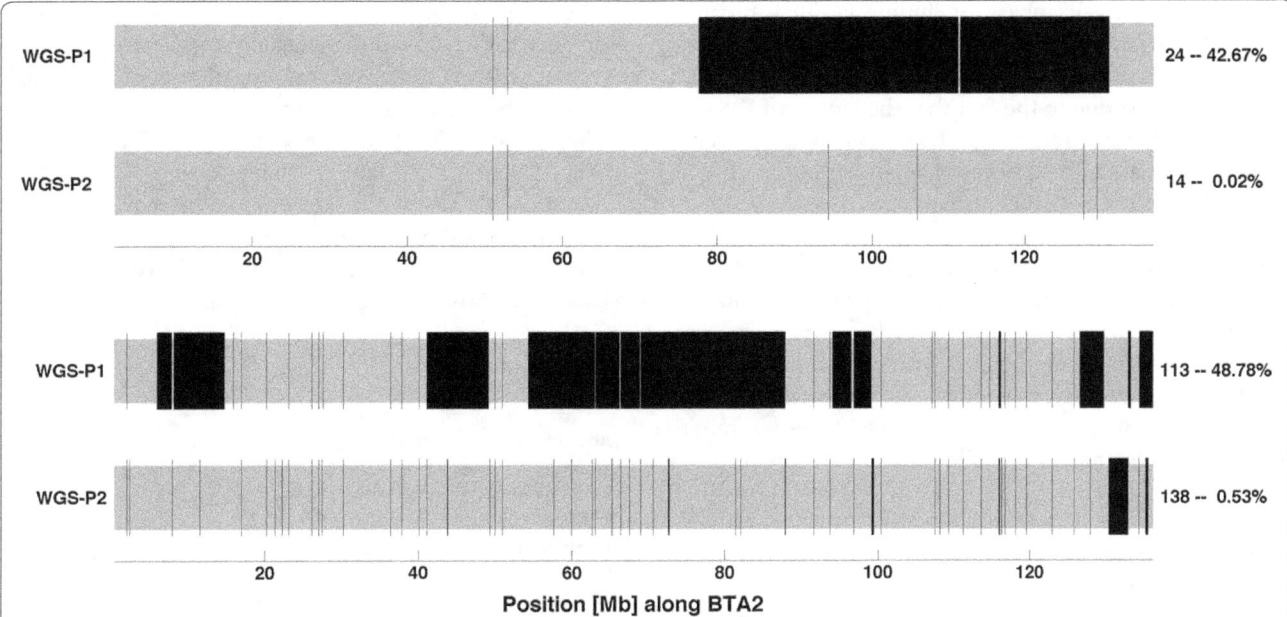

Fig. 3 WGS-P1 and WGS-P2 phases of bovine autosome 2 for two animals of the training set. Consecutive SNPs with phase in compliance with Mendelian segregation rules delimit correct segments (*in grey*); conversely, consecutive markers with phase not in compliance with Mendelian segregation rules delimit incorrect segments (*in black*). Corresponding number of switches and proportion of errors are indicated on the *right side* of each phase

showed that this could be improved from ~50 to ~99.62% of the WGS SNPs of the trusted set of variants. Correct parental origin is important for disease mapping (e.g., if it is known that the causal variant is transmitted through the maternal path), when breed origin of different haplotypes must be determined in multiple-breed crosses (e.g. [38]), when studying parental imprinting (e.g., [39]) or when estimating parent-of-origin effects for allele-specific gene expression [40]. For recent mutations in common haplotypes, parental origin and accurate long-distance haplotyping are also essential to determine whether the original or mutated version of the haplotype was inherited.

In the current study, the method was applied to improve phasing of WGS genotypes that are known with relatively high confidence (coverage $\geq 15x$) and our conclusions are restricted to this situation. Originally, the method was implemented in SHAPEIT2 to improve genotyping calling with low-fold sequencing data. Scaffolds of haplotypes obtained on larger genotyped populations and with familial information may provide even more benefits when used with low-fold sequencing data. In such a case, the scaffold would be used to improve genotype calling, to impute missing genotypes and to perform haplotype reconstruction in the reference panel. With a view to extend the method to low-coverage SNPs, additional phase information could be provided directly from sequence reads (e.g. [41]).

Improving haplotype pre-phasing has a marginal impact on imputation accuracy

The imputation accuracy achieved in our study is higher than that reported in other recent studies in cattle [25, 31, 42], both with the trusted set of variants ($r^2 = 0.9065$) or with more traditional variant filtering rules ($r^2 = 0.8907$). It is worth noting that the above-mentioned studies impute data from high-density SNP panels (777k SNPs). For instance, the ratio between number of imputed and reference SNPs on bovine autosome 29 is equal to 28.5 in [25], 46.2 in [31] and 427.1 in our study (with the trusted set of variants), thus, there are respectively 15.0 or 9.2 times more SNPs imputed from a single SNP in our study. However, comparisons are difficult, since populations and the sizes of the reference populations differ. In addition, results are often expressed as correlations (r) whereas we used squared correlations (r^2).

Surprisingly, improved haplotype pre-phasing had only a marginal impact on imputation accuracy. Imputation relies on shared identical-by-state (IBS) segments between target and reference animals on the low-density panel (here, the genotyping data). Therefore, we computed the average length of the longest IBS segment shared by any target haplotype from the phased genotype data (GEN-P1 or GEN-P2) and one of the 168 reference haplotypes (WGS-P1 or WGS-P2 phases obtained for the trusted set of variants) on all SNPs of the genotype data. The longest IBS segment was on average 43.4 Mb long for the GEN-P2 phase (including familial information) versus 26.3 Mb for the GEN-P1 phase. The good performances of the WGS-I1 scenario (based on GEN-P1 phase) could be due to the fact that the length of IBS segments between any target and the most similar reference haplotype is already sufficiently long (although shorter than with the WGS-I2 scenario).

Using additional information to improve the scaffold

A possibility to further improve phasing of WGS data and imputation accuracy could be to further enrich the scaffold with SNPs that are phased with high confidence. As an illustration of this perspective, we previously observed that for SNPs on genotyping arrays, the LD between haplotype clusters (hereafter called ancestral haplotypes—AHAP) and underlying variants was high [6]. When there is a perfect match between such AHAP and variants from the WGS (each AHAP being perfectly associated with one SNP allele), we can use these AHAP to determine the parental origin of the corresponding SNP alleles. We determined that 28% of the SNPs from the trusted set presented such a perfect association with a set of 50 AHAP and that using these haplotypes to phase these 28% SNPs resulted in a phasing accuracy of 99.9% (data not shown). Consequently, we considered that these SNPs could be added to the scaffold (resulting in a scaffold of 1,485,758 WGS SNPs of the trusted set). Phasing and imputation accuracy were improved when using this new scaffold. Parental origins were correctly assigned for 99.72% of the SNPs (compared to 99.62% previously), less switches were observed (20.83 vs. 24.29 switches per chromosome) and imputation accuracy increased from 90.65 to 90.91%. This was even more pronounced for rare variants: imputation accuracy for the rarest variants (two occurrences of the minor allele) had a median imputation accuracy r^2 equal to 94.71% compared to 86.76% with the first scaffold. These results suggest that a strategy that relies on a scaffold of variants phased with high confidence can be further extended to other sources of information as long as they provide accurate phasing information.

Conclusions

In this paper, we describe a multi-step strategy to take both LD and familial information into account when phasing WGS data. The strategy relies on the use of a 50k genotyping array, phased on a large population (including many relatives of the sequenced individuals) and using both LD and familial information, as haplotype scaffold. This strategy results in a very low proportion of mismatches with the phase obtained by Mendelian segregation rules (0.32% on average). It also results in longer correctly phased segments than a method that relies on LD only. The majority

of the errors results from single SNP errors. Imputation with such an improved pre-phasing step was slightly better than with a traditional pre-phasing step. This small difference between the two imputation scenarios may be explained by the fact that even without a scaffold, correctly phased segments are already long enough for accurate imputation. Finally, we propose an additional strategy to further improve both haplotype reconstruction and imputation of WGS data that relies on haplotype clustering based on the 50k genotyping array data.

Additional files

> **Additional file 1: Table S1.** Detailed list of the trusted set of SNPs from WGS data. Full list of the 5,185,663 SNPs referred in the current study as the trusted set of SNPs from WGS data (chromosome, position in base-pairs, identifier, reference and alternative alleles).
>
> **Additional file 2: Table S2.** Detailed list of the panel of SNPs from WGS data obtained with more traditional filtering rules. Full list of the 13,175,535 SNPs obtained with more traditional variant filtering rules and used in this study for illustrative purpose (chromosome, position in base-pairs, identifier, reference and alternative alleles).

Authors' contributions

PF and TD conceived the study, developed software, interpreted the results and wrote the manuscript and PF performed the experiments. Both authors read and approved the final manuscript.

Acknowledgements

The authors gratefully acknowledge Livestock Improvement Corporation (Hamilton, New-Zealand) for providing the material used in this study. This work was part of the TechILA research project (Grant T.1086.14) funded by the Fonds de la Recherche Scientifique-FNRS (F.R.S.-FNRS) and of the Blue Pool research project (Fonds Spéciaux C-15/72), funded by the University of Liège. Tom Druet is Research Associate from the F.R.S.-FNRS. We used the super-computing facilities of the "Consortium d'Equipements en Calcul Intensif en Fédération Wallonie-Bruxelles" (CECI), funded by the F.R.S.-F.N.R.S.

Competing interests

The authors declare that they have no competing interests.

Funding

The "Fonds National de la Recherche Scientifique" (F.R.S-F.N.R.S, Grant T.1086.14) and the University of Liège (ULg, Fonds Spéciaux C-15/72) funded the present study.

References

1. Howie BN, Donnelly P, Marchini J. A flexible and accurate genotype imputation method for the next generation of genome-wide association studies. PLoS Genet. 2009;5:e1000529.
2. Howie B, Fuchsberger C, Stephens M, Marchini J, Abecasis GR. Fast and accurate genotype imputation in genome-wide association studies through pre-phasing. Nat Genet. 2012;44:955–9.

3. Meuwissen TH, Goddard ME. Prediction of identity by descent probabili-
    ties from marker-haplotypes. Genet Sel Evol. 2001;33:605–34.
4. Browning BL, Browning SR. Efficient multilocus association testing for
    whole genome association studies using localized haplotype clustering.
    Genet Epidemiol. 2007;31:365–75.
5. Su SY, Balding DJ, Coin LJM. Disease association tests by inferring ancestral
    haplotypes using a hidden Markov model. Bioinformatics. 2008;24:972–8.
6. Zhang Z, Guillaume F, Sartelet A, Charlier C, Georges M, Farnir F, et al.
    Ancestral haplotype-based association mapping with generalized
    linear mixed models accounting for stratification. Bioinformatics.
    2012;28:2467–73.
7. Boichard D, Guillaume F, Baur A, Croiseau P, Rossignol MN, Boscher
    MY, et al. Genomic selection in French dairy cattle. Anim Prod Sci.
    2012;52:115–20.
8. Cuyabano BCD, Su G, Lund MS. Genomic prediction of genetic merit
    using LD-based haplotypes in the Nordic Holstein population. BMC
    Genomics. 2014;15:1171.
9. Cuyabano BC, Su G, Lund MS. Selection of haplotype variables from a high-
    density marker map for genomic prediction. Genet Sel Evol. 2015;47:61.
10. De Roos APW, Schrooten C, Druet T. Genomic breeding value estimation
    using genetic markers, inferred ancestral haplotypes, and the genomic
    relationship matrix. J Dairy Sci. 2011;94:4708–14.
11. Sabeti PC, Reich DE, Higgins JM, Levine HZ, Richter DJ, Schaffner SF, et al.
    Detecting recent positive selection in the human genome from haplo-
    type structure. Nature. 2002;419:832–7.
12. Voight BF, Kudaravalli S, Wen X, Pritchard JK. A map of recent positive
    selection in the human genome. PLoS Biol. 2006;4:e72.
13. Kong A, Thorleifsson G, Gudbjartsson DF, Masson G, Sigurdsson A, Jonas-
    dottir A, et al. Fine-scale recombination rate differences between sexes,
    populations and individuals. Nature. 2010;467:1099–103.
14. Abecasis GR, Cherny SS, Cookson WO, Cardon LR. Merlin—rapid analysis
    of dense genetic maps using sparse gene flow trees. Nat Genet.
    2002;30:97–101.
15. Qian D, Beckmann L. Minimum-recombinant haplotyping in pedigrees.
    Am J Hum Genet. 2002;70:1434–45.
16. Browning SR, Browning BL. Rapid and accurate haplotype phasing and
    missing-data inference for whole-genome association studies by use of
    localized haplotype clustering. Am J Hum Genet. 2007;81:1084–97.
17. Delaneau O, Coulonges C, Zagury JF. Shape-IT: new rapid and accurate
    algorithm for haplotype inference. BMC Bioinformatics. 2008;9:540.
18. Scheet P, Stephens M. A fast and flexible statistical model for large-scale
    population genotype data: applications to inferring missing genotypes
    and haplotypic phase. Am J Hum Genet. 2006;78:629–44.
19. Stephens M, Smith NJ, Donnelly P. A new statistical method for haplotype
    reconstruction from population data. Am J Hum Genet. 2001;68:978–89.
20. Druet T, Georges M. A hidden Markov model combining linkage and
    linkage disequilibrium information for haplotype reconstruction and
    quantitative trait locus fine mapping. Genetics. 2010;184:789–98.
21. Hickey JM, Kinghorn BP, Tier B, Wilson JF, Dunstan N, van der Werf JH. A
    combined long-range phasing and long haplotype imputation method
    to impute phase for SNP genotypes. Genet Sel Evol. 2011;43:12.
22. Kong A, Masson G, Frigge ML, Gylfason A, Zusmanovich P, Thorleifsson G,
    et al. Detection of sharing by descent, long-range phasing and haplotype
    imputation. Nat Genet. 2008;40:1068–75.
23. Sargolzaei M, Chesnais JP, Schenkel FS. A new approach for efficient
    genotype imputation using information from relatives. BMC Genomics.
    2014;15:478.
24. Druet T, Macleod IM, Hayes BJ. Toward genomic prediction from
    whole-genome sequence data: impact of sequencing design on
    genotype imputation and accuracy of predictions. Heredity (Edinb).
    2014;112:39–47.
25. Brøndum RF, Guldbrandtsen B, Sahana G, Lund MS, Su G. Strategies for
    imputation to whole genome sequence using a single or multi-breed
    reference population in cattle. BMC Genomics. 2014;15:728.
26. Kadri NK, Harland C, Faux P, Cambisano N, Karim L, Coppieters W,
    et al. Coding and noncoding variants in *HFM1*, *MLH3*, *MSH4*, *MSH5*,
    RNF212, and *RNF212B* affect recombination rate in cattle. Genome Res.
    2016;26:1323–32.
27. Pausch H, Aigner B, Emmerling R, Edel C, Götz KU, Fries R. Imputation of
    high-density genotypes in the Fleckvieh cattle population. Genet Sel
    Evol. 2013;45:3.
28. Delaneau O, Marchini J, McVean GA, Donnelly P, Lunter G, Marchini JL,
    et al. Integrating sequence and array data to create an improved 1000
    Genomes Project haplotype reference panel. Nat Commun. 2014;5:3934.
29. Charlier C, Li W, Harland C, Littlejohn M, Coppieters W, Creagh F,
    et al. NGS-based reverse genetic screen for common embryonic
    lethal mutations compromising fertility in livestock. Genome Res.
    2016;26:1333–41.
30. Danecek P, Auton A, Abecasis G, Albers CA, Banks E, DePristo MA, et al.
    The variant call format and VCFtools. Bioinformatics. 2011;27:2156–8.
31. Daetwyler HD, Capitan A, Pausch H, Stothard P, van Binsbergen R,
    Brøndum RF, et al. Whole-genome sequencing of 234 bulls facilitates
    mapping of monogenic and complex traits in cattle. Nat Genet.
    2014;46:858–65.
32. Harland C, Charlier C, Karim L, Cambisano N, Deckers M, Mullaart E, et al.
    Frequency of mosaicism points towards mutation-prone early cleavage
    cell divisions. bioRxiv. 2016. doi:10.1101/079863.
33. Druet T, Georges M. LINKPHASE3: an improved pedigree-based phas-
    ing algorithm robust to genotyping and map errors. Bioinformatics.
    2015;31:1677–9.
34. Delaneau O, Marchini J, Zagury JF. A linear complexity phasing method
    for thousands of genomes. Nat Methods. 2011;9:179–81.
35. Delaneau O, Zagury JF, Marchini J. Improved whole-chromosome
    phasing for disease and population genetic studies. Nat Methods.
    2013;10:5–6.
36. VanRaden PM, O'Connell JR, Wiggans GR, Weigel KA. Genomic evalua-
    tions with many more genotypes. Genet Sel Evol. 2011;43:10.
37. Miar Y, Sargolzaei M, Schenkel FS. A comparison of different algorithms
    for phasing haplotypes using Holstein cattle genotypes and pedigree
    data. J Dairy Sci. 2017;100:2837–49.
38. Sevillano CA, Vandenplas J, Bastiaansen JWM, Calus MPL. Empirical deter-
    mination of breed-of-origin of alleles in three-breed cross pigs. Genet Sel
    Evol. 2016;48:55.
39. Mott R, Yuan W, Kaisaki P, Gan X, Cleak J, Edwards A, et al. The architecture
    of parent-of-origin effects in mice. Cell. 2014;156:332–42.
40. Chamberlain AJ, Vander Jagt CJ, Hayes BJ, Khansefid M, Marett LC, Millen
    CA, et al. Extensive variation between tissues in allele specific expression
    in an outbred mammal. BMC Genomics. 2015;16:993.
41. Davies RW, Flint J, Myers S, Mott R. Rapid genotype imputation from
    sequence without reference panels. Nat Genet. 2016;48:965–9.
42. Bouwman AC, Veerkamp RF. Consequences of splitting whole-genome
    sequencing effort over multiple breeds on imputation accuracy. BMC
    Genet. 2014;15:105.

18

Genome-wide SNP data unveils the globalization of domesticated pigs

Bin Yang[1†], Leilei Cui[1†], Miguel Perez-Enciso[3,4], Aleksei Traspov[5], Richard P. M. A. Crooijmans[2],
Natalia Zinovieva[5], Lawrence B. Schook[6], Alan Archibald[7], Kesinee Gatphayak[8], Christophe Knorr[9],
Alex Triantafyllidis[10], Panoraia Alexandri[10], Gono Semiadi[11], Olivier Hanotte[12], Deodália Dias[13], Peter Dovč[14],
Pekka Uimari[15], Laura Iacolina[16,17], Massimo Scandura[17], Martien A. M. Groenen[2], Lusheng Huang[1*]
and Hendrik-Jan Megens[2*] (iD)

Abstract

Background: Pigs were domesticated independently in Eastern and Western Eurasia early during the agricultural revolution, and have since been transported and traded across the globe. Here, we present a worldwide survey on 60K genome-wide single nucleotide polymorphism (SNP) data for 2093 pigs, including 1839 domestic pigs representing 122 local and commercial breeds, 215 wild boars, and 39 out-group suids, from Asia, Europe, America, Oceania and Africa. The aim of this study was to infer global patterns in pig domestication and diversity related to demography, migration, and selection.

Results: A deep phylogeographic division reflects the dichotomy between early domestication centers. In the core Eastern and Western domestication regions, Chinese pigs show differentiation between breeds due to geographic isolation, whereas this is less pronounced in European pigs. The inferred European origin of pigs in the Americas, Africa, and Australia reflects European expansion during the sixteenth to nineteenth centuries. Human-mediated introgression, which is due, in particular, to importing Chinese pigs into the UK during the eighteenth and nineteenth centuries, played an important role in the formation of modern pig breeds. Inbreeding levels vary markedly between populations, from almost no runs of homozygosity (ROH) in a number of Asian wild boar populations, to up to 20% of the genome covered by ROH in a number of Southern European breeds. Commercial populations show moderate ROH statistics. For domesticated pigs and wild boars in Asia and Europe, we identified highly differentiated loci that include candidate genes related to muscle and body development, central nervous system, reproduction, and energy balance, which are putatively under artificial selection.

Conclusions: Key events related to domestication, dispersal, and mixing of pigs from different regions are reflected in the 60K SNP data, including the globalization that has recently become full circle since Chinese pig breeders in the past decades started selecting Western breeds to improve local Chinese pigs. Furthermore, signatures of ongoing and past selection, acting at different times and on different genetic backgrounds, enhance our insight in the mechanism of domestication and selection. The global diversity statistics presented here highlight concerns for maintaining agrodiversity, but also provide a necessary framework for directing genetic conservation.

*Correspondence: lushenghuang@hotmail.com;
hendrik-jan.megens@wur.nl
†Bin Yang and Leilei Cui have contributed equally to this work.
[1] National Key Laboratory for Pig Genetic Improvement and Production
Technology, Nanchang, China
[2] Animal Breeding and Genomics, Wageningen University, Wageningen,
The Netherlands
Full list of author information is available at the end of the article

Background

Domestication of pigs from wild boars occurred independently in Asia and Europe about 10,000 years ago [1]. Due to the biogeographic difference between wild ancestral populations, which results from 1.2 million years of separation, Asian and European pigs are genetically highly divergent [2–5]. *Sus scrofa* is native to Eurasia and North Africa, but was introduced into other parts of the world, i.e. into the Americas, primarily in its domesticated form, during the time of the European colonization in the sixteenth century, and later in Australia and New Zealand [6]. Both demographic processes, and natural as well as artificial selection, have led to the formation of a multitude of pig breeds around the world that vary in coat color, ear shape, body size, snout bluntness, behavior, growth rate, fatness, and prolificacy and other economically important traits.

In addition to domestication, crossbreeding between Asian and European indigenous pigs mediated by humans are significant landmarks in pig breeding history. Although anecdotal evidence exists even from the classical era, admixture between Western and Eastern pigs only started to become common in the mid- to late eighteenth century [7]. Introduction of Chinese pigs into Britain is documented from then and its aim was to improve the production characteristics of local pigs, which led to the creation of modern breeds such as Yorkshire (i.e., Large White), Berkshire and Hampshire [8]. In the late eighteenth century, Chinese pigs may also have been imported to America, and crossed with local pigs of European ancestry there [8], although most likely the Asian influence in American village pigs was through crosses with international breeds [9]. Reciprocally, at least since the 1840s, modern breeds such as Berkshire, Hampshire, Russian local pigs, Duroc, Large White and Landrace were introduced into China [10]. Such domestic animals were traded, loaded onto ships and released elsewhere. This is well documented, e.g., during the exploration of the Pacific by Captain Cook, who is credited for having released the first pigs on the New Zealand islands [11]. As in Europe, these imported pigs were used for crossbreeding with local breeds. However, in China, the introduction of pigs from outside and trading of pigs within China, appear to have been less widespread until recently, as is apparent from the high degree of geographic structure that remains in the Chinese traditional pig breeds [3]. Nevertheless, historical records and genetic evidence point to the contribution of European pigs to some East Asian breeds. For instance, the modern Korean Native pig is a cross between a local, traditional Korean pig and Berkshire. More recently, since the 1980s, Chinese pig breeders began programs to improve local breeds using Western stock [10] by creating synthetic breeds. In Africa, although advocated as an additional center of domestication, most of the evidence points to introgression from foreign breeds. Interestingly, Asian haplotypes predominate in East Africa, whereas European haplotypes predominate in West Africa [12].

Today, pig is a major livestock species, which in 2012 represented about 36.3% of the total meat production for human societies (www.fao.org), with major contributions from only a few international commercial breeds (i.e. Duroc, Large White, and Landrace). Nevertheless, hundreds of domesticated pig breeds worldwide [13] are still important for local meat production by small farmers. Many of these pig breeds have unique characteristics that differ from those of the international commercial breeds. Conservation of agrodiversity is one of the pillars to maintain food security, particularly in a rapidly changing world where consolidation of international plant and animal breeds is resulting in an increasingly narrow genetic basis for food production [14]. Thus, indigenous pig breeds, together with their wild relatives, are valued resources for the human society, not only for food, but also as genetic reservoirs. In addition, they constitute cultural and historical value since certain breeds are highly connected to local identity and specific agricultural practices. Finally, breed diversity can be leveraged for understanding the genetic basis of complex traits and adaptive evolution [15]. Large-scale genotyping technologies have enabled the analysis of the genetic ancestry and admixture of many domestic animals, including dogs [16], cattle [17], and pigs [18] and have also enabled the characterization of the genetic basis of phenotypic changes during domestication in chicken [19], dogs [20], rabbits [21] and pigs [22].

To date, population genetic studies using genomic data in pigs had a limited, usually regional, scope [9, 23–25]. Compared to previous generations of molecular markers, particularly microsatellites, single nucleotide polymorphism (SNP) markers allow for relatively straightforward data integration across studies since SNP genotypes can be compared unambiguously across studies. The aim of the current study was to perform a truly global integration of pig genotype data through the analysis of 1839 domestic pigs from 122 indigenous pig breeds that were collected in 29 different countries, together with 215 wild boars and 39 out-group individuals. As a result, our findings constitute a big leap in understanding the population structure, admixture, demographic history, and characterization of genetic loci involved in the domestication of pigs globally.

Methods

Samples and data

The raw Illumina 60K SNP data [26] of 3482 pigs, which include 3443 *Sus scrofa* and 39 non *Sus scrofa* suids (outgroups) (Table 1), were mainly obtained from three sources (see Additional file 1: Table S1): Wageningen University in The Netherlands (2464 individuals that encompass pig populations from Europe, Asia, Africa, Oceania, North America, international commercial pig populations, as well as outgroup suids), Jiangxi Agricultural University in China (821 individuals, which mainly consisted of pig populations from China, Russia and Ukraine), and the Autonomous University of Barcelona in Spain (197 individuals, which mainly represent pig populations from South America and Iberian pigs). Genomic SNP positions are based on the genome assembly Sscrofa 10.2 (EnsEMBL db version 83) [18].

We conducted a series of quality control procedures on the raw data using PLINK v1.9 [27]. First, we excluded the breeds with less than five individuals. For the breeds or populations with more than 20 individuals, we randomly removed one individual from a pair of highly related animals (identity by state score > 0.95), and then kept the top 20 samples ranked by the SNP call rate. Next, we removed SNPs with a minor allele frequency (MAF) lower than 0.01, a call rate lower than 90% and individuals with a call rate lower than 90%, which resulted in a dataset of 55,072 SNPs for 2093 individuals that was used to estimate ROH, haplotype diversity and effective population size. We further removed SNPs with a MAF lower than 0.05, and in high linkage disequilibrium ($r^2 > 0.2$) by using—maf 0.05 and—indep-pairwise 50 10 0.2 in PLINK v1.9 [27], respectively, and generated a dataset of 15,427 SNPs for 2093 individuals for subsequent

Table 1 Number of populations and samples by continent

Subgroup	$N_{POPULATION}$	N_{SAMPLE}
Asian Domestic	40	624
Asian Wild	8	59
European Domestic	39	596
European Wild	10	149
American Domestic	19	222
American Feral	3	36
African Domestic	2	9
African Wild	1	7
Oceania Feral	1	10
Duroc	4	79
Landrace	7	129
Large White	4	76
Pietrain	3	58
Outgroup Suids	5	39

multi-dimensional scaling (MDS), neighbor joining (NJ) tree and admixture analyses. See Additional file 2: Table S2 for further details.

Statistical analysis

Population structure

MDS was carried out using—mds-plot and—cluster options in PLINK v1.9 [27] and visualized by R programming language [28]. The NJ tree was constructed using PHYLIP v3.69 [29] based on the identical by states matrix obtained by PLINK v1.9 [27], and visualized using FigTree v1.4 (http://beast.bio.ed.ac.uk/figtree). To facilitate visualization, we randomly selected six individuals from each population to build up the NJ tree. The geographical maps were plotted using R package MAPS [30] and MAPPLOTS (https://cran.r-project.org/web/packages/mapplots/). The coordinates of longitude and latitude of each population were set according to where the pigs were sampled (see Additional file 1: Table S1). The geographical distances between each pair of breeds were computed using *distm* function in R package GEOSPHERE (https://cran.r-project.org/web/packages/geosphere/). The proportion of mixed ancestry in the populations analyzed was evaluated by the ADMIXTURE 1.22 program [31]. We evaluated different K values with the mixed ancestry model (K = 2 to 17).

Runs of homozygosity, haplotype diversity and effective population size

Runs of homozygosity (ROH) of each breed were identified using PLINK v.1.07 by a 5-Mb sliding window process across the genome with at least 50 SNPs, allowing five missing calls and one heterozygous SNP. The minimum length for ROH was set to 500 kb. ROH statistics were then transformed to F_{ROH}. We inferred haplotypes of autosomes for all individuals using SHAPEIT v2 [32]. Haplotype diversity was calculated for populations with a minimum of 10 individuals. For each population, we randomly selected 10 individuals for the analysis. The haplotype diversity of a population was measured as the average number of haplotypes in windows of 5, 10, and 15 SNPs, respectively, which is similar to the method described in [16]. LD between adjacent SNPs was measured by the genotype correlation coefficient (r^2) calculated by the—r2—ld-window 99999—ld-window-r2 0 command in PLINK v1.9. We used the same equation to fit the relationship between LD and genetic distance as previously described [33]. The SNPs used to calculate the LD within a population were filtered by applying the following criteria: a MAF higher than 0.05 and a *P* value for Hardy–Weinberg equilibrium higher than 1×10^{-6}. The effective population size was estimated according to Sved [34], based on the equation $r^2 = 1/(4N_ec + 1)$, where r^2

is the linkage disequilibrium between a pair of SNPs, N_e is the effective population size, c is the genetic distance in Morgan between a pair of SNPs, which was obtained by multiplying their physical distance and recombination rate [35]. The N_e at generation T, were obtained by the equation $T = 1/2c$, the same as described in [36].

Domestication loci

To detect loci that may have been selected during domestication, we calculated the fixation index (Fst) [37] between domestic and wild boars in Asia and Europe, separately. To avoid the influence of introgression, we used 42,808 SNPs (MAF > 0.05) in 782 individuals that have more than 90% of Asian or European ancestry in the analysis. We ranked the Fst values of genome-wide SNPs, and genes within a 100-kb region of high-Fst SNPs were identified as candidate genes that may have been involved in past selection. We selected candidate genes according to their functional relevance to phenotypes, such as e.g. behavior, development, energy metabolism, which may confer differences between domestic pigs and wild boars.

Results

Samples

After quality control, a dataset of 2093 samples representing 122 domestic pig breeds (1839 individuals), 19 wild boar populations (215 individuals) and five outgroup populations (39 individuals) was available. The 122 domestic breeds included 104 local breeds or synthetic populations and 18 international commercial populations (Duroc, Large White, Landrace and Pietrain from different countries were considered as different breeds) (see Additional file 1: Table S1). Among the 104 local breeds, 39 originated from Europe, 40 from Asia, 22 from the Americas and three from other parts of the world. The wild boars were from widespread regions around the world and the five out-group populations are *Babyrousa babyrussa*, *Sus barbatus*, *Sus celebensis* and *Sus verrucosus* from the islands of Southeast Asia and *Phacochoerus africanus* from Africa. A more detailed description of many of these samples was reported in previous studies [9, 24, 25].

Global population structure

We performed multi-dimensional scaling (MDS) analysis on 15,427 SNPs for the 2093 individuals to investigate the genetic relationships between populations of domesticated pigs, wild boars and out-group populations. The first principal component separates Asian and European breeds (Fig. 1) and (see Additional file 3: Figure S1), in agreement with independent domestication and evolution of pigs in Asia and Europe. The American, African, and international commercial populations are much

closer to European than to Asian pigs, which indicates a predominant contribution of European ancestry in the formation of these derived populations. Nevertheless, several populations are positioned in between the Asian and European main clusters. These include Oceania populations, populations from China (Lichahei and Sutai), the Korean native pig breed, Minisibs pigs from Russia and a Large White × Meishan F_1 cross (Fig. 1) and (see Additional file 3: Figure S1). The intermediate position in the MDS reflects the fact that these populations are derived from both Asian and European pigs, and we validated the hybrid nature of these populations in subsequent admixture analysis. The Lichahei and Sutai pigs from China, the LW × Meishan F1 cross, and Minisib pigs from Russia consist of approximately 50% Asian and 50% European ancestries (see Additional file 4: Figure S2).Thus, the first MDS axis represents the Asian and European ancestries.

The second axis separates domestic pigs from wild boars in both Asia and Europe (Fig. 1) and (see Additional file 3: Figure S1), which indicates that domestication and subsequent artificial selection also resulted in the differentiation between wild and domesticated populations. Regarding the international commercial pig breeds, the Duroc breed tends to cluster with American domestic breeds and to separate from other commercial breeds (Landrace, Large White and Pietrain) that tend to cluster together. These results agree with the fact that Duroc pigs were originally developed in the USA, whereas, the other international commercial breeds (e.g. Large White-England, Landrace-Denmark, and Pietrain-Belgium) originated in Europe.

The results from hierarchical clustering (neighbor joining based on identity by state distance metric) generally agree with those from the MDS analysis. An important observation is that, even on a global scale, all populations of the major commercial breeds, still cluster together, i.e. breed identity has been maintained for both commercial and non-commercial populations (see Additional file 5: Figure S3).

Regional population structures in Asia and Europe

To infer geographic region-specific details, we performed separate MDS analyses on pig populations within Asia and Europe, separately (Fig. 2). In Asia, most of the pig populations originate from China. In previous studies [3, 38], Chinese pigs were grouped into six categories that included pig types from Central China, the Yangtze River basin (East China), South China, Southwest China, North China, and Plateau (West and Northwest China), according to their external traits and geographical distributions [38]. The genetic clusters revealed in the MDS analyses are broadly concordant with this assignment

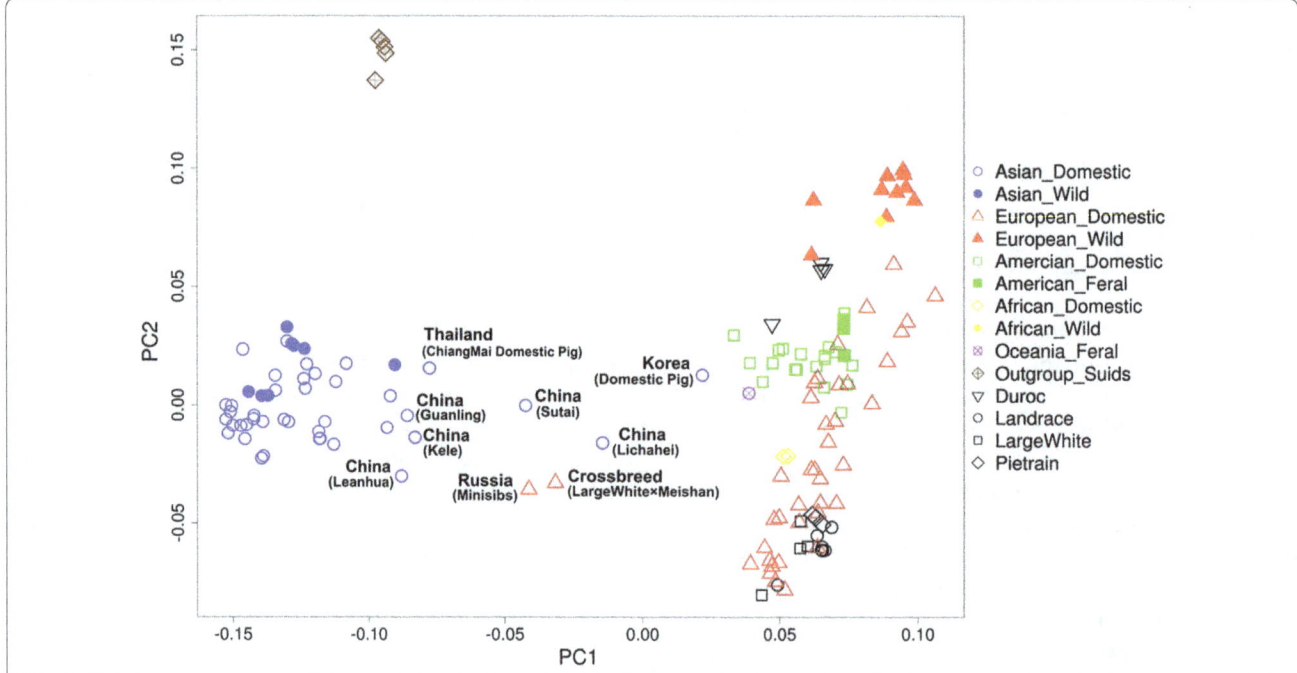

Fig. 1 Global genetic structure of pig populations in this study. Multi-dimensional scaling analysis of pig populations from the five continents. Each point represents breed-average coordinates of eigenvalues of principle components 1 and 2. Points are mainly colored based on geographic origin of breeds; *blue* Asia, *red* Europe, *green* America, *yellow* Africa, *purple* Oceania, *brown* outgroup of Suids, *black* commercial Breeds; the pig populations in the middle of the *graph* representing admixed Asian and European ancestries are annotated

into six categories (Fig. 2a, b). Pig breeds from South China and those from East and North China are located at each end of the first axis, while pig breeds from Central and West China are located in between (Fig. 2a, b). As expected under a model of gene flow between populations that is inversely proportional to physical distance, genetic distances were significantly correlated with geographical distances (Pearson correlation, *P* value = 1.5×10^{-62}) (Fig. 2c). This is in sharp contrast to the results for pig breeds from the Americas where no concordance between genetic similarity and geographical distances was observed due to the complex colonization and breeding history of American pigs [9].

In Europe, the pig breeds from Southern Europe (Italy, Spain and Hungary) and those from North and middle Europe (Netherlands, Sweden, Poland, Germany and the Czech Republic) were genetically distinct. This distinction is represented by the first axis (Fig. 2d, e). Within the UK, British Lop, Leicoma, Middle White and Welsh breeds differ from Large Black, Gloucester Old Spot, Saddleback and Tamworth breeds. However, we observed no correlation with geographical distances among pig breeds in Europe (Fig. 2f), which is consistent with previous results based on microsatellites [3]. The absence of population structure in European pigs is explained, at least in part, by the Asian introgression and subsequent

influence of highly productive "international" breeds on local pig diversity. In Europe, many 'local' or 'traditional' breeds have effectively become (partially) extinct due to such extensive crossbreeding [36, 39, 40].

Global genetic ancestries

We further examined the genetic ancestry of pig populations worldwide by varying the number of ancestries (K) in ADMIXTURE v 1.2 [31] (Fig. 3) and (see Additional file 4: Figure S2). The population structure generally agreed with the MDS results. At K = 2, the two ancestries clearly reflect Asian and European origins. The pig populations from America, Africa, Russia and neighboring countries (including Ukraine, Belorussia and Kazakhstan) are mainly of European ancestry and (see Additional file 4: Figure S2). Even the international commercial pig breeds are mostly of European origin although they have a large Asian ancestry component [23]. At K = 8, we found two distinct Asian ancestries that are represented by pig breeds from East (Meishan, CNMS) and South (Luchuan, CNLU) China. The other six ancestries are represented by European wild boars, Hampshire (UKHS) and Berkshire (UKBK), and four international commercial breeds including Duroc, Large White, Landrace, and Pietrain and (see Additional file 4: Figure S2), (K = 8). At a higher K value (K = 17),

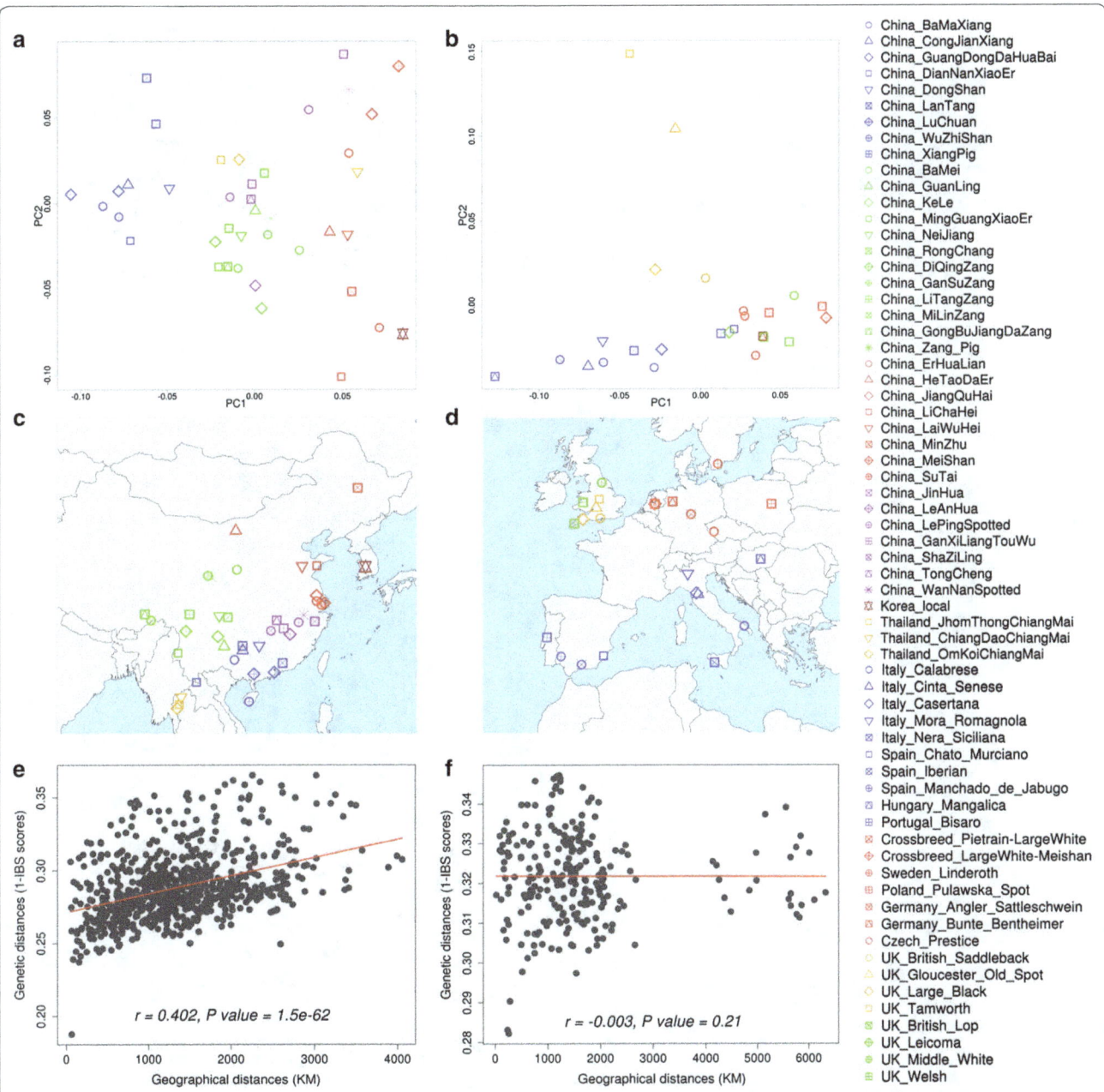

Fig. 2 Regional genetic structure of indigenous pig populations in Asia and Europe. **a**, **d** show the results of the MDS analysis of pig populations from Asia (40 breeds) and Europe (26 breeds). Each *point* represents a breed, *colors* are assigned to each breed according to their geographical distributions, which are visualized in (**b**) and (**e**) for Asian and European pigs, respectively. **c**, **f** show the correlation between genetic and geographic distances among pig breeds in Asia and Europe, respectively. The legends of pig breeds are shown on the *right*. The upper legends in the *blue box* are for Asian breeds and the legends below in *red box* are for European breeds

we found various breed-specific ancestries that reflect a recent isolated breeding history (Gansu Zang (CNGS), Meishan (CNMS), Luchuan (CNLU), Jinhua (CNJH) and Congjiangxiang (CNCJ) pigs from China, Tamworth (UKTA), Hampshire (UKHS) and Berkshire (UKBK) from Europe, and Mulefoot pig (USMU) from USA).

Admixture between Asian and European ancestries

An additional interesting pattern is the widespread admixed ancestries that we observed in pig populations across the different continents. Note that many breeds showed evidence of both Asian and European ancestries. Since these two lineages evolved independently, this admixture is a result of human-mediated activities.

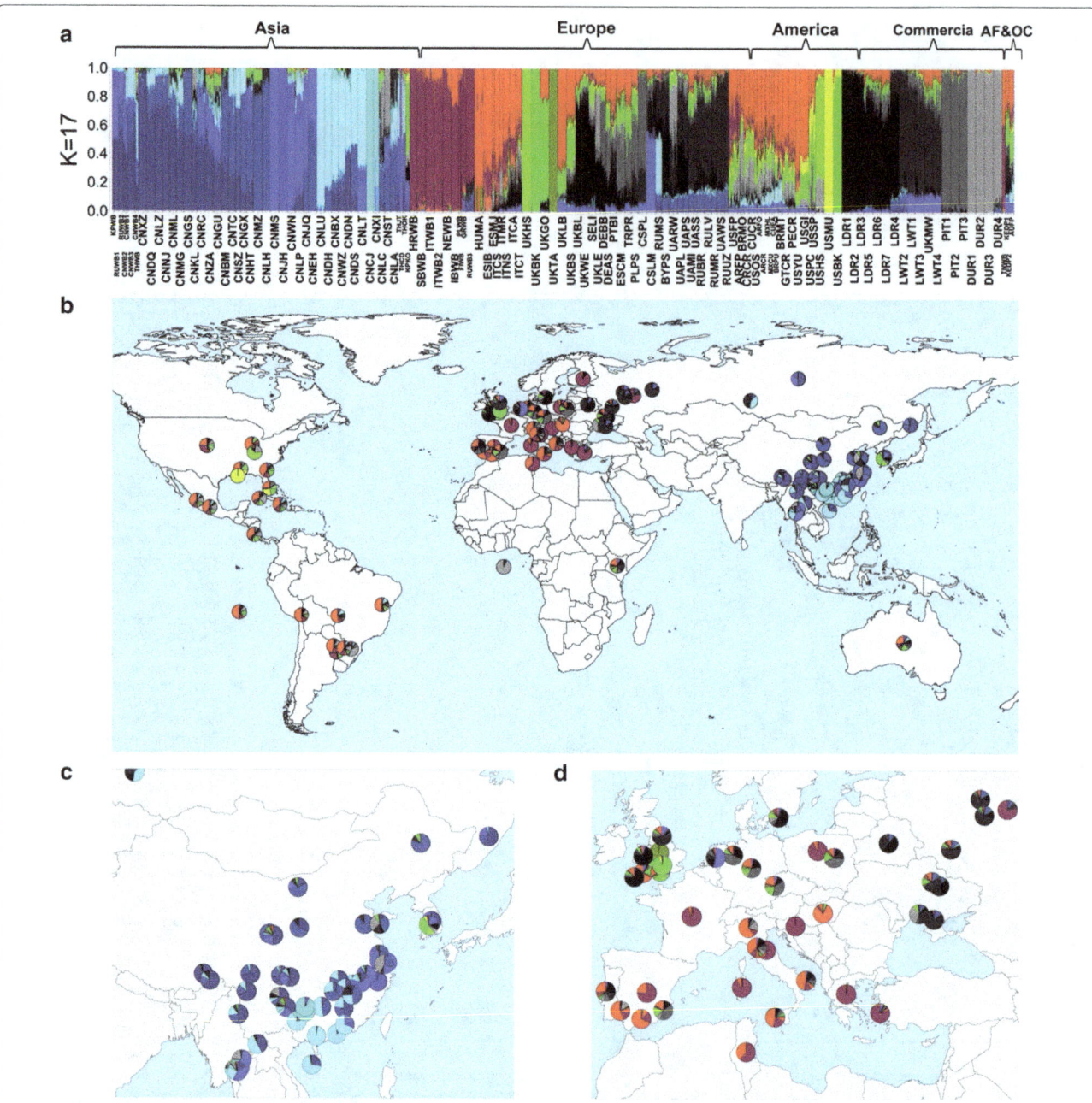

Fig. 3 Landscape of worldwide admixture of pig populations. **a** Bar plot of admixture analysis (K = 17). Each *vertical bar* stands for an individual, the *colors* represent different ancestries. **b** Worldwide map of admixture for pig populations, the *pie plots* represent different breeds, the compositions of ancestries for a breed were calculated from the averages of ancestry composition of individuals within that breed. **c, d** Regional plot for Asian and European pigs, respectively

In Europe, importation of Chinese pigs is well accredited since the eighteenth century.

In Asia, 23 (57.5%) of the 40 breeds analyzed have 5% or more inferred European ancestry (see Additional file 4: Figure S2 and Additional file 6: Figure S4), (K = 2). Most of the European introgression was inferred to be from Duroc, Landrace, Large White, Berkshire and

Hampshire breeds (see Additional file 4: Figure S2 and Additional file 6: Figure S4), (K = 13). Eight Asian breeds have more than 20% of genomic introgression from European pigs. These breeds include a Korean local breed (KPKO), a Thailand local breed (THCD), and six breeds from China (Lichahei (CNLC) from Shandong Province, Sutai (CNST) from Jiangsu Province, Kele (CNKL) and

Guanling (CNGU) pigs from Guizhou Province, Lean-hua (CNLAH) from Jiangxi Province, Minzhu (CNMZ) from Northeast China. Among these breeds with a large degree of European introgression (>20%), the Korean pig, a known East–West synthetic breed, formed the largest European ancestry group (see Additional file 4: Figure S2 and Additional file 6: Figure S4), (K = 2 and K = 13), including ancestry from Berkshire, Hampshire, Landrace and Duroc, which reflects the complex breeding history of this breed (Fig. 3a) and (see Additional file 4: Figure S2) (K = 13 and K = 17). This is largely in line with the known origin of the Korean local pigs. Sutai and Lichahei have been mainly admixed with Duroc, while Min pigs have a considerable contribution from Berkshire (Fig. 3a) and (see Additional file 4: Figure S2 and Additional file 6: Figure S4) (K = 8 and K = 17). It is interesting that the admixture with European pigs occurred mainly in Western and Northern Chinese pig breeds (Gong-bujiangda (CNXZ) and Milin Tibetan (CNML) pigs, Kele and Guanling pigs from Guizhou Province, Ming-guangxiaoer (CNMG) pigs from Yunnan province, Bamei (CNBM) pigs from Gansu province, Laiwuhei (CNLH) pigs from Shandong Province, Hetaodaer (CNHT) from Inner Mongolia and Min (CNMZ) pigs from Heilongji-ang Province); the European ancestries that are involved encompass Large White, Landrace, Berkshire or other European breeds (Fig. 3a–c) and (see Additional file 4: Figure S2 and Additional file 6: Figure S4) (K = 13 and K = 17). In comparison, the pig breeds from South and Central China, including Erhualian, Xiang, Dongshan, Shaziling, Congjiangxiang, Lantang, Jinhua, Litang Tibetan and Luchuan, show no or negligible introgression from European pigs (Fig. 3a, c).

Iberian pigs from Spain, Cinta Senese and Nera Sicili-ana pigs from Italy, and Mangalica pigs from Hungary showed little evidence of influence from Asian pigs (see Additional file 4: Figure S2 and Additional file 7: Figure S5). By contrast, there is evidence of introgression from Asian pigs for all other pig breeds from Europe, including those from Ukraine and Russia (see Additional file 4: Figure S2 and Additional file 7: Figure S5). These results confirm the widespread Asian influences in European breeds.

The North and South American samples consisted mainly of village and feral pigs from eight countries [9]. Consistent with previous studies on pigs from the Ameri-cas using 60K SNP [9], and mitochondrial DNA data [41], pig populations from rural areas have mosaic genetic compositions that consist of multiple ancestries from both Europe and Asia. The largest ancestry components were similar to Iberian pigs (ESIB), in agreement with a primigenious origin from the Iberian Peninsula. Other European components are related to Duroc, Landrace,

Berkshire, Hampshire, and European Wild boars (Fig. 3a) and (see Additional file 4: Figure S2 and Additional file 8: Figure S6). Intriguingly, a considerable contribution from pigs from both east and south China was observed in most of the American Village pigs (Additional file 8: Fig-ure S6). In general, the village pigs from Brazil, Mexico and Cuba have larger Asian components than the pigs from other American countries (Fig. 3a).

In Africa, the Tunisian wild boar shows a high degree of similarity to the European wild boar, and specifically to the wild boar from the Iberian Peninsula. A local breed from Kenya was inferred to contain both Asian and Euro-pean ancestries (Fig. 3a) and (see Additional file 4: Figure S2 and Additional file 8: Figure S6). This is in agreement with mtDNA studies, which showed that Asian haplo-types were abundant in East Africa but completely absent in the Northern African pigs (i.e. Tunisian wild boars) [41].

In Oceania, the Australian feral pigs also show admixed ancestry from Asian and European pigs (Fig. 3a) and (see Additional file 4: Figure S2 and Additional file 8: Figure S6).

The four major international commercial pig breeds, i.e. Duroc, Landrace, Large White, and Pietrain, have a considerable percentage of Asian ancestry (see Addi-tional file 4: Figure S2 and Additional file 9: Figure S7) (K = 2). At K = 8, these four breeds form four distinct ancestries. The Landrace and Large White breeds also showed a diversity of genetic ancestries related to various pig populations including Berkshire, Hampshire, South European local pigs or Asian pigs.

Genetic diversity

We analyzed runs of homozygosity (F_{ROH}), haplotype diversity, and effective population size for each pig population to assess their inbreeding history and effec-tive population size. Previous studies showed that 60K SNP data provide reasonably accurate estimates of long F_{ROH} [15]. We calculated the total length of ROH with a minimum length of 500 kbp for each individual. Consid-erable variation in F_{ROH} occurs within and across popu-lations, which reflects the complex breeding history of pigs (Fig. 4). The cumulative length of ROH ranged from 4.98 Mb for the Dutch LW × Meishan F_1 population from the Netherlands to 591.57 Mb for the Mora Romag-nola pigs from Italy, and represented between 0.2 and 20.8% of the genome. Since the Dutch LW × Meishan is an F_1 cross, it was expected to have few if any ROH. The 10 populations with the highest F_{ROH} included the Mora Romagnola (ITMR) and Cinta Senese pigs (ITCS) from Italy, the Mangalica breed from Hungary (HUMA), the Korea local breed (KPKO), the Mulefoot (USMU) and Yucatan Mini pigs (USYU) from USA, the Creole pigs

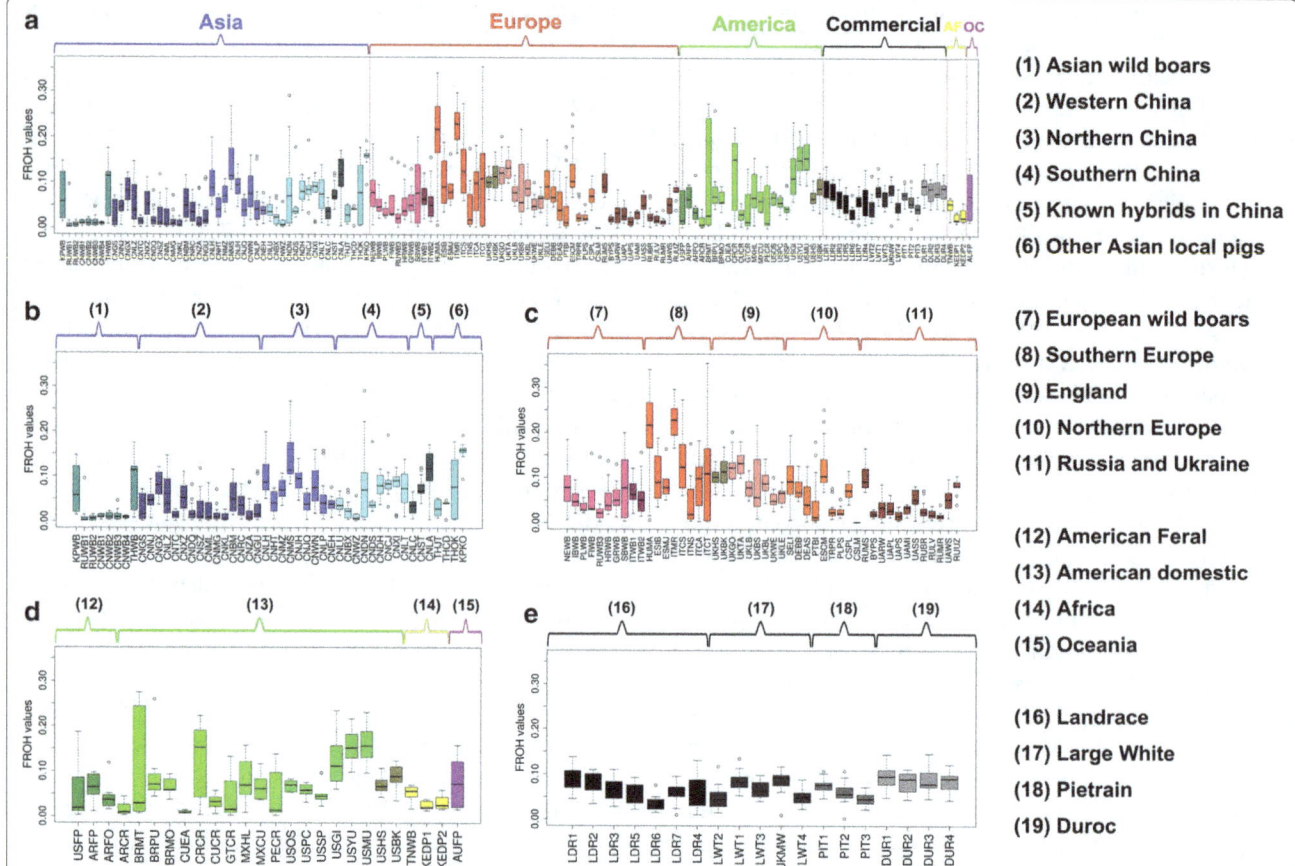

Fig. 4 Distribution of F_{ROH} for pig populations across the world. **a** Box plot showing the global distribution of total length of F_{ROH} for pig populations worldwide, each point represents the total length of F_{ROH} for one individual, each *box* represents one breed, the *colors* and the order of breeds are the same as those described in Fig. 3. Regional view of F_{ROH} distribution for pig populations in Asia (**b**), Europe (**c**), America, Oceania and Africa (**d**), and international commercial breeds (**e**)

(CRCR) from Costa Rica, the Gloucester old spot pigs (UKGO) and Tamworth pigs (UKTA) from UK, and the Leanhua pigs (CNLA) from China, which indicates that these populations have recently experienced considerable inbreeding (Fig. 4) and (see Additional file 1: Table S1). In addition, the total length of ROH was negatively correlated with haplotype diversity (Pearson correlation coefficient = -0.71, *P* value = 1.6×10^{-20}) (see Additional file 10: Figure S8). Therefore, populations with a high F_{ROH} normally have a low haplotype diversity (Fig. 4) and (see Additional file 11: Figure S9). The effective population size (N_e) for each population was estimated using linkage disequilibrium following the method described in [36] (see Additional file 1: Table S1). Considering only the populations with a minimum of 10 individuals, the estimated N_e of the past five generations is between 26 and 67. Even after accounting for a small systematic bias towards lower estimated Ne in populations that a have smaller sample size, it is clear that the N_e of indigenous pig populations is generally smaller than that of the

international commercial breeds (see Additional file 12: Figure S10 and Additional file 1: Table S1).

Loci involved in domestication

Domestication and artificial selection have resulted in a wide range of phenotypes across domestic pig breeds that differ from their wild relatives. These are related to behavior, body size, fertility, locomotion ability and adaptation to feed provided by humans. To detect genetic loci that could be involved in the transition from wild to domestic, we calculated the genome-wide fixation index (*F*st) between domestic pigs and wild boars in Asia and Europe, separately (see "Methods" section) (Fig. 5). Empirically, we considered the 428 (1%) SNPs with the highest *F*st values as potential loci under recent (domestication) selection. Only six outlier SNPs were shared between Asia and Europe, which only slightly exceeds the number expected based on re-sampling of SNPs (see Additional file 13: Figure S11). Thus, we found no evidence for specific loci being under selection during

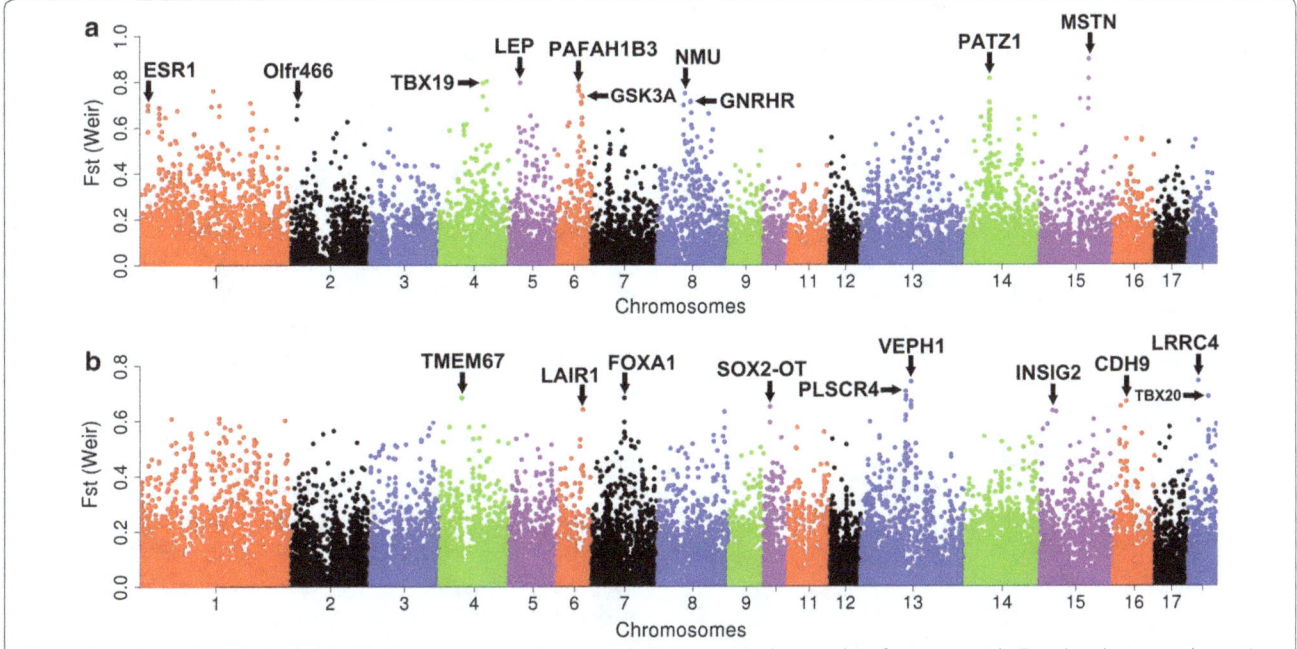

Fig. 5 Genome-wide analysis of global *F*st between domestic pigs and wild boars. Manhattan plot of genome-wide *F*st values between domestic pigs and wild boars in Asia (**a**) and Europe (**b**). *F*st values are shown on the y axis, and genomic positions on the x axis. The different chromosomes are represented by different *colors*

the independent domestication processes in Asia and Europe. We examined the genes that are located within 100 kb to the top outlier SNPs with extreme *F*st values, and made the assumption that many of the genes around the top 30 outlier SNPs are involved in functions that are associated with phenotypic changes from wild to domestic (Fig. 5; Table 2). For Asian pigs, we identified genes related to muscle development (*MSTN* [42]), energy balance (*NMU* [43], *LEP* [44] and *GSK3A* [45]), social behavior (*TBX19* [46] and *PAFAH1B3* [47]), puberty and reproduction (*GNRHR* [48], *ESR1* [49] and *PATZ1* [50]) and perception of smell (*Olfr466* [51]) (Table 2). For European pigs, we identified genes related to growth and body development (*SOX2-OT* [52]), cardiac system development (*TBX20* [53]), metabolism of protein, glucose or fatty acid (*TMEM67* [54], *FOXA1* [55] and *INSIG2* [56]), central nervous system (*LRRC4* [57], *VEPH1* [58] and *CDH9* [59]), immune system (*LAIR1* [60]), and reproduction (*PLSCR4* [61]) (Table 2).

Discussion

Pig is one of the most important livestock species for humans as a valued, global, resource for meat production and as an excellent animal model to understand the genetic mechanisms that underlie complex traits [6, 18]. Its long domestication history, originating from a large diversity of wild ancestors throughout Eurasia, and selection for economic and cultural purposes have resulted

in a large number of breeds globally, which show a wide phenotypic diversity. Our worldwide survey on SNP data from 122 breeds/populations and 215 wild boars worldwide, reveals genetic ancestries, introgression and inbreeding histories of pigs at a global scale and at an unprecedented detail. Although there are potential issues regarding ascertainment bias [40] associated with the SNP assay used in this study, admixture analyses using 60K SNP and 30 million SNPs called from whole-genome sequence data provided very similar results (see Additional file 14: Figure S12), which indicates that robust conclusions can be drawn from the 60K SNP assay data for a wide population study as presented here.

Population structure

The high degree of geographic structure observed here in the Asian domesticated pigs agrees with a previous report based on microsatellite markers [3], and differs substantially from that observed in pig populations from Europe and the Americas, in which almost no correlation between genetic and geographical distances exist [9]. The strong concordances between genetic and geographical distances for the pig populations in Asia may be attributed to the fact that pig populations within certain eco-geographical regions are more likely to have common ancestries, and that most of the breeds in Asia did not migrate over large distances. Furthermore, introgressions from European populations did not mask the identity of

Table 2 Candidate genes for domestication loci in Asia and Europe

Region	Chr	Position	Fst	Rank	Location	Genes	Notes
Asia	15	105803885	0.90	1	Intergenic	MSTN	Muscle growth/differentiation [33]
	14	51279090	0.81	2	Intergenic	PATZ1	Spermatogenesis [41]
	5	23737420	0.80	6	In gene	LEP	Growth, energy homeostasis [35]
	4	90358483	0.80	7	In exon	TBX19	Personality traits angry/hostility [37]
	6	45563650	0.78	8	Intergenic	PAFAH1B3	Development of brain [38]
	6	45609490	0.76	11	In gene	GSK3A	Insulin signaling pathways [36]
	8	58493225	0.75	14	Intergenic	NMU	Food intake and energy balance [34]
	8	69912174	0.72	20	In exon	GNRHR	Pubertal delay [39]
	1	16779942	0.70	27	In gene	ESR1	Precocious puberty [40]
	2	12631241	0.70	29	In gene	Olfr466	Perception of smell [42]
Europe	18	21362149	0.74	1	Intergenic	LRRC4	Central nervous system [48]
	13	105334978	0.74	2	In gene	VEPH1	Central nervous system [49]
	13	94430998	0.71	3	In gene	PLSCR4	Reproduction [52]
	18	42219500	0.69	5	Intergenic	TBX20	Cardiac LDL-cholesterol [44]
	4	46284264	0.69	6	Intergenic	TMEM67	Protein catabolic process [45]
	7	67285122	0.68	7	Intergenic	FOXA1	Glucose homeostasis [46]
	10	12907670	0.65	15	In gene	SOX2-OT	Vertebrate development [43]
	16	15192108	0.65	16	Intergenic	CDH9	Autism spectrum disorder [50]
	6	53526888	0.64	18	Intergenic	LAIR1	Immune response [51]
	15	27308675	0.64	19	Intergenic	INSIG2	Cholesterol synthesis [47]

most Asian breeds, at least not to a large extent. Removing the breeds with more than 20% European introgression resulted in an increased correlation between genetic and geographical distances (see Additional file: 15 Figure S13). This indicates that admixture with geographically distant populations could be a major force in breaking regional genetic-geography concordance, as has been the case in Europe. Recent breed interchanges have largely masked an underlying geographic signal. However, it is interesting to note that some breeds have remained relatively unchanged for centuries. For instance, Ramirez et al. [62] showed that the modern Iberian breed is genetically very similar to a sixteenth century Spanish pig.

Contribution of Chinese populations to worldwide pigs

The Chinese ancestries in European pigs observed in this study confirmed, on a broader population scale, the findings of previous genetic studies [2, 23, 41, 63]. These results are consistent with the historical record that South Chinese pigs were brought to England from Guangzhou in South China, the only treaty port city in China at that time, and have contributed to local British breeds, such as Berkshire and Yorkshire around 200 years ago [7, 8, 63]. Interestingly, our analyses revealed that ancestry represented by Lantang pigs from Guangdong Province is likely the major source of introgression in American pigs (Fig. 3a). The Meishan pigs of Eastern China, a breed famous for its high prolificacy,

were imported to Western countries including France, England and USA in the 1980s [64]. Meishan pigs were used in experimental crosses to study the genetic basis of complex traits [65]. Recent studies showed that many Asian alleles with favorable phenotypic effects reached a high frequency in European pigs. These included MC1R alleles that are associated with black coat color [66], an IGF2 allele for muscle growth [67], and AHR alleles for sow reproduction traits [23]. These studies underscored the importance of Asian pigs as vital genetic resources for international pig breeding and pork production.

Contribution of European ancestry to worldwide pig populations

Both MDS and admixture analysis showed that European pigs were the major contributors to pig populations in those regions of the world where *Sus scrofa* does not occur natively (America, Africa, and Oceania). These results are consistent with mitochondrial and Y chromosome polymorphisms [41]. This contribution is due, in part, to the waves of colonization by Europeans since the sixteenth century. In addition, recent increase in worldwide trading of commercial, improved, pigs throughout the globe, and the desire of local farmers to improve their pigs using these western breeds, have likely contributed to this process as well. Populations in the Americas, Africa, and Oceania tend to harbor multiple ancestries of Mediterranean countries and/

or international commercial breeds such as Berkshire, Hampshire, and Duroc (Fig. 3), which indicates a very dynamic process of global mixing of populations during several centuries.

More recently, the global process of mixing has become 'full circle' by the introduction of European pigs, themselves heavily influenced by Asian pigs, in Asia. In fact, one of the main original findings of our study is the widespread European influence in many Asian populations, the extent of which was mostly unknown until now. In Asia, we observed widespread and complex gene flow from European pigs, which indicates that many Asian indigenous pig breeds are no longer strictly Asian, but also contain a genetic component of European origin. Occurrence of European introgression in Japan [68], Korea [69] and Vietnam [70] was reported before. In China, there are over 80 pig breeds and a high diversity in phenotypes [64]. Historical documents indicate at least three waves of introgression from European pigs since the 1840s. The first wave of introgression may have occurred around the 1840s, when European pig breeds including Berkshire, Large White, Duroc, pigs from Russia, and Tamworth were brought to China by Germans and Japanese [10]. Subsequently, starting from the early twentieth century, probably since the 1910s, large-scale importation of Western European pigs, such as Berkshire in the Hebei, Sichuan, and Jiangsu provinces, and of Russian pigs in Northwest China, took place to improve local breeds. This study demonstrates that many pig breeds from West and North China contain ancestries from European pigs, notably Berkshire, Hampshire, Large White and Russian pigs, which is in agreement with historical records. Since 1937, war and civic and economic upheavals hampered systematic breeding, which may explain why most of the pig populations in China maintained their geographic identity in spite of admixture with European pigs. Since the 1980s, due to changes in Chinese policies regarding the introduction of foreign agricultural germplasms, many international commercial breeds were introduced into China, which gave rise to several synthetic breeds, such as the Lichahei from Shandong Province, and Sutai pigs from Jiangsu Province. Both breeds currently display considerable ancestry from Duroc.

Indications for conservation of indigenous pigs

Inbreeding and decrease in effective population size may reduce the fitness of a population in response to challenges from changing environments or infectious diseases. This study provides an overview on the inbreeding, demography and admixture history of pig populations worldwide. First, our analysis revealed that 40 breeds or populations have substantial cumulative ROH (>200 Mb),

and also exhibit low haplotype diversity, which indicate that these populations underwent recent inbreeding. This may reflect the fact that all domesticated and many wild populations are de facto under population management, deliberate or not. Second, we show that many of the indigenous pig breeds have smaller N_e than those of international commercial breeds. Since the commercial breeds are also the breeds that are the most admixed, this is not surprising. Finally, we found prevalent admixture of Asian and European ancestries in the indigenous pig populations, which suggests that many breeds have become less representative of the original local ancestries. The admixture of populations, particularly between East and West, has resulted in a re-shaping of the nucleotide diversity in the genomes of modern pig breeds. Because of that, only some of the current least admixed breeds may represent the original nucleotide and haplotype diversity in Europe. These results could help to make decisions on the conservation and management of pig populations. For example, Mangalica pigs from Hungary (HUMA) and Mora Romagnola pigs from Italy (ITMR) present the most extensive ROH in their genomes and the highest European ancestry, which indicate that these two breeds have undergone intensive inbreeding, and require special attention regarding conservation measures.

Genetic basis of domestication

Domestication of plants and animals has been one of the major transitions in human history. Farming practices have not only altered the human societies but the interactions with nature, especially for domesticated plants and animals. Domestication of pigs has led to dramatic phenotypic changes transforming the wild boar into pigs by altering their behavior, morphology, coat color, reproduction and physiology. The admixture and MDS analyses presented in this study confirm the close relationship between wild and domesticated *Sus scrofa* in the geographic areas where domestication took place. Therefore, the genomic regions that show a much higher than average differentiation between wild and domesticated pigs should be enriched for loci under selection during domestication. We identified a number of genes that are located near loci with extreme *F*st values and that have functions that match the phenotypic changes from wild boars to domestic pigs. For instance, domestic pigs receive a stable feed supply from humans, while wild boars need to endure starvation if they cannot find food in the wild. We identified a number of genes with functions related to energy balance and metabolism (*NUM, LEP FOXA1* and *INSIG2*), which could have contributed to the adaptation of pigs to food scarcity or abundance. Genes involved in growth (*MSTN* and *SOX2-OT*) and reproduction (*GNRHR, PATZ1, ESR1,* and *PLSCR4*) could be associated with improved meat production and reproduction traits in domestic pigs that have undergone strong artificial selection. Lastly, genes related to nervous system and behavior (*TBX19*, *LRRC4*, *VEPH1* and *CDH9*) could be associated with changes in the behavior of domestic pigs compared to wild boars. The absence of signatures of selection found in previous studies [22–24] can be attributed to the higher density of SNPs, the specific selection-detection method, or the application of specific population contrasts in those studies. While further studies are needed to validate the role of the genes that we identified here in the domestication process, our findings confirm that this long-standing genetic experiment—i.e. domestication—is continuing to yield insights into biology and evolution.

Conclusions

We present the largest population study on pigs and their wild ancestors to date, which investigates the population structure and introgression of worldwide pig populations globally. We demonstrate regional and global mixing of pig diversity, which reflect that this species has essentially followed many of the globalization events over the past centuries. Population diversity statistics such as ROH provided insight on inbreeding history and effective population sizes that allow us to recommend guidelines for breeding and conservation programs. Similar to other domesticated species, pigs represent an excellent model to study adaptation. We have identified a number of candidate genes that could have been under positive selection during domestication.

Additional files

Additional file 1: Table S1. Detailed information and parameters of population genetics for pig populations in this study.

Additional file 2: Table S2. List of number of individuals and SNPs used in each step of analysis.

Additional file 3: Figure S1. MDS plot for all pig populations with detailed breed information.

Additional file 4: Figure S2. Neighbor-joining tree of pig populations under study.

Additional file 5: Figure S3. Population structure of each population revealed by the ADMIXTURE software at K = 2, 3, 5, 7, 10, 16. We marked the grouping of pig populations on the top of the graph to improve its readability. The first layer of the legend marks the five groups: Asia, Europe, America, Commercial and AF&OC (Africa and Oceania). The second layer of the legend further denotes more specific regions in corresponding continents: ASWB (Asian wild boars), CNDM_W (Chinese western domestic pigs), CNDM_N (Chinese northern domestic pigs), CNDM_S (Chinese southern domestic pigs), ① (Chinese hybrid pigs), ② (Southeast Asian pigs); EUWB (European wild boars), EUDM_S (European southern domestic pigs), UKDM (English domestic pigs), EUDM_N (European northern domestic pigs), RUDM (domestic pigs in Russia and its neighbor countries); AMFR (American feral pigs), AMDM (American domestic pigs); LD (Landrace), LW (Large White), PI (Pietrain), DU (Duroc); AF&OC (Pigs from Africa and Oceania).

Additional file 6: Figure S4. Expanded regional plot of Figure S2 showing the scenario of admixture for pig breeds and populations in Asia.

Additional file 7: Figure S5. Expanded regional plot of Figure S2 showing scenario of admixture for pig breeds and populations in Europe and Russia.

Additional file 8: Figure S6. Expanded regional plot of Figure S2 showing scenario of admixture for pig breeds and populations in North and South America.

Additional file 9: Figure S7. Expanded regional plot of Figure S2 showing scenario of admixture for pig breeds and populations in African and Oceanian countries.

Additional file 10: Figure S8. Scatterplot of the correlation between ROH length and haplotype diversity. Note that the total length of ROH and haplotype diversity are negatively correlated.

Additional file 11: Figure S9. Distribution of haplotype diversity for pig populations across the world. Diamonds and vertical bars represent means and standard deviations of number of haplotypes respectively in 5-SNP s (A), 10-SNP (B), and 15-SNP (C) windows across the genome for each population with a minimum of 10 individuals.

Additional file 12: Figure S10. Comparison of effective population size for domestic pigs and international commercial breeds.

Additional file 13: Figure S11. Observed number of shared SNPs between the top 1% SNPs with the highest *F*st values identified in Asia and Europe does not exceed the number of shared SNPs at random. The grey bars show the distribution of number of shared top SNPs at random, the red vertical line represents the observed number of shared top SNPs.

Additional file 14: Figure S12. Results of admixture analysis using 30.4 million SNPs called from whole-genome sequence data (A) were similar to those results obtained using 60K SNP data (B). Whole-genome sequence raw data from 188 individuals mainly obtained from [4, 18, 70], were used in the analysis. The whole-genome SNPs were called using GATK best practice workflow (www.broadinstitute.org/gatk). A total of 30.4 million SNP with a MAF >0.02 and a call rate >70% were kept for admixture analysis (A). A total of 44,988 SNPs with genome positions that were concordant with those of the Illumina 60K SNPs were extracted from the 30.4 million SNP data to represent the results of 60K SNPs (B).

Additional file 15: Figure S13. Scatter plot of geographical distances among pig breeds in China against their genetic distances after removing pigs breeds with more than 20% introgression from European ancestry as revealed by admixture analysis (K = 2).

Author's contributions
LH, MAMG, HJM and BY conceived and coordinated the study. HJM, LH, MAMG, MPE, ZN, RC, LI, MS, SG, PU, PD DD, AD, OH, GS, CK, GL, AA, LBS, ATri, PA and ATra provided the samples and generated the data. LC, BY and HJM analyzed the data. BY, HJM, LH, MPE and MAMG interpreted the results. BY and LC wrote the manuscript. LH, MAMG, MPE and HJM revised the manuscript. All authors read and approved the final manuscript.

Author details
[1] National Key Laboratory for Pig Genetic Improvement and Production Technology, Nanchang, China. [2] Animal Breeding and Genomics, Wageningen University, Wageningen, The Netherlands. [3] Centre for Research in Agricultural Genomics (CRAG), CSIC-IRTA-UAB-UB Consortium, Bellaterra, Barcelona, Spain. [4] Institut Catala de Recerca i Estudis Avancats (ICREA), Carrer de Lluís Companys, Barcelona, Spain. [5] All-Russian Research Institute of Animal Husbandry named after Academy Member L.K. Ernst, Dubrovitzy, Moscow Region, Russia. [6] Institute of Genomic Biology, University of Illinois, Urbana, Champaign, IL, USA. [7] Division of Genetics and Genomics, The Roslin Institute, R(D)SVS, University of Edinburgh, Edinburgh, UK. [8] Animal and Aquatic Sciences, Chiang Mai University, Chiang Mai, Thailand. [9] Division of Biotechnology and Reproduction of Livestock, Department of Animal Sciences, Georg-August-University, Göttingen, Germany. [10] Department of Genetics, Development and Molecular Biology, Aristotle University of Thessaloníki, Thessaloniki, Greece. [11] Research

Centre for Biology- Zoology Division, LIPI, Bogor, Indonesia. [12] School of Biology, University of Nottingham, Notttingham, UK. [13] Faculdade de Ciências and CESAM, Universidade de Lisboa, Lisbon, Portugal. [14] Department of Animal Science, Biotechnical Faculty, University of Ljubljana, Ljubljana, Slovenia. [15] Animal Breeding, Department of Agricultural Sciences, University of Helsinki, Helsinki, Finland. [16] Department of Chemistry and Bioscience, Aalborg University, Aalborg East, Denmark. [17] Department of Science for Nature and Environmental Resources, University of Sassari, Sassari, Italy.

Acknowledgements

We thank Marco Apollonio from Sassari University for contributing to the sampling of Italian wild boars, and Greger Larson from Oxford University for valuable comments on the manuscript.

Competing interests

The authors declare that they have no competing interests.

Funding

This study is supported by National Production Technology System for the Pig Industry in China (nycytx-008) and Outstanding Talents and Innovation Team of Agricultural Science (2011-81) to LH, AGL2010-14822 and AGL2013-41834-R (Ministry of Economy and Science, Spain) to MPE. LI received funding from the European Union's Horizon 2020 research and innovation programme under the Marie Sklodowska-Curie grant agreement No. 656697. HJM received funding from the IMAGE project (Horizon 2020, No. 677353).

References

1. Larson G, Dobney K, Albarella U, Fang M, Matisoo-Smith E, Robins J, et al. Worldwide phylogeography of wild boar reveals multiple centers of pig domestication. Science. 2005;307:1618–21.

2. Giuffra E, Kijas JM, Amarger V, Carlborg O, Jeon JT, Andersson L. The origin of the domestic pig: independent domestication and subsequent introgression. Genetics. 2000;154:1785–91.

3. Megens HJ, Crooijmans RP, San Cristobal M, Hui X, Li N, Groenen MA. Biodiversity of pig breeds from China and Europe estimated from pooled DNA samples: differences in microsatellite variation between two areas of domestication. Genet Sel Evol. 2008;40:103–28.

4. Ai H, Fang X, Yang B, Huang Z, Chen H, Mao L, et al. Adaptation and possible ancient interspecies introgression in pigs identified by whole-genome sequencing. Nat Genet. 2015;47:217–25.

5. Frantz LA, Schraiber JG, Madsen O, Megens HJ, Bosse M, Paudel Y, et al. Genome sequencing reveals fine scale diversification and reticulation history during speciation in Sus. Genome Biol. 2013;14:R107.

6. Rothschild MF, Ruvinsky A. The genetics of the pig. 2nd ed. Wallingford: CAB International; 2001.

7. Darwin C. The variation of animals and plants under domestication. London: John Murray; 1875.

8. White S. From globalized pig breeds to capitalist pigs: a study in animal cultures and evolutionary history. Environ Hist Durh NC. 2011;16:94–120.

9. Burgos-Paz W, Souza CA, Megens HJ, Ramayo-Caldas Y, Melo M, Lemus-Flores C, et al. Porcine colonization of the Americas: a 60k SNP story. Heredity (Edinb). 2013;110:321–30.

10. Xu W. Introduction and domestication of European breeds of pig in modern China. Anc Mod Agric. 2004;1:54–62.

11. Gascoigne J. Captain cook: voyager between worlds. London: Hambledon Continuum; 2007.

12. Noce A, Amills M, Manunza A, Muwanika V, Muhangi D, Aliro T, et al. East African wild pigs have a complex Indian, Far Eastern and Western ancestry. Anim Genet. 2015;46:433–6.

13. Chen K, Baxter T, Muir WM, Groenen MA, Schook LB. Genetic resources, genome mapping and evolutionary genomics of the pig (Sus scrofa). Int J Biol Sci. 2007;3:153–65.

14. Godfray HC, Beddington JR, Crute IR, Haddad L, Lawrence D, Muir JF, et al. Food security: the challenge of feeding 9 billion people. Science. 2010;327:812–8.

15. Bosse M, Megens HJ, Madsen O, Paudel Y, Frantz LA, Schook LB, et al. Regions of homozygosity in the porcine genome: consequence of demography and the recombination landscape. PLoS Genet. 2012;8:e1003100.

16. Vonholdt BM, Pollinger JP, Lohmueller KE, Han E, Parker HG, Quignon P, et al. Genome-wide SNP and haplotype analyses reveal a rich history underlying dog domestication. Nature. 2010;464:898–902.

17. Decker JE, McKay SD, Rolf MM, Kim J, Molina Alcala A, Sonstegard TS, et al. Worldwide patterns of ancestry, divergence, and admixture in domesticated cattle. PLoS Genet. 2014;10:e1004254.

18. Groenen MA, Archibald AL, Uenishi H, Tuggle CK, Takeuchi Y, Rothschild MF, et al. Analyses of pig genomes provide insight into porcine demography and evolution. Nature. 2012;491:393–8.

19. Rubin CJ, Zody MC, Eriksson J, Meadows JR, Sherwood E, Webster MT, et al. Whole-genome resequencing reveals loci under selection during chicken domestication. Nature. 2010;464:587–91.

20. Axelsson E, Ratnakumar A, Arendt ML, Maqbool K, Webster MT, Perloski M, et al. The genomic signature of dog domestication reveals adaptation to a starch-rich diet. Nature. 2013;495:360–4.

21. Carneiro M, Rubin CJ, Di Palma F, Albert FW, Alfoldi J, Barrio AM, et al. Rabbit genome analysis reveals a polygenic basis for phenotypic change during domestication. Science. 2014;345:1074–9.

22. Rubin CJ, Megens HJ, Martinez Barrio A, Maqbool K, Sayyab S, Schwochow D, et al. Strong signatures of selection in the domestic pig genome. Proc Natl Acad Sci USA. 2012;109:19529–36.

23. Bosse M, Megens HJ, Frantz LA, Madsen O, Larson G, Paudel Y, et al. Genomic analysis reveals selection for Asian genes in European pigs following human-mediated introgression. Nat Commun. 2014;5:4392.

24. Wilkinson S, Lu ZH, Megens HJ, Archibald AL, Haley C, Jackson IJ, et al. Signatures of diversifying selection in European pig breeds. PLoS Genet. 2013;9:e1003453.

25. Ai H, Yang B, Li J, Xie X, Chen H, Ren J. Population history and genomic signatures for high-altitude adaptation in Tibetan pigs. BMC Genomics. 2014;15:834.

26. Ramos AM, Crooijmans RP, Affara NA, Amaral AJ, Archibald AL, et al. Design of a high density SNP genotyping assay in the pig using SNPs identified and characterized by next generation sequencing technology. PLoS One. 2009;4:e6524.

27. Purcell S, Neale B, Todd-Brown K, Thomas L, Ferreira MA, Bender D, et al. PLINK: a tool set for whole-genome association and population-based linkage analyses. Am J Hum Genet. 2007;81:559–75.

28. R Core Team. A language and environment for statistical computing. Vienna: R Foundation for Statistical Computing; 2013.

29. Felsenstein J. PHYLIP—phylogeny inference package. Cladistics. 1989;5:164–6.

30. Becker RA, Wilkes AR. Maps in S. AT\&T Bell Laboratories Statistics Research Report. 1993;96:93.2.

31. Alexander DH, Novembre J, Lange K. Fast model-based estimation of ancestry in unrelated individuals. Genome Res. 2009;19:1655–64.

32. Delaneau O, Marchini J, Zagury JF. A linear complexity phasing method for thousands of genomes. Nat Methods. 2012;9:179–81.

33. Amaral AJ, Megens HJ, Crooijmans RP, Heuven HC, Groenen MA. Linkage disequilibrium decay and haplotype block structure in the pig. Genetics. 2008;179:569–79.

34. Sved JA. Linkage disequilibrium and homozygosity of chromosome segments in finite populations. Theor Popul Biol. 1971;2:125–41.

35. Tortereau F, Servin B, Frantz L, Megens HJ, Milan D, Rohrer G, et al. A high density recombination map of the pig reveals a correlation between sex-specific recombination and GC content. BMC Genomics. 2012;13:586.

36. Herrero-Medrano JM, Megens HJ, Groenen MA, Ramis G, Bosse M, Perez-Enciso M, et al. Conservation genomic analysis of domestic and wild pig populations from the Iberian Peninsula. BMC Genet. 2013;14:106.

37. Cockerham BS, Wa CC. Estimating F-statistics for the analysis of population structure. Evolution. 1984;38:14.

38. Zhang Z. Pig breeds in China. Shanghai: Shanghai Scientific and Technical Publishers; 1986.

39. Herrero-Medrano JM, Megens HJ, Crooijmans RP, Abellaneda JM, Ramis G. Farm-by-farm analysis of microsatellite, mtDNA and SNP genotype data reveals inbreeding and crossbreeding as threats to the survival of a native Spanish pig breed. Anim Genet. 2013;44:259–66.

40. Herrero-Medrano JM, Megens HJ, Groenen MA, Bosse M, Perez-Enciso M, Crooijmans RP. Whole-genome sequence analysis reveals differences in population management and selection of European low-input pig breeds. BMC Genomics. 2014;15:601.

41. Ramirez O, Ojeda A, Tomas A, Gallardo D, Huang LS, Folch JM, et al. Integrating Y-chromosome, mitochondrial, and autosomal data to analyze the origin of pig breeds. Mol Biol Evol. 2009;26:2061–72.

42. Wagner KR, McPherron AC, Winik N, Lee SJ. Loss of myostatin attenuates severity of muscular dystrophy in mdx mice. Ann Neurol. 2002;52:832–6.

43. Graham ES, Turnbull Y, Fotheringham P, Nilaweera K, Mercer JG, Morgan PJ, et al. Neuromedin U and Neuromedin U receptor-2 expression in the mouse and rat hypothalamus: effects of nutritional status. J Neurochem. 2003;87:1165–73.

44. Mankowska M, Szydlowski M, Salamon S, Bartz M, Switonski M. Novel polymorphisms in porcine 3′UTR of the *leptin* gene, including a rare variant within target sequence for *MIR-9* gene in Duroc breed, not associated with production traits. Anim Biotechnol. 2015;26:156–63.

45. Waraich RS, Weigert C, Kalbacher H, Hennige AM, Lutz SZ, Häring HU, et al. Phosphorylation of Ser357 of rat insulin receptor substrate-1 mediates adverse effects of protein kinase C-delta on insulin action in skeletal muscle cells. J Biol Chem. 2008;283:11226–33.

46. Wasserman D, Geijer T, Sokolowski M, Rozanov V, Wasserman J. Genetic variation in the hypothalamic-pituitary-adrenocortical axis regulatory factor, T-box 19, and the angry/hostility personality trait. Genes Brain Behav. 2007;6:321–8.

47. Adachi H, Tsujimoto M, Hattori M, Arai H, Inoue K. cDNA cloning of human cytosolic platelet-activating factor acetylhydrolase gamma-subunit and its mRNA expression in human tissues. Biochem Biophys Res Commun. 1995;214:180–7.

48. Beneduzzi D, Trarbach EB, Min L, Jorge AA, Garmes HM, Renk AC, et al. Role of gonadotropin-releasing hormone receptor mutations in patients with a wide spectrum of pubertal delay. Fertil Steril. 2014;102:838–46.

49. Luo Y, Liu Q, Lei X, Wen Y, Yang YL, Zhang R, et al. Association of estrogen receptor gene polymorphisms with human precocious puberty: a systematic review and meta-analysis. Gynecol Endocrinol. 2015;31:516–21.

50. Yang WL, Ravatn R, Kudoh K, Alabanza L, Chin KV. Interaction of the regulatory subunit of the cAMP-dependent protein kinase with PATZ1 (ZNF278). Biochem Biophys Res Commun. 2010;391:1318–23.

51. Young JM, Shykind BM, Lane RP, Tonnes-Priddy L, Ross JA, Walker M, et al. Odorant receptor expressed sequence tags demonstrate olfactory expression of over 400 genes, extensive alternate splicing and unequal expression levels. Genome Biol. 2003;4:R71.

52. Amaral PP, Neyt C, Wilkins SJ, Askarian-Amiri ME, Sunkin SM, Perkins AC, et al. Complex architecture and regulated expression of the Sox2ot locus during vertebrate development. RNA. 2009;15:2013–27.

53. Shen T, Zhu Y, Patel J, Ruan Y, Chen B, Zhao G, et al. T-box20 suppresses oxidized low-density lipoprotein-induced human vascular endothelial cell injury by upregulation of PPAR-gamma. Cell Physiol Biochem. 2013;32:1137–50.

54. Wang M, Bridges JP, Na CL, Xu Y, Weaver TE. Meckel-Gruber syndrome protein MKS3 is required for endoplasmic reticulum-associated degradation of surfactant protein C. J Biol Chem. 2009;284:33377–83.

55. Kaestner KH, Katz J, Liu Y, Drucker DJ, Schutz G. Inactivation of the winged helix transcription factor HNF3alpha affects glucose homeostasis and islet glucagon gene expression in vivo. Genes Dev. 1999;13:495–504.

56. Yabe D, Brown MS, Goldstein JL. Insig-2, a second endoplasmic reticulum protein that binds SCAP and blocks export of sterol regulatory element-binding proteins. Proc Natl Acad Sci USA. 2002;99:12753–8.

57. Zhang Q, Wang J, Fan S, Wang L, Cao L, Tang K, et al. Expression and functional characterization of LRRC4, a novel brain-specific member of the LRR superfamily. FEBS Lett. 2005;579:3674–82.

58. Muto E, Tabata Y, Taneda T, Aoki Y, Muto A, Arai K, et al. Identification and characterization of Veph, a novel gene encoding a PH domain-containing protein expressed in the developing central nervous system of vertebrates. Biochimie. 2004;86:523–31.

59. Wang K, Zhang H, Ma D, Bucan M, Glessner JT, Abrahams BS, et al. Common genetic variants on 5p14.1 associate with autism spectrum disorders. Nature. 2009;459:528–33.

60. Tan J, Pieper K, Piccoli L, Abdi A, Foglierini M, Geiger R, et al. A LAIR1 insertion generates broadly reactive antibodies against malaria variant antigens. Nature. 2016;529:105–9.

61. Onteru SK, Fan B, Du ZQ, Garrick DJ, Stalder KJ, Rothschild MF. A whole-genome association study for pig reproductive traits. Anim Genet. 2012;43:18–26.

62. Ramirez O, Burgos-Paz W, Casas E, Ballester M, Bianco E, Olalde I, et al. Genome data from a sixteenth century pig illuminate modern breed relationships. Heredity (Edinb). 2015;114:175–84.

63. Fang M, Andersson L. Mitochondrial diversity in European and Chinese pigs is consistent with population expansions that occurred prior to domestication. Proc Biol Sci. 2006;273:1803–10.

64. China National Commission of Animal Genetic Resources. Animal genetic resources in China pigs. Beijing: China Agricultural Press; 2011.

65. Rothschild M, Jacobson C, Vaske D, Tuggle C, Wang L, et al. The estrogen receptor locus is associated with a major gene influencing litter size in pigs. Proc Natl Acad Sci USA. 1996;93:201–5.

66. Kijas JM, Wales R, Tornsten A, Chardon P, Moller M, Andersson L. Melanocortin receptor 1 (MC1R) mutations and coat color in pigs. Genetics. 1998;150:1177–85.

67. Ojeda A, Huang LS, Ren J, Angiolillo A, Cho IC, Soto H, et al. Selection in the making: a worldwide survey of haplotypic diversity around a causative mutation in porcine IGF2. Genetics. 2008;178:1639–52.

68. Murakami K, Yoshikawa S, Konishi S, Ueno Y, Watanabe S, Mizoguchi Y. Evaluation of genetic introgression from domesticated pigs into the Ryukyu wild boar population on Iriomote Island in Japan. Anim Genet. 2014;45:517–23.

69. Edea Z, Kim SW, Lee KT, Kim TH, Kim KS. Genetic Structure of and evidence for admixture between Western and Korean native pig breeds revealed by single nucleotide polymorphisms. Asian-Aust J Anim Sci. 2014;27:1263–9.

70. Pham LD, Do DN, Nam LQ, Van Ba N, Minh LT, Hoan TX, et al. Molecular genetic diversity and genetic structure of Vietnamese indigenous pig populations. J Anim Breed Genet. 2014;131:379–86.

PERMISSIONS

LIST OF CONTRIBUTORS

Chen Yao and Kent A. Weigel
Department of Dairy Science, University of Wisconsin, Madison, Madison, WI, USA

Xiaojin Zhu
Department of Computer Science, University of Wisconsin, Madison, Madison, WI, USA

Matti Taskinen, Esa A. Mäntysaari and Ismo Strandén
Natural Resources Institute Finland (Luke), Myllytie 1, Jokioinen, Finland

Aniek C. Bouwman and Mario P. L. Calus
Animal Breeding and Genomics Centre, Wageningen UR Livestock Research, P.O. Box 338, 6700 AH Wageningen, The Netherlands

Roel F. Veerkamp
Animal Breeding and Genomics Centre, Wageningen UR Livestock Research, P.O. Box 338, 6700 AH Wageningen, The Netherlands
Department of Animal and Aquacultural Sciences, Norwegian University of Life Sciences, P.O. Box 5003, 1432 Ås, Norway

Chris Schrooten
CRV BV, P.O. Box 454, 6800 AL Arnhem, The Netherlands

Amy M. Bell, John M. Henshall and Sonja Dominik
CSIRO Agriculture, F D McMaster Laboratory Chiswick, Armidale, NSW 2350, Australia

Laercio R. Porto-Neto, Russell McCulloch, James Kijas and Sigrid A. Lehnert
CSIRO AgricultureQueensland Bioscience Precinct, Brisbane, QLD 4067, Australia

Carolina A. Garcia-Baccino and Rodolfo J. C. Cantet
Departamento de Producción Animal, Facultad de Agronomía, Universidad de Buenos Aires, C1417DSE Buenos Aires, Argentina
Instituto de Investigaciones en Producción Animal - Consejo Nacional de Investigaciones Científicas y Técnicas, Buenos Aires, Argentina

Andres Legarra and Zulma G. Vitezica
GenPhySE, INRA, INPT, ENVT, Université de Toulouse, 31326 Castanet-Tolosan, France

Ole F. Christensen
Center for Quantitative Genetics and Genomics, Department of Molecular Biology and Genetics, Aarhus University, 8830 Tjele, Denmark

Ignacy Misztal and Ivan Pocrnic
Animal and Dairy Science, University of Georgia, Athens, GA 30602, USA

Jinmei Ding, Wenjing Zhao, Zhengxiao Zhai, Chuan He and He Meng
Department of Animal Science, School of Agriculture and Biology, Shanghai Jiao Tong University, Shanghai Key Laboratory of Veterinary Biotechnology, Shanghai 200240, People's Republic of China

Lele Zhao
Department of Animal Science, School of Agriculture and Biology, Shanghai Jiao Tong University, Shanghai Key Laboratory of Veterinary Biotechnology, Shanghai 200240, People's Republic of China
Shanghai Animal Disease Control Center, Shanghai 201103, People's Republic of China

Li Leng, Yuxiang Wang and Hui Li
College of Animal Science and Technology, Northeast Agricultural University, Harbin 150030, People's Republic of China

Lifeng Wang and Heping Zhang
College of Food Science and Engineering, Inner Mongolia Agricultural University, Key Laboratory of Dairy Biotechnology and Engineering, Hohhot 010018, People's Republic of China

Yan Zhang
Shanghai Personal Biotechnology Limited Company, Shanghai 200231, People's Republic of China

Graham Lough and Andrea Doeschl-Wilson
The Roslin Institute & R(D)SVS, University of Edinburgh, Edinburgh, Midlothian, UK

Hamed Rashidi and Han A. Mulder
Animal Breeding and Genomics Centre, Wageningen University and Research, PO Box 338, 6700 AH Wageningen, The Netherlands

Ilias Kyriazakis
School of Agriculture Food and Rural Development, Newcastle University, Newcastle upon Tyne NE1 7RU, UK

Jack C. M. Dekkers, Andrew Hess and Melanie Hess
Department of Animal Science, Iowa State University, Ames, IA 50011, USA

Nader Deeb
Genus plc, 100 Bluegrass Commons Blvd. Suite 2200, Hendersonville, TN 37075, USA

Antti Kause
Biometrical Genetics, Natural Resources Institute Finland, 00790 Jokioinen, Finland

Joan K. Lunney
Animal Parasitic Diseases Laboratory, USDA, Beltsville, MD 20705, USA

Raymond R. R. Rowland
College of Veterinary Medicine, Kansas State University, Manhattan, KS 66506, USA

Paul M. VanRaden, Melvin E. Tooker, John B. Cole and Derek M. Bickhart
Animal Genomics and Improvement Laboratory, Agricultural Research Service, USDA, Beltsville, MD, USA

Jeffrey R. O'Connell
University of Maryland Baltimore, Baltimore, MD, USA

Yoannah François, Alain Vignal, Caroline Molette, Nathalie Marty-Gasset, Laurence Liaubet and Christel Marie-Etancelin
GenPhySE, INRA, INPT, INP-ENVT, Université de Toulouse, 31326 Castanet Tolosan, France

Stéphane Davail
IPREM-EMM, UMR5254, Université de Pau et des Pays de l'Adour, 40004 Mont de Marsan Cedex, France

Kasper Janssen and Hans Komen
Animal Breeding and Genomics, Wageningen University and Research, Droevendaalsesteeg 1, 6708 PB Wageningen, The Netherlands

Mathieu Besson
Animal Breeding and Genomics, Wageningen University and Research, Droevendaalsesteeg 1, 6708 PB Wageningen, The Netherlands
Génétique Animale Biologie Intégrative, INRA, AgroParisTech, Université Paris-Saclay, 78350 Jouy-en-Josas, France

Paul Berentsen
Business Economics Group, Wageningen University and Research, Hollandseweg 1, 6706 KN Wageningen, The Netherlands

Donagh P. Berry, Aine O'Brien and Noirin McHugh
Animal and Grassland Research and Innovation Centre, Moorepark, Teagasc, Fermoy, Co. Cork, Ireland

Eamonn Wall, Kevin McDermott and Shane Randles
Sheep Ireland, Highfield House, Shinagh, Bandon, Co. Cork, Ireland

Paul Flynn and Rebecca Weld
Weatherbys Ltd, Naas, Ireland

Stephen Park
Identigen Ltd, Dublin, Ireland

Jenny Grose
GeneSeek, A Neogen Company, Lincoln, NE, USA

Nasir Moghaddar and Julius H. J. van der Werf
Cooperative Research Centre for Sheep Industry Innovation, Armidale, NSW 2351, Australia
School of Environmental and Rural Science, University of New England, Armidale, NSW 2351, Australia

Andrew A. Swan
Cooperative Research Centre for Sheep Industry Innovation, Armidale, NSW 2351, Australia
Animal Genetics and Breeding Unit (AGBU), University of New England, Armidale, NSW 2351, Australia

John B. Holmes and Michael A. Lee
Department of Mathematics and Statistics, University of Otago, Cumberland St., Dunedin 9016, New Zealand

Ken G. Dodds
AgResearch, Invermay Research Centre, Puddle Alley, Dunedin 9053, New Zealand

Matti Janhunen and Harri Vehviläinen
Biometrical Genetics, Natural Resources Institute Finland (Luke), Myllytie 1, 31600 Jokioinen, Finland

Juha Koskela
Aquaculture, Natural Resources Institute Finland (Luke), Survontie 9 A, 40500 Jyväskylä, Finland

Nguyên Hũu Ninh
Research Institute for Aquaculture No. 3 (RIA-3), Nha Trang, Khanh Hoa, Vietnam

Heikki Koskinen and Antti Nousiainen
Tervo Fish Farm, Natural Resources Institute Finland (Luke), Huuhtajantie 160, 72210 Tervo, Finland

Ngô Phú Thỏa
Research Institute for Aquaculture No. 1 (RIA-1), Dinh Bang, Tu Son, Bac Ninh, Vietnam

Brendan M. Duggan, Dylan N. Clements and Paul M. Hocking
The Roslin Institute and Royal (Dick) School of Veterinary Studies, University of Edinburgh, Easter Bush, Midlothian EH25 9RG, UK

Anne M. Rae
Cherry Valley Farms Ltd., Laceby Business Park, Grimsby Road, Laceby, North Lincolnshire DN37 7DP, UK

Rohan L. Fernando and Hao Cheng
Department of Animal Science, Iowa State University, Ames, IA 50011, USA

Dorian J. Garrick
Department of Animal Science, Iowa State University, Ames, IA 50011, USA
Institute of Veterinary, Animal and Biomedical Sciences, Massey University, Palmerston North, New Zealand

Bruce L. Golden
Theta Solutions, LLC, Atascadero, CA 93422, USA

Pierre Faux and Tom Druet
Unit of Animal Genomics, GIGA-R and Faculty of Veterinary Medicine, University of Liège, 4000 Liège, Belgium

Bin Yang, Leilei Cui and Lusheng Huang
National Key Laboratory for Pig Genetic Improvement and Production Technology, Nanchang, China

Richard P. M. A. Crooijmans, Martien A. M. Groenen and Hendrik-Jan Megens
Animal Breeding and Genomics, Wageningen University, Wageningen, The Netherlands

Miguel Perez-Enciso
Centre for Research in Agricultural Genomics (CRAG), CSIC-IRTA-UAB-UB Consortium, Bellaterra, Barcelona, Spain
Institut Catala de Recerca i Estudis Avancats (ICREA), Carrer de Lluís Companys, Barcelona, Spain

Aleksei Traspov and Natalia Zinovieva
All-Russian Research Institute of Animal Husbandry named after Academy Member L.K. Ernst, Dubrovitzy, Moscow Region, Russia

Lawrence B. Schook
Institute of Genomic Biology, University of Illinois, Urbana, Champaign, IL, USA

Alan Archibald
Division of Genetics and Genomics, The Roslin Institute, R(D)SVS, University of Edinburgh, Edinburgh, UK

Kesinee Gatphayak
Animal and Aquatic Sciences, Chiang Mai University, Chiang Mai, Thailand

Christophe Knorr
Division of Biotechnology and Reproduction of Livestock, Department of Animal Sciences, Georg-August-University, Göttingen, Germany

Alex Triantafyllidis and Panoraia Alexandri
Department of Genetics, Development and Molecular Biology, Aristotle University of Thessaloníki, Thessaloniki, Greece

Gono Semiadi
Research Centre for Biology- Zoology Division, LIPI, Bogor, Indonesia

Olivier Hanotte
School of Biology,University of Nottingham, Notttingham, UK

Deodália Dias
Faculdade de Ciências and CESAM, Universidade de Lisboa, Lisbon, Portugal

Peter Dovč
Department of Animal Science, Biotechnical Faculty, University of Ljubljana, Ljubljana, Slovenia

Pekka Uimari
Animal Breeding, Department of Agricultural Sciences, University of Helsinki, Helsinki, Finland

Laura Iacolina
Department of Chemistry and Bioscience, Aalborg University, Aalborg East, Denmark
Department of Science for Nature and Environmental Resources, University of Sassari, Sassari, Italy

Massimo Scandura
Department of Science for Nature and Environmental Resources, University of Sassari, Sassari, Italy

Index